Seeds of Change

Seeds of Change

The Story of ACORN,
America's Most Controversial
Antipoverty Community Organizing Group

John Atlas

Vanderbilt University Press
Nashville

Nashville, Tennessee 37235

First edition 2010

This book is printed on acid-free paper.
Manufactured in the United States of America

Cover design: John Thompson, e-volution design
Text design: Dariel Mayer

Library of Congress Cataloging-in-Publication Data

Atlas, John.
Seeds of change: the story of ACORN, America's most controversial antipoverty community organizing group / John Atlas.
p. cm.
Includes bibliographical references and index.
ISBN 978-0-8265-1705-0 (cloth : alk. paper)
ISBN 978-0-8265-1706-7 (pbk. : alk. paper)
1. ACORN (Organization) 2. Community organization—United States. 3. Community development, Urban—United States—Citizen participation. I. Title.
HN85.A3A85 2010
307.1'4097309045—dc22
2009035855

For my children,

Reuben and Becky Atlas

Contents

List of Illustrations

Preface

For forty years I worked on the front lines of anti-poverty and social justice efforts and discovered how hard and frustrating it is to make a difference. I played many roles—lawyer, executive director, board member, organizer, fundraiser, mentor, editor, public speaker, writer and publicist. I shared some of these experiences through a biweekly radio program in New York, television shows, dozens of magazine articles, and a book, *Saving Affordable Housing*. As a legal aid lawyer I helped hundreds of families threatened with losing their homes and organized civic groups like the New Jersey Tenants Organization, whose members successfully lobbied to protect renters from slumlords, unfair evictions, and skyrocketing rents. In 1976 I helped launch *Shelterforce*, a magazine for anti-poverty activists and practitioners engaged in housing and saving neighborhoods, and served as an editor and its president for thirty-three years. I have joined forces with ideologically diverse groups to promote policies that would strengthen civil society and fight poverty.[1]

In 2003, I took time off from work as a lawyer to evaluate my efforts and those of others who had dedicated their lives to the cause of democracy, equality, and justice since the late 1960s. What had we accomplished? What were the strengths and weaknesses of our efforts? What lessons could be learned that would be useful to a new generation of progressive activists, policy practitioners, and thinkers? I received a Charles H. Revson Fellowship at Columbia University and in 2004 used that opportunity to start writing a book about poverty, democracy, and politics by looking at ACORN.

ACORN was founded in 1970, about the same time I committed myself to helping poor and working-class Americans improve their lives, so its history coincided with the time frame I wanted for examining anti-poverty efforts in America. As a legal aid lawyer, I had worked with a local ACORN chapter in Paterson, New Jersey, and watched its members and their children, armed with black garbage bags, gardening gloves, and shovels, clean up a local park, removing newspapers, broken glass, and beer bottles to turn a neighborhood eyesore into a community asset. ACORN also organized a campaign to prevent lead poisoning in young low-income and minority children. I observed its members providing sound advice to families filling out tax returns, carefully showing eligible families how to obtain the federal tax credit for the working poor, a benefit supported by presidents Ronald Reagan and Bill Clinton. ACORN's largely black and Hispanic members seemed unafraid to protest and loudly confront local politicians to get what they wanted to improve their neighborhood. The organization's successes and failures, I thought, might provide valuable lessons about the subject and era I hoped to focus on.

I thought a book about ACORN would complement other books about the poor that were at odds with my own experiences. The best of them—*American Dream: Three Women, Ten Kids, and A Nation's Drive to End Welfare* by Jason DeParle (Viking Books, 2004), *The Working Poor* by David Shipler (Knopf, 2004), and *Random Family* by Adrian Nicole LeBlanc (Scribner, 2003)—document the plight of the working poor and provide a valuable, complex portrait of what it's like to be deprived in a wealthy society. But each of these writers presents poor people as mostly passive victims. Some work in low-wage jobs, while others are jobless. Some are good parents, while others neglect their children. Some are responsible citizens, while others drug addicts, criminals, or moral deviants whose actions separate them from normal society. Absent from all these books are stories of collective efforts by the working poor to lift themselves up and change public policy, like families in ACORN and those involved in New Jersey's tenant movement.

My book, *Seeds of Change*, offers a look at America's poor and challenges the assumptions of conservatives and liberals who presume that the poor are helpless victims unable to change themselves or society. ACORN reflects the American tradition of helping the poor help themselves. Its work suggests that the best prescription for reducing poverty should start, as many organizers have said, with the maxim, "If you give a man a fish, he will eat that day, but if you teach a man to fish, he will eat every night." But what if the river where you fish is polluted and the fish are dying? The hungry person who learned how to fish will need to organize or join a community group that can mobilize public opinion, demonstrate against the polluters, and sue them, as well as pressure government officials to clean up the water. In other words, we must teach people how to fight as well as fish.

In the chapters to come, I follow ACORN's organizers, leaders, allies, and opponents, weaving their stories into a tapestry that includes the broader context of American culture, democracy, and politics. I take you behind the recent headlines about ACORN and follow the lives of leaders of the organization like Maude Hurd, Beatrice Jackson, Paul Satriano, and Pearl Gilbert—black and white, poor and working class, each of whom joined after an organizer knocked on their door. These people do not seek charity. They seek justice.

You will meet others, several from elite universities, who through wisdom, sweat and toil, common sense, trial and error, and bold, brilliant strategies formed a truly unique organization, a poor people's force for individual and political transformation. You will also learn the truth behind the attacks against ACORN and allegations of its illegal activities.

Margaret Mead, the anthropologist, was only partly correct when she famously said, "Never underestimate the power of a small group of dedicated people to change the world. Indeed it's the only thing that ever has." The ACORN story also suggests that making a difference in the fight for social justice takes more than hard work and dedication. The outcome of the struggle depends on the leadership's integrity as well as the vision, tactics, and strategies employed by the small group. Unless its plans inspire the widespread participation of the working poor, significant change will not come.

Since the Boston Tea Party, every major improvement in economic, social, and political conditions has occurred when the educated elite and ordinary people join together to push for change. That's how Americans abolished slavery, established voting rights for women, ended lynching, expanded workers' rights, provided a safety net for seniors and the poor, boosted a majority of the U.S. population into the middle class after World War II, protected consumers from tobacco companies and the environment from corporate polluters, dismantled Jim Crow, and improved conditions for migrant farm workers. If America is going to dramatically reduce poverty, it will require a movement similar to those.

When I started writing this book I did not know much about ACORN's inner workings or influence. The people I followed did not accomplish everything they wanted; some made egregious errors, and some left angered and frustrated by their own or ACORN's limitations. But the more I found out, the more I became convinced that this group had something important to tell us about how to empower the poor to fish and fight.

Before I decided to write this book I asked ACORN's staff, including chief organizer Wade Rathke and executive director Steve Kest, to give me complete access to their private meetings among staff and community leaders, archives, and internal memos and to encourage ACORN's staff and leaders to talk freely with me. With some reluctance they agreed, and they kept their word. Fortunately (or perhaps unfortunately) for me, ACORN writes almost everything down. From 2004 to 2009, I read enough internal ACORN material—strategy papers, leaflets and newsletters, written constitutions, bylaws, minutes, flyers distributed at demonstrations, membership lists, internal electronic bulletin boards, annual reports, court documents, and fundraising proposals—to fill an encyclopedia.

For five years I observed ACORN's activities on local, state, and national levels. I sat in on staff meetings and private meetings with community leaders and government officials. I attended many large and small public actions organized by ACORN, as well as two of ACORN's national conventions. I am the only journalist to witness an ACORN national board meeting or national staff meeting. I was present at many of the events described in this book.

To gather material about ACORN's history, I conducted dozens of in-depth interviews with organizers and leaders of ACORN, former organizers and ex-members, elected officials, foundation executives, businesspeople, community leaders, and opponents. To get the fullest current picture, I read numerous blogs each day, with some on the left praising ACORN and all those on the right attacking it.

During this period I spent hundreds of hours hanging out with, interviewing face to face, e-mailing with, and following a dozen ACORN staff and members who were emblematic of ACORN's work. Some, including veterans Wade Rathke, Bertha Lewis, Madeline Talbott, and Brian Kettenring, allowed me to intrude into their lives to get a deep sense of ACORN's people and their day-to-day activities. This research provided me with insights into the motivations and internal dynamics of the organization. Most members and staff were cooperative and talked to me openly and frankly, including discussing some of their frustrations with ACORN. Some were resistant to talking because they correctly viewed me as invading their privacy and interrupting their daily lives.

No names have been changed. There are no composite characters. When I say that someone said, thought, felt, or believed something, the information was reported to me, reconstructed from interviews, based on diaries, or documented in newspaper and magazine articles. The notes and bibliographic references I have provided for each chapter will be useful to those engaged in the practice of community organizing, or to any reader wishing to go into more depth.

Seeds of Change

Introduction

> Through organizing, through shared sacrifice, membership had been earned. And because membership was earned—because this community I imagined was still in the making, built on the promise that the larger American community, black, white, and brown, could somehow redefine itself—I believed that it might, over time, admit the uniqueness of my own life. That was my idea of organizing. It was a promise of redemption.
>
> —Barack Obama, *Dreams from My Father*

Three weeks before the 2008 presidential election, Bertha Lewis rushed from her office to her Brooklyn apartment to catch the televised debate between Barack Obama and John McCain. Lewis, an African American, had a special interest in the debates, since during the Democratic primaries, Obama had sought and received ACORN's endorsement. Born to a teenage mother in a Florida migrant camp in 1951, Lewis had recently taken over as head of ACORN. A razor-sharp, inspiring leader, she previously led ACORN's New York chapter and had been called by *Crain's New York* magazine one of the "100 Most Influential Women of New York." *New York* magazine concurred, naming her one of the state's political "influentials."[1]

Wearing a brightly colored African dress, Lewis had spent most of the day at ACORN's New York headquarters in Brooklyn on the cell phone and at meetings, juggling her time among politicians, foundation executives, staff, and the media. Her office, like many of ACORN's 103 offices operating in cities across the United States, was humming with people, young and old, many working day and night, helping the poor fight for a better life. Though ACORN was often at the center of controversy, powerful politicians such as Bill and Hillary Clinton and Ted Kennedy and celebrities such as Roseanne Barr supported ACORN's work and spoke at its national events. Lewis was responsible for an organization with more than six hundred staff, thousands of low- and moderate-income members, dozens of coalition partners, and over a hundred chapters in forty-two states. On the day of the debate she had spent hours talking to reporters, her heart often pounding with a rush of adrenaline, denying allegations by Republicans that ACORN was involved in voter fraud.

Weary from her long day running the organization and sparring with the media, Lewis looked forward to relaxing in her living room and watching Obama do well. She struggled to stay awake. Suddenly her eyes opened wide, her brief tranquility shattered. John McCain, before millions of viewers, was warning the nation that a group called ACORN, whom he linked to Barack Obama, "is now on the verge of maybe perpetrating one of the greatest frauds in voter history in this country." ACORN, he said, may be "destroying the fabric of democracy."

She stood and yelled at the TV, "He just attacked ACORN!" She knew how ruthless Republicans could be. They had tried to destroy ACORN's reputation before, as part of the Attorneygate scandal in 2006.

She had been amused when the Republicans sarcastically attacked community organizers at their national nominating convention, mocking Obama's experience as an organizer in Chicago. Sarah Palin, in her acceptance speech for the GOP vice-presidential nomination, had declared, "I guess a small-town mayor is sort of like a community organizer, except that you have actual responsibilities." But never did Lewis imagine that ACORN would become an issue in the presidential campaign. Calls started coming from staff and members. In the tradition of a seasoned community organizer, Lewis tried to turn a bad situation into an opportunity. "Look at it this way. We finally made the big time after all these years. Hell, let's make sure they spell our name right." Vilified by McCain, ACORN had become part of the national debate. During October there were 1,737 news stories about ACORN, mostly negative.[2]

After nearly forty years of operating below the national radar, ACORN has evolved into an exceptionally successful national antipoverty group. During an era dominated by conservatives, ACORN has tackled some of America's most intractable problems—improving urban neighborhoods, increasing worker's wages, and helping low-income families buy homes. From city halls and state capitals to Washington, D.C., and Wall Street, ACORN has pressured the powerful to provide access to health care, to compensate the victims of the subprime predatory home loans, to prevent foreclosures, to register people to vote, to clean up vacant lots and turn them into parks, to improve public schools, and more. ACORN has spearheaded the living wage movement, one of the most successful grassroots organizing initiatives of the past two decades. In a dozen states (Florida, Ohio, Missouri, Colorado, Arizona, New York, California, Pennsylvania, Michigan, Massachusetts, Arkansas, and North Carolina) and 150 cities, ACORN has led campaigns to increase worker's wages. As a result, millions of Americans have gotten a raise, worth tens of billions of dollars.

Likewise, by providing free tax counseling for thousands of families, ACORN has helped make the federal Earned Income Tax Credit an effective anti-poverty program. An evaluation of ACORN's tax service program gave it high marks. The researchers found that ACORN's tax assistance resulted in almost $4 million in tax refunds to low-income families. An IRS official in Louisiana stated that the New Orleans ACORN VITA site was "amazing for a first year." In 2004 ACORN expanded its EITC assistance to fifty-one cities and generated $19 million in total refunds.[3]

Since the late 1990s, ACORN has warned about the dangers of "predatory lending" by banks, private mortgage companies, and mortgage brokers. Had policy makers heeded ACORN's warnings, the nation would have been spared the epidemic of foreclosures and the economic crisis that resulted from the meltdown of the financial sector. One study estimated that from 1994 to 2004, ACORN had redirected an astonishing $15 billion from government and corporations to improve the lives and neighborhoods of low-income families.[4]

ACORN's story is all the more remarkable because the organization has flourished even while antigovernment crusaders made the nation's poor largely invisible on the political landscape. Long after large-scale civil rights and antiwar protests ended, ACORN members continue to march, vote, lobby, and make sure the voice of the powerless is heard.

Its success has attracted enemies, many of whom were key members of McCain's conservative base. For years ACORN has been a low-level target of Bill O'Reilly of Fox News, radio celebrity Rush Limbaugh, influential conservative magazines like the *City Journal* and *National Review*, and lobbyists for the restaurant and banking industries. For example, Sol Stern in the *City Journal* argued that ACORN promotes "a 1960s-bred agenda of anti-capitalism, central planning, victimology, and government handouts to the poor." Stern said ACORN "had learned no lessons about the free-market magic that made American cities engines of job creation for more than a century, proliferating opportunity."[5]

For months preceding the 2008 presidential debates, Republican Party and right-wing echo politicians, bloggers, columnists, editorial writers, and TV and radio talk-show hosts led an orchestrated campaign blaming ACORN for widespread voter fraud. ACORN had registered nearly one million young, poor, and minority for the November 4 election who were likely to vote for Democrats. But in the process part-time ACORN hires had turned in questionable or duplicate voter-registration forms submitted in nine states, including tightly contested swing states. In October, the Associated Press quoted two "senior law enforcement" officials as saying that the FBI was investigating ACORN, seeking "any evidence of a coordinated national scam."[6] For days, Fox News ran stories on ACORN's voter-registration campaign, calling it a scandal. "All federal funding to ACORN must be stopped," demanded House Republican leader John Boehner (R-Ohio).[7]

As part of the attack, conservatives also blamed the unfolding subprime mortgage crisis on ACORN based on its support of the Community Reinvestment Act (CRA), the 1977 law that bars credit discrimination, called "redlining," in urban areas. In a September 27 editorial, the *Wall Street Journal* wrote that "ACORN has promoted laws like the Community Reinvestment Act, which laid the foundation for the house of cards built out of subprime loans" and then claimed the bailout bill would create a trust fund "pipeline" to fill ACORN's coffers. On October 14, the day before the final debate, the *Journal*'s lead editorial, titled "Obama and ACORN," described ACORN as a "shady outfit" and accused the group of being "a major contributor to the subprime meltdown by pushing lenders to make home loans on easy terms, conducting 'strikes' against banks so they'd lower credit standards."[8]

On *Fox & Friends*, *National Review* columnist Stanley Kurtz described ACORN as "a group of community organizers [who] specialize in putting pressure, really kind of intimidation tactics, on banks, to get these banks to make high-risk loans to low-credit customers. . . . They even show up at the homes of bank officials to scare them and their families. They send demonstrators into the lobbies of banks, all to get the banks to make these high-risk loans to people with low credit."[9] Fox News ran dozens of segments on ACORN in a two-week period in October, branding it a dangerous organization.[10]

Criticism was coming not just from the right. The *New York Times* and CNN repeatedly reported ACORN's troubles, including an accusation from angry ACORN supporters that the brother of ACORN's founder had embezzled a million dollars from the group and the staff had covered it up. During the week of October 6–15, CNN aired fifty-four segments mentioning allegations that ACORN submitted allegedly false or duplicate voter-registration applications in a number of states.[11]

Using TV ads, accusations by local Republican officials, and the national debate, the McCain campaign took the opportunity to link its opponent to what it called an outlaw leftist group. Despite ACORN's endorsement of Obama, he immediately distanced himself from the group. "The only involvement I've had with ACORN," Obama told the media, "is I represented them alongside the U.S. Justice Department in making Illinois implement a motor voter law that helped people get registered at DMVs." Dismayed, Bertha Lewis knew that Obama had failed to disclose the full story. For example, he had worked with ACORN on voter registration in Chicago. In addition, while he served on the board of the Woods Fund of Chicago, which funded antipoverty activism, that group had channeled $75,000 in 2001 and $70,000 in 2002 to ACORN's Chicago office. Before a television audience of more than sixty million, however, Obama had separated himself from ACORN, which had endorsed him in the primary election and helped him get votes.

Since ACORN's founding in 1970, mainstream journalists have had difficulty reporting accurately about this unique and complex group. It wasn't a charity or a social service agency or a political party. It had leaders but no charismatic public figures. It challenged powerful corporations and politicians, but it also negotiated agreements with those same corporations and politicians to win improvements for the poor. It supported parent involvement in education and the teachers' union. Its membership was composed mostly of black and Latino people, yet it mobilized people not around racial issues, but around economic justice concerns.

Although it had no public relations department, ACORN generated considerable local media attention, especially when it engaged in public protests or released a controversial report documenting corporate irresponsibility. But the attention ACORN drew during the 2008 election season was unprecedented. Some stories sympathetic to the group did appear on news programs such as *Countdown* with Keith Olbermann, *The Rachel Maddow Show*, National Public Radio, and ABC News. Lewis was talking to nationally syndicated columnists such as Clarence Page (*Chicago Tribune*) and David Broder (*Washington Post*) and appearing on Jon Stewart's *The Daily Show*. While she could no longer complain, as in the past, that ACORN was unknown to a national audience, the overall impression left by the media after the election was unfavorable.

What is ACORN? The answer begins with Wade Rathke, ACORN's savvy founder, and his dream of building an organization that would significantly reduce poverty and strengthen America's democratic process. Unlike so many public interest groups created or expanded during the 1970s, Rathke's group started not in Washington, D.C., but in the South, in Arkansas. The group began to take off in the mid-1970s, when many of ACORN's original staff—having graduated as did Barack Obama from Ivy League schools—committed themselves to organizing the nation's least advantaged citizens. Stirred by the students who flocked to the South in the early 1960s to support the civil rights movement, they hoped to build a new political force.

Unlike many idealistic young men and women of that era, they did not chill out or drop out. Nor did they join the Democratic Party or become political campaign operatives or take well-paying jobs at one of the liberal public policy organizations that proliferated inside the Washington Beltway. They won't be found at exclusive cocktail parties hobnobbing with former secretaries of state, cabinet members, and Democratic Party bigwigs. Instead, they live on modest incomes and work primarily as behind-the-scene organizers rather than as public figures.

Many of the low-income members of ACORN, mobilized by its young idealists, are ordinary people who have made extraordinary changes. They have stepped beyond their private lives and become leaders. In Little Rock, Albuquerque, Chicago, Philadelphia, New York, New Orleans, and other places, they work with friends and neighbors to stand up for their rights. ACORN's organizers have been mostly middle class and college educated, its members poor and street smart.

ACORN's real power has stemmed from these members. When Lewis took over, these poor and working-class volunteers, mostly black or Hispanic, numbered more than 400,000. To support their organization, they have paid annual dues. Many have emerged from the rank and file to help lead ACORN.

Unlike many other large associations, ACORN has not depended on one famous leader. There has never been a Jesse Jackson, Gloria Steinem, or Ralph Nader in ACORN. Its champions are many and their personalities varied. Most are unknown outside their neighborhoods, but to the poor and moderate-income families living in the Flatbush section of Brooklyn, the Lawndale section of Chicago, the Ninth Ward of New Orleans, and the hundreds of other neighborhoods where ACORN organizes, they are heroes and heroines. Some were involved with their churches, schools, or unions before they joined ACORN, but most of them have never been leaders until an ACORN organizer contacted them. ACORN organizers taught these leaders and tens of thousands of low-income Americans how David can defeat Goliath.

The ACORN story illuminates an important tale about how community organizing can enhance democracy, advance progressive politics, and reduce poverty. It shows America how ordinary people can improve their own lives while making their country a more livable society. ACORN's problem solving concentrates on mustering what ACORN considers poor people's most important source of power—the poor themselves. Thousands of nonprofit groups around the country help the poor. Some provide charity and social services, the classic form of do-gooder noblesse oblige. Others advocate on behalf of the poor, but without input from the poor themselves. And some, like ACORN, have organized the poor to fight for themselves. Among the thousands of community groups around the country, ACORN has stood almost alone as a national force, with the ability to win major reforms at the neighborhood, city, state, and national levels.

The history of ACORN dispels the myth that the only way we can help the poor is through soup kitchens, charity, and social services. ACORN's people have never accepted the notion that the United States can meaningfully improve the lives of the poor through kindness and compassion alone. They don't give out grocery bags at food pantries. Rather, the people in this story energized the poor so they could clean up their communities, build homes, and increase wages.

Rathke has shown that when it comes to fighting poverty, what counts are structure, philosophy, strategy, and size. By the end of the 1990s, ACORN's basic structure was in place: a national organization with local chapters, with dues-paying members drawn from the poor, working class, and middle class of all races and ethnicities, and capable of acting locally and nationally on many issues, not just one. As Lewis took the helm, ACORN's size and reach resembled those of a large labor union, as well as of influential advocacy groups like the NRA and the Sierra Club. Leaders of organizations trying to increase their effectiveness studied ACORN to learn from its experience.

Its feet-on-the-ground pragmatic and progressive philosophy contrasts with more ideological groups on both ends of the political spectrum. It has applied the art of compromise, but only after its strategies and tactics pushed the limits by mobilizing its members through voter registration and confrontation, politics and protest, negotiation and collaboration. ACORN's leaders have been willing to join partnerships with its enemies. They believe that the perfect is often the enemy of the good.

This book is above all about hope and power. Americans are still stirred by Martin Luther King's "I Have a Dream" speech because we share our country's spirit of what is possible, even in the face of adversity. The spirit of hope and the power that comes from community organizing is ACORN's moral bond with Barack Obama, who went to work in Chicago with a group similar to ACORN after graduating from Columbia University. In his 1995 memoir, *Dreams from My Father*, Obama tells what motivated him: "Change won't come from the top, I would say. Change will come from a mobilized grass roots. That's what I'll do. I'll organize black folks. At the grass roots. For change."[12]

During his primary campaign for president in 2008, Obama challenged detractors who accused him of being what he termed a "hope-monger." Obama said his opponents' view was that "if you talk about hope, you must not have a clear view of reality." Hope, Obama said, is not "blind optimism" or "ignoring the challenges that stand in your way." But "nothing in this country worthwhile has ever happened except when somebody somewhere was willing to hope." To make hope a reality requires the power of people, Obama added, pointing to his public life: "I've won some good fights and I've also lost some fights because good intentions are not enough, when not fortified with political will and political power."[13]

"That is how workers won the right to organize against violence and intimidation. That's how women won the right to vote. That's how young people traveled south to march and to sit in and to be beaten, and some went to jail and some died for freedom's cause."[14]

ACORN's success, along with the election of Obama, suggests the need for a public philosophy that redefines the appropriate relationship among government, the private sector, and ordinary people. Just as President Barack Obama's agenda is pushing America to rethink these issues, ACORN's history has confirmed that Americans need a new direction. In a country suspicious of state intervention, ACORN's experience shows that we require a government not just off our backs, but also on our side, and that an activist government, when combined with a well-organized, vigorous civil society, can and should be a vital force in the struggle for a just and sustainable society.

ACORN's high-stakes confrontations reflect the continuing struggle for the soul of the United States. At the dawn of the Obama era, the nation is holding its breath, trying to decide what kind of society we want to be. Business interests and conservative ideologues threatened by ACORN's agenda, which opposes unfettered free-market solutions to U.S. problems, continue their attacks. Obama is both a mainstream politician and an activist at heart and, like President Franklin D. Roosevelt, has to balance those two impulses. But since the times make the president, Bertha Lewis believed ACORN could help stir an upsurge of activism that might help make Obama a better president—as the depression-era activism made FDR a better president and made it easier for him to accomplish New Deal reforms. Obama's election provided an opening for progressive groups like ACORN to advance their agendas. But Lewis also had to cope with the aftershocks of the attacks by the Right and internal tensions caused by the transition in leadership from its founder to the newly elected yet untested Lewis. This book is also a cautionary tale about what can happen to a community based anti-poverty group when it becomes very effective at fighting for social justice.

Chapter 1

Wade Rathke and the Roots of ACORN

I would not lead you into the Promised Land if I could,
because if I could lead you in, someone else would lead you out.
—Eugene Debs

Power is the ability to achieve a purpose.
Whether or not it is good or bad depends upon the purpose.
—Martin Luther King Jr.

Early on the morning of May 25, 1970, a determined young man packed his belongings—his clothes, his wife's clothes, and his only piece of furniture, a rocking chair—into his 1967 Datsun station wagon. He slid into the front seat and began a 1,500-mile trip from Boston to Little Rock, Arkansas, uncertain of his future but convinced he could transform American politics. He planned to help the poor by organizing them into a powerful political force.

At twenty-one, Wade Rathke had already come a long way. Two years earlier, he had been a sophomore at Williams College. Like many students during that era, he had joined the radical activist group Students for a Democratic Society (SDS) and agitated against the Vietnam War. But Rathke found the Williams students elitist, the professors dull, and his courses irrelevant to his aspirations. In January 1968 he dropped out and headed south to New Orleans, his hometown, to organize resistance to the war. His father, Edmann, an auditor who lived in a middle-class neighborhood of New Orleans, was furious. "You were an Eagle Scout," he cried. "Now you're a traitor and a dropout!"

Rathke was disturbed but unmoved by his father's tirade. He didn't live at home and did not want his father's money. To get by, he worked as a busboy, then as a print dryer, and finally as a lift-truck driver. He volunteered as a draft counselor and organized college demonstrations against the war. Yet after six months Rathke found himself as restless and frustrated as he'd been at Williams. He was tired of advising pampered college students on how they could avoid military service. The students "were not the blacks, Puerto Ricans, and working families, many of whom I had worked with and who were really suffering in America." Rathke was not, as he later put it, "interested in setting up a service bureau for upper-middle-class college kids."

Like many activist students in 1968, Rathke believed that the times were ripe for world-shattering change. The antiwar movement had become so powerful that it forced President Lyndon Johnson not to seek reelection. Yet, Rathke felt, the hopes of 1968 were not coming to fruition, partly because many antiwar leaders had contempt for or were indifferent to working-class people.

In August 1968, five days after his twentieth birthday, Rathke married his high school girlfriend, Lee, a secretarial school graduate. Uncertain about what he should do next, he defaulted to a conventional route and headed back to Williams. On the way, he attended a national SDS meeting in Ann Arbor, Michigan, and watched in dismay as the group tore itself apart.[1] A leader of a faction of SDS, called the Progressive Labor Party, talked of unions seduced by "false consciousness"—meaning that workers persisted in supporting the capitalist system that oppressed them—and challenged those attending to start a worker-student alliance. Rathke shook his head in disbelief.

Later he told his wife that the speakers were a bunch of spoiled students who never worked a day in their lives. "The idea that workers were looking for alliances with students, and that students would lead them to the Promised Land, was bullshit," Rathke thought; these student activists were completely disconnected from reality. He sensed that their politics, unlike his own, lacked the vital element of hope. That was his last SDS meeting. A rangy redhead with a long lean face and a prominent Adam's apple, Rathke wore denim shirts and cowboy boots, as if to show the other activists in the North that this Louisiana boy was not one of them. He could have been mistaken for a country-and-western singer.

Back at Williams during the fall of 1968, Rathke set up a draft-counseling center and organized a three-day shutdown of the campus to support a sit-in at the administration hall by African American students. Eventually, though, he imagined a different path—an antiwar movement not simply set on ending the war but growing into a force for fundamental change, addressing issues like economic inequality, the shortage of jobs, and city slum conditions.[2]

But that fall, organizing the poor and working class would have to wait. Running short of cash, Rathke trudged fruitlessly from factory after factory, warehouse to warehouse looking for work. After several weeks he landed a job with a federally funded antipoverty program in North Adams, Massachusetts, not far from Williams. The program advised welfare recipients regarding their rights. When Rathke read an article in the *Nation* about a plan to reduce poverty, the rigor of its arguments intrigued him. The authors, Frances Fox Piven and Richard Cloward, urged leftist activists to help the poor get on the welfare rolls. They noted that throughout history, only when the poor used disruptive protest tactics did they succeed in significantly improving their lot. Their break-the-bank strategy would require adding millions to welfare, which in turn would "precipitate a profound financial crisis," since cities lacked the funds or the staff to accommodate the spiraling number of desperate people seeking financial assistance. This strategy, Piven and Cloward predicted, would force mayors and governors to lobby for a guaranteed adequate annual income for the poor.

Soon after Rathke started working at the antipoverty community center, he joined several staffers on a bus trip to Boston to attend a rally for the National Welfare Rights Organization (NWRO). Rathke stood on the Boston Commons that summer day with several hundred others listening to NWRO leader George Wiley urge the crowd "to join our crusade for welfare rights." Wiley, a black man in his late thirties, cut a formidable figure with his large Afro and his billowing African dashiki. A former leader of a civil rights organization, the Congress of Racial Equality (CORE), with a PhD in chemistry, he had created the NWRO in 1966. Wiley wanted to achieve economic gains for welfare recipients comparable to the rights won in the civil rights movement in the South. In their influential article in the *Nation*, Piven and Cloward had shown that for every family on the federal welfare program Aid to Families with Dependent Children (AFDC), at least one other family was eligible but not enrolled. These activist sociologists advocated mobilizing the poor in racially tense big cities in states that were of crucial electoral importance to Democrats, the party then in power. By picketing outside welfare offices for more food, clothes, and money, they argued, the poor would pressure mayors and governors into lobbying Washington for increased benefits and possibly reform the welfare system with a national minimum income for poor families.

Partly spurred by federally funded antipoverty programs, Wiley as well as Cloward and Piven had noticed that small local welfare rights organizations were hatching in Los Angeles, Chicago, Cleveland, Baltimore, and other cities, their intent to encourage the poor to apply for welfare. Wiley modified the Cloward-Piven plan by focusing his organizers on those who were already on welfare but had not received all the benefits they were eligible for. Within two years, tens of thousands of single minority mothers in hundreds of local demonstrations disrupted welfare offices, demanding an end to the arbitrary eligibility restrictions and stingy payments. One egregious rule allowed a social worker to deny aid to a mother if the worker believed—no proof required—that a man was living in her home. This arbitrary rule also discouraged a father from living with and supporting his children.

Conservative critics claimed that expanding the welfare rolls would create a "culture of dependency." Even Wiley's liberal critics believed the answer was more jobs, not more welfare. (Sen. Robert Kennedy, running for president on an antiwar and antipoverty platform in 1968, shared this view.) Civil rights leader Whitney Young, director of the Urban League, said it was more important to get one black woman into a job as an airline stewardess than it was to get fifty women on welfare. At the rally Rathke attended, Wiley responded to his critics: "Many theorists say we need to get people off the dole, find more jobs, cut costs, solve poverty. That's fine. But I say, any welfare reform that doesn't leave poor people better off, is no reform at all." His voice rising, he continued: "What we're doing is getting the people involved in demanding rights as human beings from a system that treats them like animals."[3]

Wiley believed that NWRO's success would in large part hinge on his ability to recruit and train skilled organizers who could energize welfare mothers. Attending the rally was one of Wiley's early recruits and the head organizer of the Massachusetts NWRO chapter, Bill Pastreich, a young white man with hawk eyes that gave him an almost predatory appearance. Before joining NWRO he had served in the Peace Corps and had been forced by his host country in Latin America to leave because he had organized a number of rent strikes. He went on to study community organizing in a Syracuse University training course based on the methods of Saul Alinsky, the guru of community activism, then worked for César Chávez's United Farm Workers. Just before the NWRO rally, the *Boston Globe Magazine* had run a profile of Pastreich titled "The Organizer."[4]

Pastreich knew about Rathke's antiwar organizing and approached him at the rally with an offer: "We need you to open up a welfare rights office in Springfield, Massachusetts." Rathke replied, "Let me think about it." He saw in Wiley a charismatic leader with a hopeful strategy, and he wanted to work for him. Even though it would be only a summer job, he and his wife, Lee, agreed that the welfare rights movement had more potential to change things than did his work at the local antipoverty agency. He called Pastreich, trying to leave him with the impression that he was an experienced organizer. "I don't know much about your welfare rights group," Rathke said, "but let me take a look at Springfield to see if it's ripe for organizing." In fact he knew nothing about organizing poor people and years later would say, "I wouldn't have known if a neighborhood in Springfield was ripe for organizing if it bit me on the ass." Pastreich was not fooled, but he knew Rathke was smart, had organized students, and had that fire in the belly that, with good mentoring, helped turn young idealists into effective activists.

"How soon can you do that?"

"I'll check it out next weekend," Rathke promised.

When Lee came home from work, Wade told her about his plan to visit Springfield that coming weekend, August 15, 1969. "I got tickets to the Woodstock Festival," she protested.

"But I promised Bill I would go check out Springfield," Wade answered. "There'll be other rock concerts." Looking back, Rathke would think of Woodstock as a symbolic moment that separated the political activists from the mostly tie-dyed and beaded cultural ones.

Rathke hitched an hour and a half ride from Williamstown to Springfield, where he bedded down in a sleeping bag on the porch of Wally Foster, the editor of Springfield's underground newspaper. Early the next morning, Saturday, Rathke confidently canvassed community centers, black churches, and public-housing projects. He knocked on doors, enjoyed talking to the people he met, and managed to identify neighborhoods where significant numbers of poor people lived. He had always imagined himself embedded in a cause consistent with his deeply held values about equality, which could change the lives of the poor for the better.

Back home, Rathke let Pastreich know that he would accept his unconventional job offer, which turned out to be more like accepting a mission.[5] As Rathke quickly learned, NWRO was not going to pay him; he would have to hustle money from friends in the antipoverty agencies. In the summer of 1969, he moved to Springfield, which would prove the first stop on a lifelong road.[6]

Pastreich's plan for building an uprising in Springfield exploited a little-known provision in the welfare laws. Although federal and state government funded the welfare program, counties and cities implemented it and were required to provide for the "special needs" of the recipients. If a family needed clothing or furnishings, for instance, the law compelled the Welfare Department to give that family a check to cover their cost. Pastreich instructed Rathke to hire some organizers, find some community leaders, and then "flood the welfare offices by applying for more benefits."

As Rathke walked through the poor neighborhoods of Springfield, he kept in mind his decision to recruit blacks, Puerto Ricans, and whites simultaneously, because "if you brought in blacks first, then you would have a tough time with whites or Puerto Ricans later." At a large housing project that Rathke targeted as the main locale to canvass, he found the people he needed, including Barbara Rivera, a white welfare recipient; her Puerto Rican husband; and Roger Brunelle, a social worker at a Springfield community center. They agreed to help Rathke locate leaders, who in turn would help them find people on welfare. None of these initial recruits had any experience in community and political action—for example, in the civil rights movement or in union or church activism—but they were angry about the low welfare grants and wanted to improve their lives. In six weeks, with Rathke's seat-of-the-pants training, they became leaders in the community and ready to put NWRO's scheme into effect.

The welfare rules entitled a family of three to three chairs, a family of four to four, as well as linens and household furnishings. Rathke and his recruits went door knocking in the low-income neighborhoods of Springfield, asking residents what they had and what they lacked. Entering an apartment, they would ask, Where's your fourth chair? Your third bed sheet? Your missing pillows and pillowcases? Rathke, charming with his southern drawl, would point out, "You have a right to these things." Upon leaving, he'd give the family a flyer inviting them to an upcoming welfare rights meeting.

Many welfare recipients were attracted to the campaign. It was simple to understand, it appealed to their self-interest, and it encouraged them only to exercise their legal rights. Rathke's pitch added to the appeal. In one-on-one organizing, he projected confidence, with sad eyes that conveyed empathy and deep respect for the poor.

At the meetings, women filled out the proper forms to apply for welfare benefits and paid their one-dollar dues to the NWRO. Right after the meetings, fifty to sixty women would take buses to the welfare office in Springfield, where they presented caseworkers with their properly completed applications specifying the chairs, sheets, pillowcases, and school clothing that they were entitled to. Rathke accompanied them, but the women did the talking, sometimes the shouting. Some of the caseworkers were sympathetic, others were intimidated and even frightened, but all were overwhelmed by the load of paperwork set in motion by the NWRO campaign. The applicants would make it clear that they would be back in two weeks to pick up their checks. The next day another busload would arrive. Within two weeks, word spread in the housing projects, and soon hundreds were filling out forms to get welfare for the first time, and others to get money for their special needs.

The actions got the city officials to pay attention and negotiate with the new members of a loose group called the Springfield Welfare Rights Chapter of NWRO. Rathke and the group reached an agreement with the city Welfare Department to designate a pick-up day when all the mothers could go to the department to obtain their checks. Eventually, two hundred mothers would arrive to apply for welfare on a pick-up day, while another hundred were collecting their checks for school clothing for their children or for furniture.

Rathke quickly gained a reputation as one of NWRO's best organizers. Pastreich said to him, "Maybe you do know what you are doing."

Rathke replied, "I thought you knew what you were doing when you hired me." "Hired" continued to be a misnomer, since like most NWRO organizers, Rathke was expected to live off the land. He worked out a deal with Teddy Sylvester, director of an antipoverty program, to pay him eighty dollars a week to organize for NWRO. Lee Rathke supplemented their income working as a bank teller and secretary. Some NWRO organizers lived on small donations or depleted their savings. Pastreich spent four thousand dollars of his savings in the first year he organized in Boston. Rathke commandeered free stationery, flyers, and NWRO buttons.

Rathke also recruited volunteers to help him organize. His best prospects were students from schools of social work, VISTA volunteers from the federal community service program, and employees from community–action programs and government antipoverty agencies. "All these training programs and so forth are fine," Rathke would say, "but people need to organize to get some power and money now. Help them get it!" He would smile, argue, guilt trip, and captivate his potential recruits. His pool of recruits was not out of the ordinary for the late 1960s. Across the country, staffers of hundreds of government-funded antipoverty programs were helping the NWRO, either overtly or covertly. Some risked losing their jobs, because NWRO's confrontational tactics had alienated many government officials, especially those who opposed all antipoverty programs.

These tactics were about to backfire in Springfield. Empowered by their NWRO experiences, the hundreds of women who got special clothing allowances for their children during the summer of 1969 launched a drive to obtain winter clothing for adults. What they and Rathke did not know was that the city's welfare director had had enough of what he considered Rathke's antics. So many clients had flooded his office at 760 State Street with demands for clothing, furniture, and housing money that he feared the system would burst. When he heard of the group's planned sit-in to demand winter clothing, he consulted the city's attorneys and discovered that while the recipients had a right to children's clothing, they had no legal right to winter clothing for adults. He planned to fight back.

Rathke relished the prospect of the upcoming battle. A sharp-witted student, he had been suspended from high school several times because of clashes with authorities he thought were in the wrong.[7] When his high school guidance counselor explained to his parents that their son's self-righteousness and sarcasm were provoking school authorities again and again, Wade's father, Edmann, knew exactly what she meant, having himself been counseled many times by his supervisors at Chevron's accounting department to stop questioning his bosses and to curb his sarcasm and criticism of others. Edmann Rathke was certain that his behavior had blocked his career advancement.

Now Wade Rathke was eager to take on Springfield's welfare director, Lawrence Durkin, whom he viewed as a genial and decent individual but also as a functionary in an evil system. Rathke organized his sit-in for October 15, 1969, Vietnam Moratorium Day. (That day, ten million Americans in town squares and college campuses across the country would speak out against the war.) Schools had been closed down because of a teachers' strike, so students from the Black Student Union at Springfield College, who were looking for a way to link their opposition to the war to poverty issues, were available to support the welfare mothers.

On the morning of the fifteenth, the unsuspecting director opened the welfare office doors as usual. At eleven o'clock, Rathke and 250 women and students moved down the street toward the office. They held signs reading, "More for the poor, less for the war." Durkin locked the door to the building and called police to guard the entrance. When Rathke, the welfare mothers, and the college students reached his street-level office, Durkin allowed ten women to enter. They demanded sixty-five dollars for each mother to buy a winter coat and boots. Durkin replied that such an outlay was against the state's policy. As the women outside the office grew restless, an NWRO leader snuck in a back entrance and unlocked the office door; Rathke and hundreds of welfare recipients flooded inside. When the police arrived, they smartly pushed past the women who had voted to get arrested and seized the male students first, roughed up Rathke and dragged him to the police van, then directed the women toward the front door. The police told them that once outside, they would be arrested and placed in police vans. But as the women left the building, the vans pulled away; to avoid arresting hundreds of women welfare recipients, the police had tricked them into vacating the building.

Barbara Rivera and other leaders started a picket line in front of the welfare office, demanding that the police release Rathke and the others. But when Vera Smith, the chair of the Hill Welfare Rights Organization, saw the police pushing one of the leaders in the back, she crashed through a glass door and into the welfare office. Although other welfare rights demonstrators stayed disciplined, someone in the gathering crowd threw a rock at the paddy wagons, and a riot ensued.

The incident touched off two days of unrest in Springfield and the destruction of property worth millions of dollars. As a few people set stores on fire in slum neighborhoods, looters barely kept ahead of the spreading flames and smoke. Thirty demonstrators, mostly students, were arrested. The mayor imposed a three-day curfew. From his cell, Rathke heard the fire sirens, the squawk of two-way radios, the sound of cop cars racing up and down the street. He wondered what had gone wrong.

Although Rathke was released and charged with simple trespassing, none of the families obtained money for winter coats, and many citizens, including some families on welfare, angered and scared by what they saw as a "welfare riot," turned against Rathke and his organization.[8] At first Rathke felt devastated. The protest was a complete debacle, he thought, and he wondered if he would have to rebuild the organization from scratch. He approached the first organizational meeting after the riot with some trepidation, because he was not sure how people would respond. To his amazement most of those Rathke had organized felt empowered. Just a few weeks after the riot, they organized another demonstration at the courthouse in which almost a hundred people participated.

Meeting turnout never faltered after the riot. In the Puerto Rican community the older men led the way back to the meetings, arguing that they had won with NWRO before, and they owed loyalty to the organization now. Rathke was exhilarated. He helped the group organize a successful campaign around free school lunches for poor children. His success spilled over to poor families who were not on welfare and not in an NWRO chapter but, emboldened by its actions, applied for and received benefits. (One of the black students who was inspired by the events, Ken Wade, stayed active in civil rights and thirty-four years later became the CEO of NeighborWorks America, a nonprofit corporation that runs a multimillion-dollar grant and training program that supports a national network of 240 affordable housing and community-development organizations.) Three months after Rathke moved to Springfield, he had mobilized more than two thousand whites, Puerto Ricans, and blacks into six neighborhood welfare rights groups. After six months, the human flooding of the welfare offices had succeeded far beyond his expectations; members were receiving several million dollars in benefits from the Welfare Department.

Rathke felt as if the revolution was coming and these people were leading it. To his colleagues he referred to the mothers as "a strong conflict group, essential to social change." His experiences, including the riot, had taught him a great deal about strategy, tactics, action, anger, and courage. His work reinforced his belief that the poor needed power to deal with their own affairs. It deepened his respect for the people he organized, whom he learned to trust and rely on. Most of all, it reinforced his belief that one important resource for poor people was their ability to disrupt.

After Pastreich left to build NWRO's Connecticut affiliate, Rathke moved to Boston to become the head organizer for the Massachusetts group. By then, he and the other NWRO activists had built local chapters in almost every major city in the country; NWRO's membership had grown to 22,000, and its influence on welfare recipients well beyond that number. During the 1960s the number of mothers and children enrolled on the federal welfare program doubled to nearly ten million, and benefits rose from $338 per month for a family of four to $435 per month. Between 1965 and 1971, the welfare population in New York City alone swelled from 538,000 to 1,165,000. The NWRO deserves some of the credit (or blame, critics would say) for this increase—directly, by organizing its members to demand relief, and indirectly, by promoting the notion that even poor jobless people have rights to benefits from the government if society can't produce enough jobs and child care to allow mothers to enter the workforce.

To many Americans, this dramatic increase in the number of women on welfare during a period of prosperity was a scandal. Some white voters, angry at the uprisings and looting in the nation's black ghettos, called the looters "worthless welfare cheats." Richard Nixon, in the 1968 presidential race, had promised to bring law and order to the cities and to reduce the welfare rolls.

To Wade Rathke, Bill Pastreich, George Wiley, and the other organizers and leaders of the National Welfare Rights Organization, the increase in recipients and spending on welfare was not a disgrace but the righteous victory they had planned. Despite Richard Nixon's rhetoric about welfare, Daniel Patrick Moynihan, Nixon's chief domestic advisor, was promoting a guaranteed national income plan that called for $1,600 per year for a family of four—far less generous than NWRO's plan, which sought $5,500. Some NWRO leaders believed momentum was on their side, and it was just a matter of time before they could force Nixon to support NWRO's sweeping reform plan.

One night in the winter of 1970 in his small apartment on Rutland Square in Boston's shabby South End neighborhood, Rathke sat in his kitchen drinking coffee with his colleagues around a wooden table. They talked about alternative strategies. Rathke, now twenty-one, felt NWRO's success at increasing the welfare rolls had been overshadowed by the backlash against these same poor families, by middle-class Americans whom Nixon called the nation's "silent majority." His mood was pensive. He had been reflecting on his experiences and drawing on his deep knowledge of America's populist history and social movements. He rose from the kitchen chair (a recent purchase from Goodwill), refilled his cup of black coffee, and said, "Welfare rights might be at a dead end."

Rathke began formulating a more audacious strategy to help the poor. He still believed in the welfare rights cause, but he thought making the United States a more just society would require an advocacy group that helped the working poor and the middle class as well as welfare mothers. According to his analysis, centrist and right-wing politicians had succeeded in convincing the broad middle-class majority that their pocketbooks paid for welfare rights. The potential allies of the poor—especially white working-class families—had become their enemies. This would limit NWRO's capacity to make major reforms.

NWRO leaders like Johnnie Tillman, a welfare mother of six from the Watts section of Los Angeles, disagreed with Rathke. They insisted NWRO stay the course. With Nixon publicly behind (but privately scornful of) Moynihan's idea to eliminate welfare with a guaranteed income, NWRO would now focus on exerting political pressure on the Nixon administration to make sure the minimum guaranteed was closer to $5,500 than $1,500.

To achieve this goal, the NWRO needed to move into the South, and George Wiley thought Rathke was his man to implement the expansion. NWRO leaders chose New Orleans and Little Rock as bases of southern operations. In New Orleans, they could lobby U.S. senator Russell Long, the chair of the Senate Finance Committee, which oversaw welfare legislation, a Democrat who was both a segregationist and a New Dealer. In Arkansas, their target would be Rep. Wilbur Mills, the chair of the House Ways and Means Committee and the most powerful architect of social and economic legislation in the country.

But Rathke had his own plan. Convinced that the base of welfare mothers and their children was too thin to support the heavy political weight needed to change the nation, he offered Wiley this deal: "I'll go south, but you've got to let me organize a larger organization, beginning in Arkansas. We can't build a large poor people's organization where the next-door neighbor to the welfare recipient was just as antagonistic to welfare as anyone else. We have to break out of the single-issue welfare campaigns to build a majority constituency where the next-door neighbors are in it together and not fighting each other." Wiley agreed and raised $5,500 from a foundation for Rathke's six months' salary and expenses.

Arkansas was hardly a bastion of liberalism. In 1957, its governor, Orval Faubus, famously defied a court order to desegregate a Little Rock public high school by commanding National Guard troops to prevent the admission of nine black youngsters. Unions had little power in a state whose so-called right-to-work laws restricted workers' bargaining rights. Former ACORN workers Madeleine Adamson and Seth Borgos accurately summed up Rathke's risky adventure: "With a Southern heritage of racial separation, a conservative political environment, and a negligible history of community protest, Arkansas offered an acid test for this experiment."[9]

By contrast, Rathke looked to Arkansas's populist past for inspiration. In the 1930s, the Industrial Workers of the World, a militant union known as the Wobblies, agitated among the lumber workers, and the interracial Southern Tenant Farmers' Union stirred up the sharecroppers, who advocated for fair cotton prices. Rathke liked the variety of settings in Arkansas which he could organize—the ranch and farm towns in the west and north; the cotton plantation communities of the Mississippi Valley; and the small city of Little Rock—135,000 people.

He also appreciated the state motto, "Regnat populus"; after four years of high school Latin, he knew that it meant "The people shall rule." Despite the aluminum companies, milk producers, oil and timber companies, utility companies, and remnants of a plantation system that controlled the rich resources of Arkansas, he thought he could use the slogan to help him organize. In the middle of his first big campaign, Rathke would introduce the name of his group—Arkansas Community Organization for Reform Now, or ACORN.

Chapter 2

Stepping onto a Larger Stage

> At the highest level of politics, there is no one who now reliably speaks for the people, no one who listens patiently to their concerns or teaches them the hard facts involved in governing decisions. There is no major institution committed to mobilizing the power of citizens concerning their own interests and aspirations.
>
> —William Greider, *Who Will Tell the People*

Wade Rathke did not speak in abstractions about the class struggle, but instead talked about the economic issues of immediate concern to the poor, like housing, clothing, jobs, and money. As a model he looked to America's populist past—a tradition of common people mobilizing against wealthy and powerful financial and corporate interests—from the abolitionists who helped end slavery, to the Progressive era reformers in the early 1900s who cleaned up urban slums and sweatshops, to the labor activists who organized unions.

He was particularly attracted to the agrarian revolt that spawned the Non-Partisan League, one of the most successful state-level reform organizations in the nation's history. Emerging at the tail end of the Populist revolt, which was one of the largest mass movements in U.S. history, it mobilized southern and Midwestern farmers to battle the railroads, grain companies, bankers, and politicians. Rathke's grandfather had emigrated to North Dakota in 1916, in the midst of that revolt. The farmers united against an unresponsive state government controlled by banks, railroads, and big grain dealers. The Non-Partisan League's populist platform called for state-owned grain elevators, a state-controlled hail-and-fire insurance company, and a state bank. In 1919, the Bank of North Dakota, located in Bismarck, became the only state-owned bank in the nation, providing much needed access to credit for farmers. Members of the Non-Partisan League paid six dollars in dues, later raised to sixteen dollars biannually, and promised to support League candidates for public office. Wade Rathke would never forget the importance of charging members dues.

His political consciousness was also informed by early twentieth-century muckraking journalists like Ida Tarbell, who forced John D. Rockefeller to break up his oil trust into smaller companies. Rathke had more than just an intellectual connection to the muckrakers; his father was an auditor for Chevron, one of America's giant oil companies, once a part of Rockefeller's oil trust.

Rathke and Alinsky

Rathke's modern model for empowering the powerless from the bottom up was Saul Alinsky. Rathke studied Alinsky's books, *Reveille for Radicals* and *Rules for Radicals*, how-to manuals for activists. Alinsky believed in the radical American idea that democracy is for ordinary people. In the 1940s, he developed his basic model in the Back of the Yards, the old Chicago stockyards neighborhood made famous in Upton Sinclair's classic muckraking novel, *The Jungle*. There, he recruited local leaders from the churches, block clubs, sports leagues, and unions that formed the Back of the Yards Neighborhood Council, the first of what Alinsky would call the People's Organization. Alinsky guided them to identify common interests that brought together into a large organization previously hostile ethnic groups of Serbs and Croatians, Czechs and Slovaks, Poles and Lithuanians. The council pressured, demanded, and negotiated with government officials and businesses on bread-and-butter issues such as better garbage collection, improved schools, fresh milk for children, and more jobs.

From the 1930s through the early 1960s Alinsky's community organizing work resulted in important local victories. In Rochester, Chicago, and other cities, Alinsky and his protégés built effective organizations that targeted slumlords, got big companies to provide jobs to ghetto residents, and forced municipal governments to improve public services in neglected neighborhoods. His first book, *Reveille for Radicals* published in 1946, got considerable attention, but he was considered a *community* organizer whose ideas applied effectively only at the local political level. The groups that Alinsky helped organize in various cities had no political ambition or agenda beyond their own communities.[1]

In 1965, the publication of Charles Silberman's *Crisis in Black and White* brought Alinsky another wave of public attention. Silberman described Alinsky's organizing work in Chicago's Woodlawn slum, where he taught black residents how they could make themselves an effective political force. Alinsky's group organized a boycott of white merchants who overcharged neighborhood consumers, and they forced slumlords to clean up their properties.[2] Alinsky believed that if you want to help improve the lives of people, you need to help them organize for power. He derided charity, philanthropy, and do-goodism. Based on his early experiences, Alinsky developed a method of gaining power that others could duplicate, no matter what their objectives. It had five essential elements:

1. Voluntary associations need paid, well-trained, professional organizers.
2. Working behind the scenes, the organizer's job is to build a democratically run community group. Individual participation alone can give the powerless a sense of their own dignity.
3. To encourage participation, the organizer has to appeal to people's self-interest around concrete winnable issues.

4. To win victories, groups need to use a variety of tactics, notably dramatic public confrontations. ("Keep your enemy off guard," Alinsky warned. He would use nearly any method for making authorities miserable—rent strikes, demonstrations, marches on city hall.)[3]
5. To sustain a group over time requires more than boycotts, protests, and picketing. The organizers have to recruit leaders and raise money by building upon formal relationships with community institutions, especially churches and unions.

Rathke also studied the work of Fred Ross, an Alinsky coworker who organized in the barrios of California, New Mexico, and Arizona. Like Pastreich from NWRO, Ross rejected the Alinsky model's call to organize the leaders of churches and unions to serve as the natural foundation for groups. Ross found greater success organizing house-to-house on specific issues of concern to community members. Instead of pulling together local churches, Ross went door-to-door and held house meetings similar to coffee klatches, a practice adopted by the NWRO. In 1960, Ross and César Chávez successfully applied the house-meeting, issue-organizing approach to the effort to organize farmworkers.[4]

Rathke noted that grassroots organizing had reached a state of uncertainty throughout the country. Community organizing needed a model that could change the United States by tackling issues that reached beyond the borders of cities and local neighborhoods. Unlike most antipoverty activists, Rathke believed that primarily focusing on local targets would not succeed on issues such as affordable housing and better jobs, because the leverages of power were at the state and national levels. If community organizers were to make a significant difference in the lives of the poor, they had to ratchet up their efforts, raise their sights, and help build a national movement that was greater than the sum of the myriad local groups fighting slumlords, welfare bureaucrats, and utility companies.

Rathke envisioned a national, multiracial, neighborhood-based operation that would address a range of problems facing low- and moderate-income people. In building ACORN, Rathke hoped to retain what was effective in his welfare rights experience—winnable campaigns, dues, direct action, strategic use of the press—while incorporating part of the old Alinsky model. "You can win stoplights from here to eternity," Rathke would tell young recruits, "which is what many community organizations around the country have excelled at, but unless your organization addresses the question of who has the power to control what happens in a neighborhood, a city, a county, or a state . . . then all your organization will achieve is a proliferation of stoplights in low to moderate neighborhoods. Obviously, ACORN's goal is much more."

Rathke noted that 70 percent of the population of Arkansas earned less than $7,000 per year and determined that, in that context, "if you fashion a program that will attract people who earn, say, $8,000 or less, then you're appealing to a very large majority."

A Different Breed

While Rathke was a product of the New Left, he was estranged from many of its student and antiwar leaders, especially those who were the sons and daughters of liberals or were "red-diaper babies," as the children of radicals and communists were called. Their parents were disproportionately northern, professional and secular, and supported Adlai Stevenson and the United Nations. Rathke had entirely different roots. His father grew up in Orange, California, volunteered for the Navy, and attended Millsaps College in Jackson, Mississippi, where he met his wife to be, Cornelia Ratliff. Cornelia was a native of Drew, Mississippi, and worked as a junior college administrator. Both parents believed deeply in America as a meritocracy. Rathke recalled his mother repeating homilies like, "If you keep your nose clean, work hard, and do well in school, then I don't care what your race is or your family background—in America, you'll succeed."

Shortly after serving in World War II, Rathke's father, Edmann, was hired as a bookkeeper by Chevron, which before long relocated him and his wife to Wyoming. Soon after Wade was born there in 1948, the Rathkes moved to a Chevron-owned oil camp at Wilson's Creek, Wyoming, and then to company camp five miles outside Rangely, a town in northwestern Colorado, where Wade's brother, Dale, was born. Next the family moved to New Orleans, then to Irving, Kentucky, and in 1955, after Chevron promoted Edmann to field auditor, back to New Orleans. In his first seven years, Wade lived in seven different cities or towns.

After renting a house in a working-class neighborhood on the west bank of New Orleans, Rathke's father bought one of the first houses in a sandy, treeless New Orleans subdivision called Oak Park, built on swamp fill near Bayou St. John not far from Lake Ponchartrain. But every summer until Wade was thirteen years old, between June 15 and Labor Day, the family traveled the West as Edmann audited the books of every pumping station, tank farm, wellhouse, and other Chevron facility from New Mexico to North Dakota. Wade never had the chance to become rooted in one place—good preparation for life as a traveling organizer.

In 1960, the year Wade Rathke would start junior high school in New Orleans, many white student activists were arriving in the South to fight segregation, and white politicians were campaigning against the 1954 Supreme Court decision that struck down the concept of separate but equal education. When the federal court ordered the New Orleans school system to desegregate, most parents, including Wade's, paid close attention to the events surrounding six-year-old Ruby Bridges. Ruby's mother enrolled her in the New Orleans elementary school system, and a U.S. marshal escorted her to Frantz Elementary School; all the school's white parents pulled their children out to protest integration, and Ruby spent her first year in a class of one. She showed up at school every day, initially to find angry, threatening mobs outside her classroom. Her father lost his job, and her grandparents lost their place as tenant farmers. The Rathkes sympathized with Ruby Bridges and opposed segregation, although they were politically conservative. But with the New Orleans school system in chaos, they thought the schools would close down and so enrolled Wade and Dale—to the brothers' horror—in the school where they attended church. The schools did not shut down, and the next year both boys went to their neighborhood public school, F. W. Gregory Junior High School, where Wade was elected president of the student council.

For high school, Wade enrolled in Benjamin Franklin Public High School. He had scored in the ninety-ninth percentile on the Iowa Basic Skills Tests and well over 120 on the IQ test. An experimental school founded in 1957 for children of "high academic potential," Ben Franklin High had stirred up considerable controversy because in 1963, it was one of the few integrated schools in the South. (For Wade, an integrated school meant growing up with black friends like his football teammate Edgar Taplain.) Wade graduated near the top of his class, but at Williams College he was astonished to discover that half his classmates had graduated from prep schools, and none were from the South. His decision to go to Williams was somewhat whimsical; he knew very little about the school, except that it had an excellent political science department and was, he mistakenly thought, near Boston. These sophisticated children of the rich and privileged made him feel, he said, like a "green-behind-the-ears hick."

In the summers of 1966 and 1967, Rathke's father lined up a job for him as a roustabout on an offshore oilrig. His schedule was to work from 6:00 AM to 6:00 PM for fourteen straight days and nights, living on the rig, then have seven days off. Wade fixed lines and leaks, cleaned, painted, and put out fires—dirty, noisy work, occasionally arduous and a few times dangerous, especially when he had to work in the middle of severe rainstorms.

Wade worked with crews of men from all over the South and West—Texas cowboys, Mississippi rednecks, and Louisiana coonasses, many of whom had fought in the Korean War or had children Wade's age fighting in Vietnam. The polls in the South and Southwest showed 70 percent of the people supported the war, yet in face-to-face conversations with Wade, not a single man said he wanted his son going to Vietnam. Wade would say to them, "I'm not for this war; it looks like bad stuff." The rugged men would look him in the eye and say things like, "Wade, listen, I don't want a goddamn piece of this war." Or, "I didn't support my kid going, I just want him back alive." Or, "You do whatever you can do to stay out of this goddamn mess."

His encounters taught him that people are more complex than he had realized. Unlike many young left-wing activists at the time who said that "unions block the path of revolution" or induce "false consciousness" (based on a Marxist theory that institutions in a capitalist society mislead the proletariat about the nature of capitalism and their own oppression), Rathke would never view union and blue-collar workers as his enemies. If they were misguided about school integration or the war in Vietnam or the welfare system, that didn't mean they were evil people or that they couldn't change their views.

Arkansas

Soon after Rathke arrived in Arkansas in the spring of 1970, he hired his first organizer, Gary Delgado, a tall, handsome African American native of Brooklyn with a big Afro who wore dungarees and long-sleeved sky-blue workshirts. Delgado had begun his organizing career working for the National Welfare Rights Organization during the previous hot, humid summer in a small black northeast Washington, D.C., neighborhood. His first time out, he knocked on the doors of sixty-one families: fifty-nine people came to his first meeting. He thought he was "an organizing god."

Rathke went door-to-door with Delgado in Little Rock for six weeks with, as he would later say, "a pit in my stomach the size of a grapefruit." Gloria Wilson was his first test. He knocked on the door of her small bungalow in Little Rock's South End neighborhood. To the east lay the expressway and an access road a hundred feet away. The same distance to the west was a low-rise public housing project. The twenty-one-year-old Rathke asked Gloria, only two years older but a single mother with a couple of kids, what problems she faced. Gloria said she was on welfare and didn't like it. Welfare payments were too low and she couldn't get a job. She was determined to surmount the stereotype of the welfare mother: "I'm not who the welfare system thinks I am." Rathke kept telling her, "Yes, these are the kinds of things an organization like ACORN could handle if we could organize people to act." He convinced Wilson that day to join him and start knocking on the doors of her neighborhood.

Door knocking was his test of whether someone was ready to lead. Gloria Wilson, along with Carolyn Harris, two African-Americans and Sue Hodge, who lived in Silver City Courts, a white housing project in North Little Rock, became part of a group of young women in a hurry who saw themselves caught in the welfare system because of bad luck, bad choices, and babies to feed. Wilson was soon elected the chair of the South End organizing committee.

Rathke and Delgado, an excellent organizer, found five neighborhoods of low-income residents in addition to the South End and completed some research for the first Arkansas campaign. With the help of a volunteer lawyer, they found in an Arkansas welfare manual a statement that poor people had a right to obtain furniture—not money to buy furniture, as in Massachusetts. So in Arkansas they would launch a campaign for more furniture.

A campaign to get the state to provide more furniture for families might have seemed like just more welfare rights activity, hardly consistent with the bold vision of building a multiracial, multiclass organization capable of transforming U.S. politics. For Rathke, however, it was a first step, a staging area from which to mount larger campaigns that would attract people who earned at or just below the state's median income. He was familiar with this kind of campaign, and he wanted to jump-start his organization. He knew that ordinary people would fight for small, winnable things such as furniture. These battles won, they would move on to larger, more significant issues—higher-paying jobs, affordable housing—that would appeal to a larger constituency.

Several barriers stood in the way of winning more furniture for welfare recipients in Arkansas: Gov. Winthrop Rockefeller, who was unwilling to spend more money on welfare, and a tightfisted state welfare department. ACORN needed allies, but Rathke was afraid that the state's emerging black middle class, many of whom owed their jobs to the governor, would not support his campaign. He deliberately recruited white women on welfare to knock on doors in a neighborhood that George Wallace, the segregationist former Alabama governor, had carried when he ran for president two years earlier. Rathke figured that blacks would join an organization that had white members, but that white poor people would be reluctant to join a group that was already mostly black. So organizing white people first would become an ACORN rule.

For weeks Delgado knocked on doors, spoke at churches—a new experience for a nonpracticing black Catholic from Brooklyn—and attended house meetings, at which he arrived early to ensure getting dinner. Scrounging meals became a regular practice; some of the mothers treated him like a son. One muggy morning at the east end of Little Rock, Delgado held his first organization meeting, hoping that three or four dozen people would attend. He was thrilled when 125 showed up. It was time for the next step.

On a hot sunny day in the summer of 1970, dozens of women, including Gloria Wilson and her friends and family, appeared at the county Welfare Department to demand furniture. Over the next four days, Rathke, Delgado, and several staff volunteers mobilized an additional four hundred welfare recipients, mostly black mothers, to march to the welfare offices. The events were widely covered by TV and the press, which spent much time and print speculating on who organized the demonstrations, on the interracial nature of the group, and on the militancy of its leadership.

At a subsequent demonstration on the grounds of the governor's mansion, the group's members and organizers, including Rathke and Delgado, were themselves impressed with the importance of their efforts when they noticed several state secret service agents keeping an eye on them. That event made the front pages of the two major dailies. The sheer vibrancy of the campaign lifted the spirits of Delgado and the other organizers.

Meanwhile, Rathke had hired Peter Hobby to organize a support group, Citizens for the Abolition of Poverty, for this welfare rights campaign. Because Hobby happened to be the son of the pastor of Second Presbyterian Church in Pleasant Valley, the most powerful and respected Presbyterian minister in Little Rock, his involvement instantly neutralized the governor, a tactic Rathke would use repeatedly in the future. Soon after the demonstrations, the reverend and his son Peter inspected the homes of several welfare recipients and issued a press statement condemning the "inhumanity of a state where children are forced to sleep on the floor" for lack of beds and other furniture.

Rockefeller's office called to negotiate. At the opening session, Gloria Wilson sat quietly through the early negotiations with the governor and his aides, which were not going well. Frustrated, she spoke of the desperate needs of those on welfare: "We have to choose between feeding our kids or buying a decent bed." She pulled off her wig to make the point that she was losing her hair because of the stress of being on welfare, screaming, "Something has to be done." As Rathke would later say: "An organizer can't ask someone to do that, nor would it ever occur to an organizer to think of such a move. It was a dramatic moment and jarred the governor, helping the negotiations."[5] Even so, the talks stalled because the governor did not want to give in to Rathke's demands. The public actions continued.

After the first series of demonstrations at various places, Delgado looked on with disbelief every day when Rathke returned to his office, the back room at the Arkansas Council of Human Relations, leaned back in his chair, propped his boots on a desk, and waited confidently for the governor to call. Finally, he did, and ACORN had its first victory. Rockefeller created a new state agency, Furniture for Families, charged with collecting and distributing used furniture to welfare recipients. According to the *Houston Post*: "A 22 year old, ex-SDS member, organized a group of welfare mothers in a successful effort to resurrect the rusted remnants of southern populism."[6]

With her sister Dora, her brother Bill, and a few neighbors, Gloria Wilson went door-to-door passing out information about ACORN. They all wore the ACORN badge with pride. Dora remembered getting her first badge and Gloria telling her what the letters stood for and how proud she was when she said those words. Wilson remained active with ACORN for many years and twenty-three years later, still a member, was elected to Little Rock's municipal governing council.

After ACORN had agitated with Rockefeller on issues ranging from school lunch programs and public housing conditions to lower utility rates, the governor began to view Rathke's group as a potential ally. As the gubernatorial race between Rockefeller and Dale Bumpers heated up, a Rockefeller aid asked ACORN to register black voters in exchange for a lump-sum payment of five thousand dollars, an offer Rathke refused because ACORN was nonpartisan in the race between Rockefeller and Bumpers. Yet a few days later, a local political operative associated with Rockefeller gave Rathke three thousand dollars in a brown paper bag. ACORN remained neutral in the race, but Rathke used the money to hire staff and buy free textbooks for the children of his new members. ACORN was too new to endorse candidates and get involved in politics. After Bumpers won without ACORN's backing, Rathke, looking to network with the new governor's supporters, took a small group of ACORN leaders to the new governor's hotel victory celebration, telling the leaders, "It's free food, plenty of contacts, and it looks like we backed a winner all along."

With the campaign's success, Delgado also got an education about Southern culture. To pay back the mothers for all the meals they had fed him he invited seven black leaders to dinner on him at a place of their choice. When he asked where they wanted to eat, they said the bus station. "Why?" he asked. One woman captured all the leaders' feelings: "The food is served cafeteria style, so we can get anything we want. Plus, it's not too expensive, and because it used to be we couldn't eat there and now we can."

ACORN or NWRO

But success brought organizational tension between ACORN and the local NWRO chapter. The older welfare rights leaders like Barbara Hampton, a local leader, didn't trust Gloria Wilson and her cohorts, new leaders who had cast their lot with Rathke. While thirteen neighborhood groups voted to switch from NWRO to ACORN, two groups, one led by Hampton, voted to stay with NWRO. Hampton, one of the welfare mothers who originally agreed to have Rathke come to Arkansas, called a press conference in early February 1972. "Rathke is a middle-class white," she said. "He never had stomach cramps from hunger. How is he going to get the message over of the needs of poor people?"

Hampton went on to level criticisms that would be repeated by future ACORN opponents. "ACORN has taken credit for the achievements of the NWRO in Arkansas. ACORN has become a middle-class-type lobbying group. . . . It only uses poor people or welfare mothers to do the demonstrations. . . . Paid organizers do all the work in the name of poor people, but not with poor people. . . . ACORN's desire for power is greater than its concern for poor people." These were the first but not the last attacks on Rathke by black leaders and activists.[7]

Another NWRO leader referred to Rathke as "an ego-tripping white dude from Louisiana." Although by the early 1970s black power was no longer on the rise, many white liberals and left-wing activists were intimidated and cowed when confronted by black nationalists. Rathke recoiled at the criticism but didn't lash back, even though it could destroy his credibility. He moved quietly away from the condemnation, remaining confident that the future of ACORN did not depend on the opinions of a few welfare rights leaders who, he thought, lacked a base and the ability to organize one.

With his youthful self-confidence, partly due to a Manichean view of the world in which he was one of the good guys, Rathke took these attacks in stride. Also, he was most concerned with how to broaden ACORN's constituency to include other than the welfare poor.

The same self-confidence that made Rathke's staff and others work to impress him would later turn at times to arrogance, leading him to quickly dismiss and publicly criticize those he disagreed with. For example, he wouldn't hesitate to criticize activists who received media attention for being leaders when in fact they had few followers. Rathke's quick tongue damaged both him and ACORN, alienating not only those he criticized, but also his staff, funders, and other activists.

Rathke had seen many antipoverty groups win victories and create enduring change, then fall apart when their organizers left. He believed a lasting organization not only required a professional staff but also should represent the interests of working-class and even middle-class families, as well as the poor. He left NWRO, his sponsoring organization, when it became clear that its national leadership rejected his idea of expanding the group's service base beyond welfare recipients. George Wiley, however, remained a Rathke supporter and until his tragic death in a 1973 boat accident, viewed Rathke's idea of serving a broader constituency of working-class groups as the future of community organizing.

Rathke had brought ACORN to life. In addition to the Furniture for Families victory, ACORN under Rathke's leadership had organized Vietnam veterans to obtain state benefits, unemployed workers to change the unprincipled practices of employment agencies, and property owners trying to save their neighborhoods against blockbusting and freeway construction. Yet when a group of white rural farmers asked ACORN to help them fight the Arkansas Power and Light company (AP&L), their request gave Rathke pause; although the prospect played into his desire to build a broader populist movement, organizing a middle-class group was outside his experience. AP&L planned to build a generating plant on the banks of the Arkansas River about three miles from the farmers' homes. They were worried that the plant's pollutants might destroy their livelihood. But AP&L, a wholly owned subsidiary of a giant regional utility holding company, seemed too powerful an opponent for the newly formed ACORN to take on. Rathke made an apparently quixotic decision to help the farmers. When Steve Kest, an Ivy League student from New York, and John Beam, the son of an air force officer, who had just returned from traveling in Chile, decided to join ACORN to fight poverty, though, the odds changed; ACORN had a fighting chance.

Chapter 3

ACORN's Model T

> [The campaign against AP&L was] the first time that the source of local discontent had been explored to its corporate roots.
> —Wade Rathke

In 1969, when Steve Kest, a high school senior, received his acceptance to Harvard, he was determined to use his education to make a difference in the world. The oldest of three children, he grew up in an upper-middle-class family in White Plains, New York, twenty-five miles north of New York City, but he had been stirred by the students who went South in the early 1960s to support the black lunch-counter sit-ins and West to help César Chávez galvanize the Chicano farmworkers.

When Kest arrived at Harvard in fall of 1970, he found the tail end of the antiwar movement and its transformation into sectarian infighting dispiriting, elitist, and unproductive. He was looking for something that allowed him to engage with a broader constituency on a wider range of issues. At the end of his sophomore year, Kest found an organization that seemed to match his interests. He wrote Wade Rathke, who had been organizing in Arkansas for the past year, to ask if he could use a summer intern. Within a month, Kest was doing research to support ACORN's local organizing campaigns. Although polite and low-key, he had little respect for authority. His intelligence and attention to detail made him a good researcher. His high energy and wry sense of humor would make him a good college organizer.

Rathke, a college dropout, tried to convince Kest that he was more valuable in Arkansas than at Harvard and that, like Rathke, he should drop out. Kest did take a year off from school and became ACORN's research department in Little Rock. Rathke almost convinced him to quit Harvard altogether, but Kest's father called Rathke with an offer: "You've had him this long, and I won't stand in the way, but let him finish school and then you get him back."

In 1973, when Kest first heard about Arkansas Power & Light's (AP&L) plan to build a 2,800-megawatt coal-burning power plant on the banks of the Arkansas River, he saw both a danger and an opportunity. Situated a scant three miles from the farms of the families of Jefferson County, this was going to be no ordinary plant, as Kest's research uncovered. The power station's four huge smokestacks would spew 469 tons of sulfur dioxide, 14 tons of particulate matter, and 291 tons of nitrogen oxides into the air daily—more pollutants than any power plant in operation in the United States. At a billion dollars, the plant was the single largest private investment ever undertaken in Arkansas.

Rumors quickly spread among the farmers and others who lived in the area that the plant's high pollution levels would cause life-threatening harm to surrounding families, poison the water supply, and damage buildings and equipment. The Arkansas State Department of Planning warned that the plant would be "possibly the worst single source of air pollution in the world." In rural Arkansas, the contaminants would settle on the rich, productive land where farmers grew rice, soybeans, and cotton. With an eye toward expanding ACORN's constituency, Kest found scientific studies that demonstrated that even low levels of sulfur dioxide in the air could damage cotton and bean crops, destroying the Jefferson County farmers' livelihoods.

To take advantage of this organizing opportunity, ACORN needed a smart organizer and it found one in John Beam. He too was caught up in the activism of the day. A graduate of Northwestern University, he had organized food co-ops and then spent six months traveling in South America. In Chile just before a military coup overthrew President Salvador Allende, Beam had been unable to organize cooperatives and decided to leave. "Had I been successful," he later recalled, "I might have ended up buried in a wall like those young men in the movie *Missing*." Back in the United States in 1973, he read an ad in a radical underground newspaper: ACORN was looking for organizers. With very little organizing experience, Beam was thrust into a campaign to pressure AP&L to stop building its proposed plant.

The son of an Air Force officer, Beam was a disciplined organizer. At an old school building in Jefferson County, he held a meeting of three dozen farmers who lived in the area. A heavy-set farmer stood up and said, "I don't believe this here power plant belongs to Arkansas Power & Light Co. I think it belongs to some New York concern." Another farmer told the gathering, "I'm definitely against it because they can't burn coal without hurtin' us." A third said to his neighbors, "We're trying to organize a group here, to find out just how that power plant is going to affect us . . . our land . . . our environment . . . our livestock . . . our buildings and machinery." They agreed to form an ACORN chapter to be called the Jefferson County Improvement Association. Martin Kirby, a reporter for the *Arkansas Democrat*, attended one of the group's meetings and observed:

> These farmers were no sharecroppers. Most of them were medium-well-off landowners, typical middle-class Arkansans. Very few were even in working clothes. They were the type who would go to their graves believing in the righteousness of racial segregation and who could afford to send their children to the nearby segregationist private school. Still they sounded the typical ACORN themes: they were the underdogs, victims of powerful, self-serving interests; only collective action would get results; they were going to demand that their elected state and national representatives join with them in their cause or regret it.[1]

One of the farmers summarized the key ingredient: "It takes numbers. You've got to have numbers to make a showing."

The farmers Beam organized came up with the clever idea of AP&L paying a security deposit. A delegation of ACORN farmers delivered a petition signed by a thousand area residents asking the company for a $50 million "deposit in reverse." Like a renter's deposit, it would serve as a guarantee against any damages suffered by the farmers from the plant's operations. Despite publicity and pressure, AP&L not only refused to put up a deposit, but also ignored the farmers' concerns.

Then Kest discovered two facts that he thought would force AP&L to concede to ACORN's demands: first, AP&L was a wholly owned subsidiary of Middle South Utilities; second, Middle South's largest stockholder, with $8 to $10 million worth of stock, was Harvard University. Armed with the "Harvard connection," the ACORN farmers shifted the battle over the power plant construction from Arkansas to Harvard Yard, delivering a letter to Harvard president Derek Bok on November 5, 1973, that asked the university to aid the group in its battle against AP&L. Would university officials meet with ACORN to discuss the possibility of using part of the profits from its Middle South stock to finance an independent study to examine the dangers the new plant posed to the environment? The letter also asked Harvard to support ACORN in its petition to the Arkansas Public Service Commission (APSC), the government regulatory agency that had final approval authority over the construction of the plant, and to use its influence as a major stockholder in Middle South to "persuade" the utility to establish the "deposit in reverse" fund and not to build the plant without effective pollution controls.

Rathke and Kest calculated that asking Harvard for support was a long shot. The utility company was a good investment, and although Harvard's students and faculty had protested the university's stock holdings in the Gulf Oil Corporation operated in the Portuguese colony of Angola, the school had never faced a request by an outside activist group. If Harvard agreed to ACORN's request, it would set a precedent: any activist group could pick out a company in which Harvard owned stock and ask the university to play a leading role in opposing its policies, citing the ACORN case.

President Bok, who had never heard of ACORN and didn't believe its request merited a response, hoped to bottle it up in committees he had appointed. On November 9, 1973, Steven B. Farber, an assistant to Bok, forwarded ACORN's materials to the chair of the group that would make the final decision and asked him to review the documents and determine whether the "complicated questions" raised by ACORN should be referred to a student-faculty-alumni committee for consideration. For the next two months, Harvard dragged its feet, reviewing documents submitted by the utility company, ACORN, and a Harvard Board of Trustees committee set up to examine both sides.

Meanwhile, Kest had obtained the support of a few campus groups, including the New American Movement and Harvard Ecology Action. Sophomore Ruth C. Streeter, a spokeswoman for Ecology Action, said her group would supply money for ACORN and would begin a petition drive. Kest also made sure that the Arkansas press covered the story, leading the state's new governor, Dale Bumpers, to come out in support of ACORN's request that Harvard study the plant. Less than a week after President Bok tried to suppress ACORN's request by referring it to various committees, Governor Bumpers, speaking at the National Governors Conference in Boston on November 14, promised that Arkansas Power & Light's controversial coal-burning power plant would not be built "until every technology available has been used" for pollution control.

Rathke convinced Bill Kitchen, a former ACORN staff member, to go to Cambridge for a few weeks to organize student and faculty support for ACORN'S position. On November 19, Kitchen presented Bok with a petition signed by 1,741 undergraduates asking the president to use Harvard's influence to ensure that the proposed power plant would be environmentally safe. The school's daily newspaper, the *Harvard Crimson*, chronicled the whole episode, including several stories by student reporter Nicholas Lemann (later a prominent journalist and dean of the Columbia University School of Journalism). The coverage made it difficult for university officials to ignore ACORN's request.

After two months and no action from Harvard, in February 1974, ACORN's staff invited nineteen colleges and universities that owned stock in Middle South Utilities to join its fight against the power plant. Another Harvard committee commissioned yet another study on the plant and promised a decision one way or the other on Harvard's support for ACORN within another two months. In March, Kitchen announced that five colleges and universities owning AP&L stock—Princeton, Cornell, Vanderbilt, the University of Wisconsin, and the University of North Carolina—had agreed to scrutinize the plant's environmental impact statement, news that elated ACORN's farmers, who continued to pressure AP&L.

Rathke, Kitchen, and Kest, however, felt ACORN was losing momentum. On April 20, 1974, the Arkansas Public Service Commission (PSC), which regulated private utilities, scheduled its licensing hearings on Arkansas Power & Light's proposed plant. Time was running out for ACORN when late in the spring, Harvard published a four-page statement that called on AP&L to "re-examine its plans with respect to the problem of sulfur dioxide and other emissions" and urged the utility to reconsider installing the additional emission controls ACORN had advocated. Though not all the farmers had hoped for, the letter carried weight both with the PSC and with AP&L.

The research submitted by ACORN to the PSC combined with ACORN's activists and the pressure from Harvard led PSC, the final arbiter, to cut the size of AP&L's proposed plant by half and to mandate pollution-control devices. Although the AP&L never issued a statement saying that it had abandoned the project because of this stricture, the plant was never built, a dramatic and surprising victory for ACORN and a pivotal moment in its history.

ACORN's accomplishment reflected a departure from the makeup and strategies of other antipoverty groups. With a new constituency of white rural farmers, ACORN had become a cross-class, multiracial group that could organize blacks and whites, the welfare poor and family farmers, into one activist group. Further, it had proved that it could win on issues distinct from those of the welfare rights movement. Immediately after the AP&L victory, Rathke understood that ACORN had achieved an additional breakthrough. By taking a local battle statewide and then to Harvard, ACORN had broken with a tradition that limited community-organizing efforts to local issues and campaigns.

In still another community-organizing precedent, Rathke said later, "for the first time, the source of local discontent had been explored to its corporate roots." He believed big corporations were largely responsible for the persistence of so much poverty in a country with such enormous wealth, but it was hard to make that point in practice. Now, he said to his staff and anyone who would listen, ACORN had succeeded in doing so.

Replicable Model

After its victory against AP&L, news of ACORN spread across Arkansas, and its chapters multiplied. Rathke would soon create an Arkansas governing council made up of elected representatives from a half-dozen regional areas. ACORN was on the map, not only in Arkansas, but also beyond, setting the stage for expansion into other states. By 1975, ACORN had expanded statewide in Arkansas, and opened chapters in Texas, and South Dakota, a state with a tradition of agrarian populism in which U.S. senator Jim Abourezk had invited Rathke to organize. In Arkansas, ACORN waged a statewide campaign to lower utility rates for the poor, make lower-priced generic drugs available, and reform the property tax laws to tax intangible property—stocks and bonds (the last would earn ACORN the permanent enmity of the Arkansas banking and finance industry). ACORN established two spin-off organizations: a consulting firm made up of ex-staffers that would do research for ACORN, and a training institute that would not only train organizers but also serve as a tax-exempt entity that could receive charitable donations.

Although ACORN already published a newsletter sporadically, in 1976 Rathke set up two corporations to purchase the *Arkansas Advocate*, a small liberal bimonthly magazine, and a self-sustaining noncommercial FM radio station in Arkansas that would feed into local organizing. The magazine folded within two years when Rathke failed to develop a sufficient subscription base. Undeterred, he confidently wrote that given a low- and moderate-income constituency, "we are probably a lot closer to envisioning a radio network than we are a newspaper division." The radio network never materialized, but Rathke created two southern-based radio stations, KNON and KABF, that still broadcast from the small storefront offices built by community volunteers. Most importantly, Rathke was certain he had a replicable model for building local chapters neighborhood by neighborhood across the country, an organizing version of the assembly line that he was convinced he could set up in any low-income community.[2]

Using Rathke's model, by the mid 1970s ACORN had organized more than five thousand families in Texas, South Dakota, and Arkansas—60 percent white, 40 percent black, most with incomes no higher than seven thousand dollars a year. Its budget expanded to $250,000, enough to hire twenty staff, most of them organizers. Although the ACORN model would change over time, certain elements established by the mid-1970s endured. For organizing drives, every organizer would follow a detailed protocol that in Rathke's experience had proved successful. First, the organizer analyzes the demographics, politics, issues, and leadership of the neighborhood, city, and state. This fact gathering includes meeting with community leaders and driving through a neighborhood, often called a "windshield tour." Next, the staff and a local organizing committee develop a set of issues discovered through knocking on doors and signing up dues-paying members. While the first Arkansas neighborhoods were often smaller, the typical ACORN neighborhood eventually comprised 1,500–2000 households. The goal was to systematically knock on every door in the community over a six- to eight-week period and sign up 10 percent as dues-paying member families.

In the early 1970s, dues for member families were one dollar per month or ten dollars per year if you paid in advance. In the tradition of labor, Rathke wanted neighborhood residents to financially support their own organizations, a funding imperative that differed from that of most community-organizing and antipoverty groups. The point of collecting dues was not simply to raise money for ACORN's operations, but also to give members a sense of ownership of the organization, and the right to participate and make decisions about its issues and strategy. Members were not "clients" or "recipients" who were supposed to be grateful for someone else's largesse. Rathke later emphasized the importance of dues in a 1978 interview with the *Christian Science Monitor*: "ACORN lives or dies based on its membership's willingness to organize and pay their dues. . . . It doesn't matter if I or the governor or anyone else thinks we're doing great. If the membership stops paying dues we're out of business."[3]

From the start, Rathke understood that although ACORN would raise funds from foundations, its confrontational culture meant that only a small fraction of the nation's philanthropic sector would support it. Initially, ACORN was widely viewed as a responsible civic group trying to improve the community. As ACORN gained recognition, often because of its in-your-face actions, it lost much of its Mom-and-apple-pie appeal. Public officials began complaining about ACORN's tactics, among them North Little Rock school superintendent: "I have nothing against people getting what they supposedly justly deserve, but [ACORN's] tactics are not necessary or desirable."[4] At the beginning of 1974, ACORN received a civic award for its good work from the Little Rock U.S. Jaycees Foundation luncheon; at the end of 1975, because of criticism from business and political opponents, the Jaycees barred ACORN leaders from their luncheon.

By the early 1980s, ACORN organizers were being taught that within two months, they should invite people who show an interest in taking action to a community meeting; there, the group elects temporary officers and with the guidance of the organizer identifies the issues to take action on. If the city has several chapters, as Little Rock did, a citywide executive board coordinates the neighborhood groups. Members are encouraged to come to meetings, participate in decision making, and engage in demonstrations. "There are two kinds of power, money and people," Rathke always said at training sessions. He then quoted Nicholas von Hoffman, a one-time Alinsky organizer, who recalled the time "we moved 10,000 people in Chicago and it wasn't enough to beat the Daley machine." The best organizers understood that one can never mobilize enough people when trying to wrest concessions from the establishment.

Above all, for Rathke, this replicable model was not an assembly line for unskilled workers but an art form that required well-trained, skilled professionals—a fundamental challenge that had perplexed all community-organizing groups, including Saul Alinsky's. Like Alinsky, Rathke understood a key factor that religious and other charity groups have sometimes failed to comprehend. To help the poor, one needs to empower them. And to empower them one needs to build a large organization capable of overcoming well-financed opponents whose self-interest will lead them to oppose efforts that promote equality and opportunity for the poor.

The Importance of Professional Staff

Rathke also understood that his vision required more than well-meaning volunteers. ACORN needed paid full-time professional staff. At first, finding and retaining staff was easy. Rathke could rely on young people—mostly children of blue-collar workers from Arkansas, Texas, and Louisiana—caught up in the momentum of the antiwar, antipoverty, and civil rights movements or on VISTA volunteers like Carolyn Carr, a recent graduate of Marquette, and Sue Hanna, a dental hygienist.

By 1980, Rathke's dilemma was how to recruit and keep talented organizers committed to hard work and to advancing the interest of ACORN's members, while keeping salaries within ACORN's slim budget; Rathke also philosophically opposed high salaries for a group that was going to raise money from poor people.[5] Organizing for ACORN was not a cushy job, and salaries were low compared even to those of other nonprofits. Rathke told a reporter that his organizers made only $37.50 a week after taxes to avoid resentment from the people they organized. There was no overtime, no comp time. Almost all ACORN's members, including the elected leaders, even though they were poor, made more than ACORN's staff. (The low pay left ACORN open to the criticism that only middle-class people subsidized by their parents could afford to work for the organization.)

Rathke's model also required organizers to deal with a dilemma similar to the one that some nongovernmental organization staff and Peace Corp volunteers face today in third-world countries: how to encourage people with little hope in the future and unaccustomed to engaging in the democratic process to build participatory institutions in their own communities; additionally, in ACORN's case, how to train local leaders to accomplish goals. Rathke had adopted the Alinsky organizing model, which put decision making in the hands of the local members, who chose what issues to undertake and elected their own leaders. The organizers trained and developed the leaders, and the leaders then took the lead while the organizer remained subtly in the background.

As Alinsky advised in *Rules for Radicals*, "much of the time . . . the organizer will have a pretty good idea of what the community should be doing," but the community will reject an organizer who tries to dominate through the force of argument. The approach rather was to use "guided questioning" and rely on "skillful and sensitive role playing." Alinsky admitted that this strategy was manipulative in the same way "a teacher manipulates, and no less, even a Socrates. As time goes on and education proceeds, the leadership becomes increasingly sophisticated. . . . [The organizer's job] becomes one of weaning the group away from dependency upon him. Then his job is done."[6]

The line between manipulation and empowerment is often thin. Whichever strategy prevailed in Arkansas, within three years of organizing there, ACORN had established an enviable record. The group had exposed a property-tax system overwhelmingly biased against low-income property owners and led a successful effort to reform the property tax system to increase the taxes of the wealthy and decrease the taxes of low-income Arkansans. ACORN's Unemployed Worker's Organizing Committee had led a campaign that forced the state's labor department to take action against abuses by employment agencies. ACORN had pressured local officials to build parks, put up stoplights, and improve drainage systems. A newly organized ACORN's Vietnam Veteran's Organizing Committee had pushed a bill through the Arkansas General Assembly that gave vets free college tuition. ACORN had forced the Fort Smith city directors to amend a sewer proposal, saving low-income families $150 each. ACORN won the right to have public representation at the University of Arkansas Medical Center. The organization had built tenants' groups that gave renters some power to improve their living conditions. It had also won a free busing service for schoolchildren; elected city directors, school board members, justices of the peace, and state legislators sympathetic to the needs of ACORN members; challenged the real estate interests in Little Rock to stop blockbusting; and fought the Wilbur Mills Expressway, which would run through low-income neighborhoods in Little Rock.

From the outset, Rathke committed to a strategy common in the civil rights and labor movements but rare among antipoverty and community-organizing groups, that is, exercising the power of voters in a democracy to accomplish goals. A campaign to stop the racially harmful practice of blockbusting gave ACORN the opportunity to experiment with this tactic.

Chapter 4

The Innovation of Electoral Politics

It makes no sense to spend an afternoon confronting an elected official who is not doing the job he is supposed to be doing and ignore the same official—or his job—come November.

—Wade Rathke

Enough is enough. We will wait no longer for the crumbs at America's door. We will not be meek, but mighty. We will not starve on past promises, but feast on future dreams.

—ACORN People's Platform

To most community organizers and antipoverty groups, electoral politics was the antithesis of grassroots organizing. Wade Rathke disagreed. He thought political participation could help the poor win victories and maybe extend ACORN's reach nationwide. ACORN would suffer its share of defeats. Yet the higher goal of expansion would match even Rathke's lofty expectations.

He began to test his theories in the white working-class section of Oak Forest, an older declining Little Rock neighborhood, where it fought against an insidious real-estate practice, blockbusting. Realtors combed a neighborhood, warning homeowners that blacks were moving in. Panic would set in, followed by fire sales of homes and plummeting property values. Realtors and speculators would acquire the homes cheaply, raise the price, and sell them to black families at a steep markup.

Between June and December 1972, ACORN organizers like Carolyn Carr signed up black and white homeowners in Oak Forest to fight back. Soon signs popped up on dozens of front lawns saying: "We Like It Here—This housing is Not for Sale. ACORN." Organizers emphasized that this anti-blockbusting crusade was not anti-black but designed to protect a working-class neighborhood; they isolated and exposed anyone trying to make the issue white versus black neighborhoods. ACORN slowed the panic selling but did not wipe out the blockbusting entirely. Another section of Little Rock, the predominantly black area near Central High School, in 1972 needed a public park for neighborhood children to play in. ACORN pressured the city to locate a beautiful park along the Arkansas River and, to ensure the safety of the children, to put up a stoplight at a busy intersection, improve street drainage, and round up stray dogs.

Despite these victories, Little Rock continued to starve the poorer neighborhoods of city services. The Central High neighborhood suffered from rundown homes and the threat of an expressway to be routed right through a residential section. Rathke understood that to combat those issues took considerable political clout. Unlike most community organizers and antipoverty groups, Rathke did not condemn involvement in electoral politics as the antithesis of grassroots organizing. To increase the power of neighborhood groups, ACORN set up a Political Action Committee (PAC) made up of its leaders and kicked off a Save the City campaign aimed at reversing the decline of Little Rock's neighborhoods. ACORN invited all the candidates for Little Rock's school board to attend the kick-off rally and present their platforms; ACORN's PAC chose to back Doug Stevens and Bill Hamilton, both committed to ACORN's program: free textbooks, abolition of school fees, inclusion of special education programs, and more funding for Little Rock's low- to moderate-income areas.

ACORN's foray into electoral politics carried substantial risks. A loss would brand ACORN as weak and ineffective, and there was no spinning the results—ACORN's candidates would either win or lose. Furthermore, no school board candidate had ever won a citywide election without winning the wealthy Fifth Ward, where several board members lived but lower-income wards were not well represented. Undaunted, Rathke urged ACORN to go "toe to toe against the establishment." Hamilton lost, but Stevens made election history: he lost the Fifth Ward but won the election. Inspired by this success, some ACORN members decided to run for office themselves.

The head organizer of the International Ladies' Garment Workers Union, Carolyn Carr's friend Art Martin, agreed with this decision. When ACORN members decided in 1974 to run for seats on the Pulaski County Quorum Court, Arkansas's largest county government authority, ILGWU members joined them. The Quorum Court, with more than four hundred members, was responsible for the county budget but was not a well-known institution. ACORN's leaders saw running a slate of candidates for the court as an opportunity to maneuver tax dollars toward the needs of low- and moderate-income citizens. In a low-key campaign, 250 ACORN and ILGWU candidates ran a low-key campaign meeting face-to-face with voters; 195 were elected. Of the two newspapers covering the story, one called ACORN "subversive" and the other praised its election success as "a victory for grass-roots power."

Stunned by ACORN's victory, the Democratic Party establishment fought back. The county judge and chair of the Quorum Court resisted ACORN's efforts to exert citizen control of Pulaski County's budget by ruling that a dozen of the ACORN members were not qualified to serve. During the process of budget approval, he miscounted votes, manipulated meetings, and when ACORN's representatives boycotted a meeting so that the group lacked a quorum, he pushed the budget through over their protests.[1] Despite the Democratic Party's resistance, though, the Quorum Court became a more democratic body. Issues important to ACORN's members and followers were at least debated, such as funding services to low-income areas at the same level upscale areas enjoyed.

The electoral experience in Little Rock led Rathke to believe he had discovered a secret ingredient to gain power for the poor. He often told the staff and members:

"It makes no sense to spend an afternoon confronting an elected official who is not doing the job he is supposed to be doing and ignore the same official—or his job—come November."

ACORN began running more candidates for office, and attacks on the group escalated. In June 1976, state representative Boyce Alford of Pine Bluff called ACORN a "possible threat to capitalism and democracy." George Wimberly, Little Rock's mayor, accused the group of being "secretive," according to the *Arkansas Democrat*.[2] Most telling, the state Democratic Party establishment, fearful of ACORN's growing influence, passed a constitutional amendment, bitterly opposed by ACORN and the ILGWU, that reduced the Quorum Council's seats from 400 to 15, making it harder for ACORN members to win election to those seats. Despite the new law, ACORN members won 4 of the 15 seats.

Rathke touted these victories publicly as proof not only of ACORN's organizing power but also of its skill at translating that power into electoral victory. Privately, though, he began to have doubts about the advantage of running ACORN members for political office: "Winning alone, they [ACORN's members] are often dwarfed and isolated by the majorities, and accountability to the membership and public is sometimes an issue despite the merit of their individual contributions. In running individual members . . . the organization fears in some cases it has built politicians rather than power, despite the influence and access achieved."[3]

A Risky Inside-Outside Strategy

By 1976, although unaware of the tactics emerging among religious Right leaders like Jerry Falwell, Rathke was executing a plan similar to theirs. Just as the religious Right organized outside the Republican Party to influence it, ACORN would organize outside the Democratic Party, building chapters, winning on local issues, lobbying, marching, and voting. Financial and political independence would allow ACORN to sway both Democrats and Republicans.[4]

Rathke faced the same conundrum that social movements like populism confronted at the end of the nineteenth century. As Rathke came to see it, if ACORN were to play a role in pushing the country leftward and toward an agenda that would uplift the poor, it had to expand beyond Arkansas, Texas, and South Dakota and overcome the localism of its organizers and leaders. He envisioned leaping beyond the local by building his own national network. His vehicle was the innovative use of electoral politics.

On a sunny spring day in 1976, at his Little Rock office on West Fifteenth Street, Rathke sat down at his desk, an old door supported by a sawhorse at each end. With a window fan circulating the warm air, he typed an internal organization memo, "The 20/80 Plan," which began: "ACORN has an organizational and professional responsibility to demonstrate the potential of community organizing as a mechanism for social change." On six single-spaced pages, he spelled out a bold plan to expand ACORN from chapters in three states to chapters in twenty by 1980—just four years away. Rathke argued that ACORN could use the presidential campaign to build ACORN's national stature. He even had the audacity to contemplate ACORN running a presidential candidate with support from public campaign financing, which had been introduced in 1974 in the wake of Watergate. Raising $5,000 in twenty states in contributions of less that $250 would trigger a matching grant from the Federal Campaign Commission; Rathke's idea was that "the feds would pay for the 20/80 plan."[5]

ACORN would also use the 1968 Voting Rights Act that facilitated voter registration, along with the Democrats' new rules in caucus states, where, as Rathke wrote in the memo, "the entire ball game is based on organizational strength." Further, if ACORN succeeded in electing delegates to the Democratic Convention, the organization could influence the selection of the presidential nominee and the Democratic Party platform. But where did Rathke expect to find the money and people to organize new chapters in seventeen states, recruit members to run as delegates, and win?

Rathke anticipated the risks of his strategy, which he outlined in his memo. A membership split might occur involving especially members who leaned Republican. The campaign would cost an enormous amount of money and staff time. Also, since ACORN was a nonprofit organization, the IRS could harass it, even though such activity would be perfectly legal—it was not a tax-exempt 501(c)(3) nonprofit. Rathke wrote that ACORN should expect a push back from corporations and their allies, as well as from those who would brand the group a bunch of communists.[6]

Rathke's memo met with mixed reactions. John Beam, a veteran of the Little Rock election campaigns, was opposed to the 20/80 plan because he thought the Democratic Party would prove untrustworthy. Others opposed the plan because they believed that no amount of work would reform the Democratic Party or, worse, ACORN's leadership would be co-opted by the party. Many organizers and leaders were concerned that the plan would cause conflict within the organization and drain money and time away from organizing. On the latter point, Rathke retorted that the plan would increase ACORN's coffers, although he supplied only speculative evidence to support that position.

To address the concerns of those who feared internal division, Rathke borrowed an idea from the Progressive era's Non-Partisan League: ACORN could shape its platform from existing and common organizational issues and people could run for convention delegates not as Democrats or Republicans but as ACORN members. Among staffers who agreed with Rathke's plan, Zach Polett, one of the recently recruited Harvard grads, argued that the Quorum Court campaign proved ACORN's effectiveness in using elections. Mary Lassen, another recruit from Harvard and the Missouri head organizer, wanted more black and women leaders in ACORN; she said the campaign could build alliances with other progressive forces—labor, women's groups, minorities.

Rathke agreed to run uncommitted delegates in both Republican and Democratic primaries and made it clear that ACORN's campaign was about pushing issues of concern to the poor, not about endorsing a candidate. ACORN organizer Gary Delgado, who had left the organization, came back to oversee the platform development and later noted that this practice reaffirmed an organizing principle of staying within the experience of the membership, as well as a reluctance to develop positions that might be termed "ideological."[7]

The final decision on strategy rested with the newly created National Executive Board of sixty leaders selected by the members from ACORN's three areas—Arkansas, Dallas–Fort Worth, and Sioux Falls, South Dakota. Responsible for matters beyond the scope of the individual city and state boards, its members at their first meeting elected the first ACORN president, Steve McDonald, a soft-spoken, bespectacled Vietnam veteran disabled by multiple sclerosis. McDonald always wore a suit and tie, in contrast to the casual dungaree-clad organizers around him. He had joined ACORN in 1971 as a member of the Vietnam Veterans' Organizing Committee, a group organized by ACORN to advocate for the interests of veterans.

Rathke made sure that at that meeting, the new leaders debated the question of whether ACORN should build stronger local chapters based on local issues or expand by engaging in national issues and campaigns. Rathke wanted to make sure ACORN did both, again departing from Alinsky, who was suspicious of large organizations and espoused strict neighborhood autonomy. Rathke wanted a national organization made up of local chapters with a measure of local autonomy and the ACORN name attached to each. Alinsky's local organizations each had its own identity and never joined a common national campaign.

In contrast to Alinsky, Rathke thought that if ACORN was to grow, he had to foster a membership whose identity transcended local loyalties and who believed that the growth of ACORN nationally equaled organizational health. Some leaders on the national board, fearful of expansion, opposed diverting resources from their local operations and using those resources in ways that would entangle ACORN in divisive national issues. Others, including McDonald, countered that neighborhood problems were inseparable from policies made in Washington, D.C., and commented at the national board meeting that "neither could be tackled without an organization wielding national power."

Urged on by Rathke and other senior staff, McDonald insisted that for ACORN to "organize the unorganized," it had to expand. A majority of the board agreed. The outcome of that debate established ACORN's commitment not just to specific places or to neighborhood organizing, but also to a utopian ideal of organizing all low- and moderate-income people throughout the United States. Soon afterward, Rathke began dispatching his Arkansas-trained organizers first to New Orleans, then to St. Louis, Houston, Memphis, and Detroit.

The Power of Big Business

Rathke and the others in ACORN didn't see it coming, but they were swimming against the tide of powerful political and economic trends that emerged in the 1970s. It was an inauspicious time for people to try to build the type of activist, progressive antipoverty organization Rathke had in mind.

ACORN wanted government regulation and spending to solve its members' problems. Its vision, tactics, and methods were anathema not only to big business, but to the ideological and religious Right and their corporate-sponsored think tanks, as well as to ACORN's potential allies on the left.[8] The growing power of business interests would be ACORN's major obstacle. From the late 1940s through the early

1970s, the United States had experienced a dramatic increase in per capita income and a simultaneous decline in the gap between the rich and the poor. The incomes of the bottom third, even the bottom half, of the class structure rose faster than incomes of those at the top. Pushing to maintain these trends, progressives like United Automobile Workers president Walter Reuther and others in the left wing of the Democratic Party had been making proposals since World War II to renew and expand the New Deal and engage in national economic planning. Reuther advised Presidents Kennedy and Johnson to champion a bold federal spending program for full employment that would include government-funded public works and the conversion of the nation's defense industry to production for civilian needs.[9]

Both presidents rejected Reuther's advice, partly because they were concerned about alienating sectors of business who opposed Keynesian-style public spending and economic planning. Reuther's base, the union movement, was also shrinking. Johnson's announcement of an "unconditional war on poverty" in his 1964 State of the Union Address pleased Reuther, but the details of the plan revealed its limitations. The War on Poverty was a patchwork of small initiatives that did not address the nation's basic inequalities.[10]

Meanwhile, with competition from Germany and Japan increasing, major U.S. corporations mounted an assault on the postwar New Deal social contract. The enemy was the labor movement and the rising living standards of the poor and working class.[11] The plan was not a secret. An editorial in the October 12, 1974, issue of *Business Week* pointed out the biggest problem corporate America would face: "It will be a hard pill for many Americans to swallow—the idea of doing with less so that big business can have more. . . . Nothing that this nation, or any other nation, has done in modern economic history compares with the selling job that must be done to make people accept this reality."

But large corporate interests would soon gain allies in the religious Right, the Republican Party, and even the moderate wing of the Democratic Party, especially from the new young Turks known as neoliberals.

ACORN Grows

By 1978, ACORN had chapters in twelve states. (In terms of expansion, Falwell's Moral Majority had an advantage over Rathke's ACORN: an existing local network of evangelical Christians and preachers.) Although some of the new chapters—Georgia Action, Carolina Action, and the Citizen's Action League from California—were independent organizations that shared ACORN's goals and agreed to affiliate, Rathke had to build most chapters from scratch. For these, he strategically selected states that would hold a Democratic primary or a statewide caucus. In a primary, voters cast their ballot for a particular candidate; party members gather, hear speeches, and engage in discussion before voting for a candidate—a good forum for a group like ACORN that could mobilize people.

Of this era, as Gary Delgado wrote in *Organizing the Movement*:

> By keeping in regular contact with its groups, ACORN was able not only [to] replicate its organizational model, but to use centrally gathered research on what has become standard targets—banks, utility companies, and specific federal regulatory agencies—in a number of localities. It's possible to mount almost the same campaign in Missouri and Arkansas against Southwestern Bell's proposed pay phone hikes, and the generic drug bill drafted by Arkansas ACORN in 1975 could be the basis for similar efforts in Texas and Missouri in 1977–78.

An ACORN convention planned for Memphis, to be held near the 1978 Democratic Party midterm convention, would test how the 20/80 campaign was doing. Would it be a Rathke folly or pragmatic evidence to support his vision of the organization as a national presence?

On December 9, more than a thousand ACORN members from around the country met for the first time as they marched in the freezing rain outside the party's convention site. Said Elena Hanggi, who would become ACORN's president in 1983: "It was our first chance to really see the potential of the organization. We were surprised at how much the same we were even though we were from all over the country . . . [and] many Democrats were falling over themselves to speak at our convention." ACORN members demanded changes in the Democratic platform that reflected concerns about affordable housing, jobs, energy costs, and health care.

In the six-month period leading up to the nominating conventions for the 1980 presidential election, Dewey Armstrong, ACORN's first political director, along with Gary Delgado and Carolyn Carr, coordinated ACORN's organizers as they worked in their local communities and fashioned a national platform to present to both parties.[12] Divisions emerged between low-income and working-class members on whether to support higher welfare payments or higher wages for work. Some were for easing union-organizing efforts; others (from the South) were anti-union. Some were for nuclear power; some were against it.

On July 1, 1979, at ACORN's second national convention and platform conference, delegates met in the gym at Washington University in St. Louis and finalized ACORN's policy program, the "People's Platform." It reflected bread-and-butter issues in nine areas: energy, health care, taxes, housing, community development, banking, jobs, income, and rural issues. While members were in favor of local control of school spending, they avoided controversial issues such as integration by busing, fair housing, and the ERA. Rathke's introduction was moving but contained no manifestos, no overarching philosophy; Delgado criticized the platform as "a hodgepodge of progressive notions with no underlying ideology" that avoided the issues of race and sex.[13] But the "hodgepodge" platform was consistent with the vision of Rathke, Kest, and others, who saw ACORN as a pragmatic membership-driven organization, a vision that would serve it well. This proved prudent, as over the next three decades, as the socialist Left collapsed, the populist ACORN would survive and grow.

After ACORN's members overwhelmingly passed the "People's Platform," 200 of the 1,500 delegates marched to the suburban home of S. Lee Kling, the chair of President Carter's campaign finance committee, where they planted nine boards in the lawn whose labels corresponded to the planks in the platform. Next came inconclusive but sympathetic meetings with Democratic operatives, aides, and candidates, including Rosalyn Carter, Hamilton Jordan, and Edward Kennedy. ACORN also presented its positions to the Republican Platform Committee in Detroit and to the delegates assembled there.

As the Democratic National Convention approached in 1980, Rathke had nearly achieved his goal of expanding ACORN to twenty states, partly by exploiting the ubiquitous media coverage of the presidential nominating process and its central place in U.S. political life. From the ghettos of Detroit and Philadelphia and Sun Belt trailer parks in Arizona and Nevada to the Texas barrios and subdivisions of Iowa, ACORN had taken root in forty communities, where members worked to increase affordable housing, defeat urban renewal plans, oppose toxic chemical threats, and stop tenant evictions. During the 1980 primary season, forty-two ACORN members were elected as delegates to the Democratic National Convention.

At the convention, ACORN waged a protracted struggle with the Democratic Party to put poor people's issues at the top of its agenda. Rathke tried to build on grassroots support to push policy change at the top: the Massachusetts and California ACORN activists met with Kennedy, who had waged a primary fight for the presidential nomination against Jimmy Carter, and got his support for ACORN's resolution on low- and moderate-income representation. But ACORN could not gain the support of Carter and the Democratic Party regulars, who did not trust outside groups, certainly not one like ACORN that used confrontational tactics. ACORN also had difficulty getting the support of other liberal activist groups. Typical was the statement of the Texas Women's Political Caucus, which initially chose not to support ACORN because its platform did not support the Equal Rights Amendment. Although ACORN's executive board would support the ERA in 1980, a number of women's groups, reflecting the single-issue politics of the day, remained lukewarm to ACORN's platform.

In an attempt to meet one of ACORN's demands, the Democrat National Committee agreed to establish the ACORN Commission, chaired by Houston representative Mickey Leland and including ACORN members Elizabeth Martinez of Bridgeport, Connecticut, and Charles Crews of Jacksonville, Florida. The commission held hearings in six states on ACORN's proposals for increased participation and representation for low- and moderate-income people on the Democratic Party's National Committee, yet when the commission presented its recommendations to that committee in Philadelphia in 1982, it gave only lip service to the idea of greater inclusion of low- and moderate-income people. Martinez denounced the Democratic plan as offering "just a few crumbs," with nothing approaching ACORN's proposed quotas for representation.

Using Elections

Measured by ACORN's effect on the outcome of the election or concessions wrenched from the Democrats, the 20/80 campaign was a disappointment. ACORN's forty delegates made barely a ripple among the four thousand other delegates, and

ACORN remained far from the centers of power. Rathke took a longer view, though. His strategy had helped consolidate and expand ACORN's membership and had brought leaders from around the nation into a unified group with a shared set of goals. That ACORN's campaign had influenced, however slightly, an institution as large as the national Democratic Party, he told members, "demonstrated the value of a tightly knit national organization." A question remained. Would Rathke and ACORN's other leaders continue to use political primaries and conventions to raise issues and build a national antipoverty organization?

Rathke had taken antipoverty work and community organizing into more unprecedented tactical terrain. ACORN's increasing use of elections and partisan politics was a radical departure from the community-organizing tradition. No theorist involved in community organizing had ever looked to partisan electoral politics as a tool for change. Rathke correctly felt that to provide more than band-aids for the poor, an organization needed power, and power was proven on Election Day. "Victories are won on the streets," Rathke would say, "but they are ratified at the polls."

The reasons other groups took a hands-off position on electoral politics were many. Most couldn't win at the polls because they lacked the money or followers. Others feared losing their tax-exempt status or their funding, or they were steeped in the Alinsky tradition of community organizing—that groups should focus on specific issues and avoid endorsing candidates, running candidates, or getting close to a political party. Alinsky thought that the risks of direct participation in the campaigns of specific candidates outweighed the benefits. Like the public interest organizer Ralph Nader, he assumed that efforts to bring community groups into partisan electoral battles only sapped an organization's strength, co-opted its issue focus in a cult-of-the-candidate mentality, and alienated its members. A group may have members who are Republicans, Democrats, and Independents, so partisan electoral activity could be diversionary and divisive. Alinsky and his disciples, as well as Nader (who two decades later would change his mind), urged their groups to let the candidates fight it out, then attack the winner with protest demonstrations, large meetings, letter writing, and lawsuits.

Rathke understood that shunning elections was a tactical blunder and that eschewing electoral politics allowed groups to claim to speak for the poor while never proving that they had a base and followers. The nonelectoral approach implicitly threatened public officials with defeat, but it was an empty threat. When politicians caught on, they took the groups' demands less seriously—which is precisely what happened to Ralph Nader's organizations in the 1980s and 1990s when he lost his clout as a public advocate.

Beyond understanding the connection between partisan politics and power, politics added to ACORN's ability to grow in size and scope. From the very beginning, Rathke measured ACORN's potential power in terms of expanding the group's body and reach. Like a businessman calculating his year-on-year increases in overall sales to determine if business was growing, Rathke measured ACORN's annual growth in numbers: local neighborhood chapters, cities with chapters, members, organizers, dues, and funding.

As important as electoral politics was to ACORN, however, it had to identify the pressing problems the poor faced and figure out effective ways to help solve them. In the 1970s, the country was experiencing what economists called "deindustrialization."[14] In many communities where ACORN planned to organize, factories closed down and well-paying jobs were replaced by jobs in the expanding low-paid service sector. During ACORN's door-to-door neighborhood organizing drives, many people complained about low-wage work with no benefits, no future, and no unions. In neighborhood meetings, members trying to get off welfare by working in part-time health care and other service-sector jobs raised their hands to ask other members and organizers if ACORN could help. ACORN's staff would check the phone book for unions who might help, and at the next meeting the report would be: "Hey, no answer," or "The union wasn't interested." In the mid 1970s, though only about 20 to 25 percent of the U.S. workforce was unionized, unions didn't have active organizing departments.

Jobs and income should be an important focus of ACORN's work, Rathke decided, and in 1976 he wrote a memo that introduced one more unprecedented component to his community-organizing model. If successfully implemented, it might solve some of the problems facing these workers and improve ACORN's numbers, measured in victories, members, dues, and funding—in other words, ACORN's power. It would also transform ACORN into an unrecognizable form.

Chapter 5

Organizing a Union in the 'Hood

Since the founding of ACORN, Rathke had thought long and hard about labor unions. He read every book he could find in the library on the subject, among them the autobiography of United Auto Workers (UAW) leader Wyndham Mortimer, *Organize! My Life as a Union Man*. Mortimer's book recalled his exciting days as an organizer for United Auto Workers (UAW) in the 1930s, where he had played an important role as an organizer in forcing General Motors to recognize the UAW as the sole representative of the General Motors workers. "The greatest hope of American labor," he wrote, "is in the rank-and-file membership, the men and women who pay the dues and who maintain the unity and solidarity at the bench, the lathe, and the assembly line."[1]

Inspired by these words, Rathke tinkered with the idea of organizing unemployed workers, especially teenagers and young adults.[2] He assumed correctly that most poor urban youngsters coveted the income they could earn for summer jobs. In the early 1970s, he recruited several unions to help him lobby Little Rock and other cities to provide unemployed youths with summer jobs. ACORN also pressured unscrupulous private employment agencies to stop discriminating against blacks.

Rathke next considered organizing a full-fledged ACORN union. Such a drive had no precedent. Some community-organizing groups, such as the IAF and Citizen Action, followed the path of Saul Alinsky, who had always tried to work with labor (but never to organize unions), whenever possible bringing union activists and leaders into his organization as part of his leadership group. Envisioning an umbrella organization of existing groups, Alinsky brought together neighborhood associations, small businesses, and the Catholic Church, as well as labor unions. Rathke wanted to go further and create independent unions affiliated with ACORN. Although he recognized the difficulty of organizing unions—union membership had been declining for more than a decade—Rathke believed he could organize just about anything.

In December 1976, several months after Rathke had issued his 20/80 memo, he wrote a memo to the staff and leaders that began: "The primary thrust of ACORN has always been the community. The issues of everyday life are central. We concentrate on . . . low-to-moderate-income people for 16 hours a day. We compete in these time spaces with the media, sleep, and church, among other things. We cannot beat sleep or church. . . . Over the long haul, we have to impact with a heavier and more organized hand [on] other areas of membership concern." He went on to recommend the development of "independent unions" as a way to help people where they worked. Unions affiliated with ACORN rather than the AFL-CIO would bring financial stability to ACORN via more dues-paying membership, he argued, and ACORN'S community organizers could simply transfer their skills to union organizing. Overhead would be minimal since ACORN already had office space. Household workers, sugarcane workers, small farmers, fishermen, and clericals—all workers who were without union representation—were waiting to be organized. Many staff responded as they had to his 20/80 expansion plan: he was pushing ahead too fast. Rathke responded, "No, we simply did not have sufficient resources . . . to develop a staff and membership, which could produce these surges of growth even earlier." In 1978, Rathke convinced the ACORN National Board to found the United Labor Unions (ULU) to organize workers whom existing unions were neglecting. With just a few experienced ex-organizers from welfare rights, a small amount of funding, and numerous legal and jurisdictional obstacles ahead, Rathke started union locals in New Orleans, Boston, and Detroit.

Madeline Talbott

In Detroit, not only would ACORN test its union-organizing theory, but also Madeline Talbott would test herself as a head organizer. Talbott stood out among the talented recruits from Harvard signed up between 1973 and 1977, who were among the pioneers to shape ACORN. Others included Seth Borgos, who succeeded Steve Kest as ACORN's research director; Steve Holt; Meg Campbell; Mary Lassen; Steve Bachman, who became ACORN's attorney; and Zach Polett, ACORN's longtime political director. They became aware of ACORN through Steve Kest or the AP&L campaign. Most of all they were inspired by Rathke's vision and what he had accomplished. These recruits joined Beam, Carolyn Carr, and other young organizers, many from elite universities, including Steve's younger brother Jon and Fran Streich. They built ACORN's statewide organization in Arkansas and chapters in South Dakota, Texas, Louisiana, Tennessee, and Missouri. They were all smart, ambitious, and capable of implementing the complicated art of organizing, ACORN style.

Madeline Talbott grew up in the fifties in a family that moved around the country with the postings of her father, a colonel in the Army Corps of Engineers. Her mother attended college, modeled clothes, rode horses, worked as a private detective, and during World War II was assigned by the navy to break Japanese codes. Both parents were politically moderate Kentucky Democrats who supported Lyndon Johnson and the war in Vietnam. They took the notion of citizenship seriously and were pleased when their daughter joined a teenage civic group headed by two activist Protestant ministers.[3]

In the fall of 1968, Talbott entered Harvard, a tall woman with long, dark hair who chose preppy Villager and Lady Bug outfits. Unlike many of the coeds in the Cambridge area, she stayed away from marijuana, bell-bottom blue jeans, and peasant blouses. Yet in the spring, she watched SDS take over the administration building. The cops came and busted some heads and arrested several students. The incident provoked a huge meeting in the football stadium, where Madeline and hundreds of students voted to strike and set up picket lines around campus. She stashed the preppy clothes, put on a surplus army jacket and jeans, and joined the strike.

Unlike other student activists, Madeline never adopted a Marxist political ideology. She considered radical groups to be "too elitist, too dismissive of regular ordinary people, or too rigid and too in love with their own vision of the working class rather than the real people." By the middle of her sophomore year, she felt isolated at Harvard, estranged from the campus activists, as well as from most of her old friends, who did not share her politics. When a dorm mate, Diane Gold, called out in the dorm hallway for someone who spoke Spanish and was willing to work at a community center in nearby Chelsea, Talbott signed up.

During the fall of 1969, she went door to door in the low-income Puerto Rican section of Chelsea to invite mothers to meetings about starting a day-care center. Although Talbott found it difficult to get many of the women to the meetings, she delighted in her friendship with them. The women fed her, cared for her, and contrasted sharply with the students she knew at Harvard, where she did not feel at home; a close-knit, caring community was just what she needed.

That summer, while working in the Chelsea community center, for the first time she saw poor people wield power; the occasion was a demonstration led by one of Wade Rathke's organizers at the Massachusetts Welfare Rights Organization. Later that summer, she felt powerful herself when she helped her Chelsea mothers win their day-care center. "I was hooked," she recalls. "I became completely enchanted with my work. I had never seen poor people act with such courage before, and after the summer I longed for more of that feeling again."

After working in Chelsea, taking a year off, finishing her junior year, and then spending two years in Ethiopia with the Harvard Africa Volunteer Project, Talbott returned for her senior year at Harvard and began to think about a job.[4] At a fall seminar on community organizing, Steve Kest came to recruit Harvard students to ACORN. He dwelled on ACORN's campaign against Arkansas Power & Light, which many students knew about because it involved the university and was a frequent topic in the *Harvard Crimson*.

Talbott liked what she heard about ACORN but assumed that it would be difficult to get a job at such a great organization. When she went to the Harvard career office toward the end of her senior year and paged through some binders of nonprofit job notices, she happened upon one from ACORN. It listed a weekly salary of forty-five dollars. At that low rate of pay, she figured, there would be jobs available.

Her next step was an exploratory trip to Little Rock, where John Beam picked her up at a bus stop. She stayed with Beam and his girlfriend, Polly, but couldn't interview with the head of ACORN, Wade Rathke, who was out of town. The next day she went with Beam to visit an ACORN member and collect dues. After a few days of bombarding Beam and the rest of the ACORN staff with questions, she returned to Cambridge and applied for the job. When she hadn't heard from ACORN in two weeks, she followed up with a letter and soon afterward received an envelope with ACORN as the return address. She anxiously opened it and read the terse letter: "Everyone was very impressed with you. You're hired. Organize, Wade Rathke."

Talbott and the other new recruits moved to the picturesque Arkansas backcountry, where they trained under Rathke's supervision and learned how ACORN helps the poor.

Talbott arrived as ACORN's head organizer in Detroit in 1978, less than a year after the $350 million Renaissance Center opened downtown. The center's glistening glass-and-steel towers, a showpiece of modern urban architecture, stood on land where the radiating spokes of the city's main boulevards met the majestic Detroit River. The Center was a project of an interracial business, union, and government coalition called the New Detroit forged by Henry Ford II and Max Fisher, an oil magnate and Republican fund-raiser. In the wake of Detroit's 1967 riots, Ford, Fisher, and their partners had invested millions in the new complex, hoping it would spark a rebirth that would bring new life to Detroit's crumbling downtown and decaying, crime-ridden neighborhoods.

Madeline threw herself into a variety of community campaigns. As usual, she started with the critically important organizing drive. She identified low-income areas by census data; noted the areas of substandard housing; located the City Hall, the Chamber of Commerce and other potential places of confrontation; identified issues in which the local press had shown an interest; and drove to look at geographic areas, usually identifiable neighborhoods that her instincts told her were ripe for organizing. She talked to the staffs of other political and community groups, civil rights organizations, social service agencies, and schools and came up with a list of community leaders. In Detroit, like most cities, numerous groups were involved in the community and resented outsiders that came in and became involved in their issues. So knowing the leaders of a community gave her a chance to neutralize potential business and political opponents as well as adversaries within the nonprofit antipoverty community.

As part of her research effort, Talbott studied the history of various issues and looked at how deeply potential rivals were involved in them. Experience had taught her that, regarding such rivals, she needed "to avoid them, freeze them out, and not tread on 'their' issue until after you have built your base." Nonetheless, many local leaders grumbled about ACORN "coming into our community." Although some had a legitimate concern for the poor, many were more interested in protecting their political turf. The problems facing the poor in Detroit were and remain intractable, and most low-income neighborhoods need all the help they can get.

Talbott also completed a survey that identified leading liberals and progressives who could become allies in an organizing campaign. According to the ACORN manual, such people "give you . . . legitimacy in the area, since you are initially talking to them about the possibility of organizing rather than the fact of it. The suggestions [other liberals and progressives] make also give us the mandate to be there." As to other groups, Talbott knew to guard against being used if a group's goals were not in ACORN's interest.

After a few months of research, Talbott was ready to find a set of pressing problems, scour the area for potential local leaders, sign up dues-paying members and, most important, develop a polarizing issue that separated the poor from others. By 1979, a year after Talbott arrived in Detroit, one fact was very clear to her. Whatever the expectations of New Detroit, the attempt to improve the entire city would not work. The public and private investments generated by the New Detroit in the central business district were not trickling down or out to ordinary Detroiters like Pearl Gilbert, a disabled black worker who lived in an old decaying neighborhood far from Renaissance Center. "Improvement" meant living next to a six-foot pile of dirt spread over bricks and rotting wood, the dangerous remnant of an abandoned and wrecked home where her children played instead of in a park. The city had spent millions of federal dollars on destroying empty homes, but little money on building new low-income housing or better police protection.

Pearl Gilbert was too poor to move, and when Madeline Talbott came knocking on her door, she had been petitioning city officials to clear the vacant lot. At first she was ignored. When Pearl persisted, she was told that the weeds on the lots were cut down only once every seven years. Pearl was a fighter, but acting alone, she could accomplish nothing. She had resigned herself to the neighborhood's squalor.

Pearl invited Madeline into her living room, where Madeline told her about ACORN, emphasizing that it was an organization controlled by its membership. "What you and the members want determines what ACORN does. In other neighborhoods," Talbott said, "we got tax reductions, more police, stoplights, parks, whatever the neighborhood wanted to do to improve."

"Can you help me with abandoned homes, get the city to cut these weeds down?" asked Pearl.

"If you and your neighbors want that, we'll start with that," said Madeline.

Pearl joined up and worked with Madeline and the other ACORN staff, and together they forced the city to cut down the weeds. Encouraged, Pearl agreed to spearhead an ACORN organizing drive. She began to tell her neighbors, "One person standing alone can easily be pushed down, but a lot of people backing you up can get you some action." She also understood a core idea of ACORN organizing: polarize the issues to get the person you are organizing angry. ("You know damn well city hall would deal with abandoned houses if they were in a rich man's neighborhood.")

With Pearl providing the leadership, ACORN got the lot cleaned up. Next they took on a General Motors development plan that would displace more than three hundred low-income black families. Through persistent protests and appeals to federal housing officials, ACORN won a commitment from the city council to pay each displaced family four thousand dollars to help them relocate. ACORN cleared out vacant homes, cleaned up dumping sites, and successfully lobbied the city council to overturn a mayoral veto, which meant that $1.2 million in federal funds for loans and grants came into the hands of urban homeowners. ACORN also halted utility rate hikes and lobbied Michigan utility companies to charge lower rates to the elderly and poor. Talbott was a tough but diplomatic charmer. Her intense but persistent, pleasant manner made her an effective negotiator. Most of all, she wanted to win.

Referring to Talbott's work, Victor Livingston of the *Detroit News Magazine* noted that with her high, commanding forehead and thin nose, she resembled an emerging young actress, Meryl Streep. Regarding her work, he wrote that ACORN "attracted media attention somewhat out of proportion to its size—but perhaps not out of proportion to its impact on urban communities. For all her work, Talbott's annual salary was $6,700.[5]

Keith Kelleher

When Madeline Talbott and Wade Rathke offered Detroit ACORN volunteer Keith Kelleher a job, he leaped at it. A 1978 graduate of Fordham University, he had moved to a Jesuit Volunteers Corps community that provided services to the poor on the city's southwest side. He was excited about immersing himself in the Detroit community, having grown up in Irish working-class neighborhoods in New York, where his extended family included many cops. A jack-of-all-trades at a local food bank during the week—driving trucks, picking up and delivering food to parish and community food banks, and writing grant proposals—at night and on the weekends he was involved in anti-nuke and peace movement activities at the nearby Catholic Worker house, where a Jesuit priest served as his mentor. Kelleher gave out leaflets to support the United Farmworkers' grape boycott and walked a picket line for locked-out newspaper workers on strike in the southwest suburbs.

ACORN sent Kelleher to New Orleans for training. His first on-the-job session took place on a typical hot and sticky October day. His trainer, ACORN head organizer Therese Bouie, gave him some pointers about the neighborhood, the issues, and how he should approach people at the door. She drove Kelleher to a neighborhood bordered by a levee where, she said, folks might be mad about some recent flooding. Kelleher emerged from the car with his clipboard in hand and his sweaty t-shirt sticking to his body. As he went door to door, several young men across the street eyeballed him suspiciously, whispering and pointing. In the early afternoon, he proceeded nervously, knocking on doors. No one answered at the first six doors. Kelleher marked his forms with their addresses and put a note by the house numbers to come back if he had time at the end of his three hours. Does this door-to-door stuff really work? he wondered.

At the seventh house, the front door was open and voices came from inside. He knocked on the wooden screen, and a young child came to the door. When Kelleher asked to speak to the head of the house, the child ran to the back of the house yelling, "Mama, there's a *white man* at the door!" A few moments later, a frowning middle-aged woman appeared. Kelleher thought, "Uh-oh . . . she's not happy."

He launched into his pitch, shouting loudly through the screen door: "Hi, my name is Keith and I'm with the community organization ACORN. We're just going door to door in the neighborhood today to see what the problems are. What do you see as the big problems in the neighborhood?" He had his ACORN button on, but ACORN was still new in New Orleans in 1979 and had little name recognition in the neighborhood.

"Huh, what?" She seemed thrown off by his loud, rapid delivery.

"Uh, the neighborhood . . . " He stumbled, forgot his rap, and stood there in silence as he racked his brain for what to say next. So he started again, ending with, "Some folks were talking about the fact that the flooding was out of control."

"You got that right," she said, and proceeded to complain about how she and her husband had worked all their lives, saved and bought a house, but that when it rained, the neighborhood turned into a swamp. "With all the taxes I pay, we don't need this neighborhood looking like a swamp!"

Kelleher remembered to polarize the issue. "You think the richer neighborhoods of the city flooded like yours?"

"No way!" she said. "They dry as a bone in them rich wards, because they got nice houses and good drainage while we're stuck with that!" She pointed at the pools of water in front of her house.

"Well, that's why folks are joining ACORN," Kelleher said. "To get rid of flooding like that. ACORN works on bigger issues, too, like high utility bills, ah—"

She cut him off. "How do you join?"

He couldn't believe it. She was interested in joining! "ACORN's a membership organization," Kelleher said. "Just like a church or a union, people pay dues of one dollar per month, only ten dollars per year. That helps pay for the costs of the campaigns like the flooding. Let me show you the card."

She took the clipboard card out of his hand and started filling out the card as he showed her newspaper articles about other victories. She gave him her ten-dollar dues with the membership card, carefully counting out a five-dollar bill and five ones into his palm. Kelleher filled out the member portion of the card and tore it off for her wallet, put the money under the membership card on his clipboard, and gave her a flyer about an upcoming neighborhood meeting. "If you need a ride, call the number on the flyer."

He would later tell friends, "I was high as a kite. I signed up a member." The thrill of success drove him to the next doors, envisioning hundreds of dues-paying members, arms locked, marching on the Board of Sewerage demanding drainage like the rich wards, hundreds of people singing and chanting, confronting the police, and pushing through as the television cameras rolled.

This carried him for two and a half hours. He signed two more members and had some solid callbacks who said they wanted to join and gave him a specific day to come back.

Therese pulled up in her Toyota and asked if he signed up any members.

"Only three paid. But I got a couple of callbacks who say they want to join."

"Three!" she exclaimed. "That's impressive, especially for a first timer. Most trainees are lucky to get one."

McDonald's and Burger King

Kelleher was hooked. When he returned to Detroit, ACORN recruited him as a union organizer. It was an inauspicious time to go union organizing. A declining union movement represented only 24.1 percent of American 21 million workers; the lure of a union-free environment in the South and abroad had led to plant closings and wage and benefits concessions. Kelleher would soon find himself in the middle of an unprecedented drive to organize workers.

Former St. Louis ACORN's head organizer, Dan Cantor headed ACORN's fast-food union organizing campaign. He had his eye on a variety of rapidly expanding low-wage jobs—home care, janitorial, and hotel and restaurant work. America was becoming a nation of short-order cooks, with McDonald's employing more than twice as many people as U.S. Steel. Public sector unions, such as the American Federation of State, County and Municipal Employees (AFSCME) and the American Federation of Teachers (AFT), were successfully organizing government workers, but private service sector workers were mostly ignored. The AFL-CIO trade unions disregarded the low-wage private sector and stuck to organizing the dues-rich construction and auto, steel, and manufacturing industries. Into the gap stepped ACORN. With financial backing from the United Auto Workers, Cantor set up his office next to ACORN's headquarters in the downtown YWCA. The fast-food industry was the major nonunionized, labor-intensive industry in the United States. Madeline Talbott thought Detroit ACORN's union drive would prove even more controversial than her community work.

Kelleher joined ACORN's organizing drive at the Greyhound Bus Station Burger King in downtown Detroit. A year earlier, in 1979, Cantor and his United Labor Unions organizers had walked into Burger King, ordered burgers and fries, and talked with the cashiers about unionizing. Organizing committees were soon established, and the rank-and-file leaders met with other workers at their homes and workplaces. Then came the pressure. Walking past eroded buildings along garbage-strewn streets, Cantor organized a picket line of teenagers, mostly African American, who marched toward the Burger King. Plant closings had tossed many of these high school students' parents out of work, and with unemployment at 16 to 38 percent for black teenagers, they believed that these low-skilled service jobs might be their best legitimate opportunities—they needed these jobs to add to the family income. Holding signs that read, "Union rights are human rights," they chanted, "No more threats, no more lies, we want the right to organize."

On February 22, 1979, the Burger King workers voted 25–23 for the union in an National Labor Relations Board election, ACORN's first victory in Detroit. That Burger King was the first fast-food franchise unionized in the United States. Kelleher was thrilled, until he heard that management had challenged five ballots. The NLRB ordered another election.[6]

Meanwhile, with the backing of the United Auto Workers, ACORN aimed a union drive at three inner city McDonald's owned by black businessman Ralph Kelly. ULU quickly signed up employees on union authorization cards, the first step in winning union representation. Nearly all the employees were between sixteen and nineteen and black. Some were the children of autoworkers, while others relied upon the meager wages they earned at McDonald's to supplement family income. Cantor filed for an election with the National Labor Relations Board.

McDonald's fought back with its own version of a community-labor strategy. The company challenged ULUs right to have an election, then illegally fired union activists—"troublemakers"—and planned celebrations and parties to show the workers that McDonald's was a good employer, unions were unnecessary, and that the workers might lose benefits if they voted for the union.

McDonald's also reached out to the city's power brokers and played the race card. On April 23 and 24, New Detroit organized two secret meetings of representatives from seventy black community groups, nearly all of which were funded by New Detroit. The media was excluded. They came to hear members of a black McDonald's owners association blast ACORN's organizing drive. Leaders of New Detroit called ACORN's organizers "outsider agitators" who were exploiting black Detroiters for their own selfish purposes. Questioning ACORN'S motives and its commitment to low-income Detroiters, the New Detroit group claimed that fast-food restaurants meant increased jobs for many black youths. The fast-food business in Detroit had become an industry where black storeowners prospered. Kelly, who owned the three targeted McDonald's, opposed ACORN's union organizing because, he claimed, "it will mean higher prices, fewer job opportunities for young blacks." New Detroit's vice president and the head of its so-called Self Determination Committee, Paul L. Hubbard, who was at the meeting, told the *Detroit News* that ACORN was "antithetical" to the committee and promised that community groups "threatened by ACORN" would get funding and expertise.

Hubbard told the press that "there was a unanimous feeling that steps should be taken to get ACORN out of the city," and paid ACORN an unintentional compliment: "They have a good knack for using young and older people, people who don't have political knack." Hubbard explained that New Detroit's "concept of community self-determination is that people in the neighborhoods should organize their own activities and choose their own issues. But with ACORN, the leaders choose the issues. . . . They use a figurehead in the community and they program that person to run the ACORN agenda." (He failed to mention that his group often manipulated agendas and picked which people would get New Detroit's money.) Another member of the committee said, "The unionization drive was the work of an organization whose training literature exhibits racist overtones."[7]

Radio personality Bill Johnson, who attended the meeting, explained to the *Detroit News* why New Detroit opposed ACORN: "ACORN comes in and provides the expertise and gives direction. Actually, it's a pretty good method. But New Detroit, with its grants to community groups, tries to see *itself* as the focal point in terms of community organizing. And ACORN makes it difficult for them to control community organizing. ACORN is able to generate a lot of support in the face of established organizations because these organizations haven't been doing anything. It's the fault of these organizations if ACORN is successful. ACORN is just filling the void."

But opponents who saw ACORN as interfering with the community's self-determination were not completely wrong. To some businessmen ACORN was just another group coming into their community and trying to establish a power base for its own selfish reasons. While the black businessmen were looking for their place in the sun, a few businessmen sympathetic to ACORN wondered, Why don't they unionize some white-owned Burger King or McDonald's?

Kelleher and Cantor's immediate concern was the revote ordered by the NLRB in Burger King campaign. With the other organizers in their windbreakers and sneakers Kelleher and Cantor continued to work day and night, certain that sixteen of the twenty-nine workers at the Burger King would vote for a union. Finally, Cantor went to the Federal Building for the vote count with ULU chief organizer Mark Splain, a former welfare rights organizer. The *revote* went 28-1 against the union.

After the votes were counted, Burger King's attorney looked at Dan Cantor and gloated. Cantor looked back and cursed, advising the attorney in Yiddish, "Go eat whale shit!" ACORN had misplayed the racial politics, focusing too narrowly on the economic issues instead of race. Kelleher, the newcomer, was stunned and humiliated. He went home, sulked for a few hours, blamed the workers and the organizing committee members, but mostly blamed himself for not working hard enough or smart enough. He doubted if he had what it took to be a union organizer. But he wanted to get even. With whom he would get even and how was not exactly clear—perhaps with a McDonald's victory.

Just a few days before the McDonald's election, restaurant management, on what it dubbed McHappy Day, brought in a star Houston Oiler, running back Earl Campbell, to give a pep talk about why it was unnecessary to have a union. Campbell's union—the National Football Players Association—lambasted him publicly for doing so. Support for the union dropped from two-thirds signed up on cards to one-third. On May 2, 1980, McDonald's workers voted down the union, 104–46. Management had charmed, cajoled, badgered, and bullied them into opposing the union. Kelleher and Cantor were young, naive, and ill prepared for the McDonald's juggernaut.

Outclassed, outspent, and outgunned by McDonald's management, ACORN's union organizers had learned the foolhardiness of taking on, as their first organizing drive, the fast-food industry, backed by the money from a multinational corporation. The Detroit ULU decided to organize smaller companies that would be more subject to community pressure—companies that hired bus drivers, home nurses who changed bedpans, janitors who mopped floors, and cleaning women who scoured toilets.

Victories began to build. Although the fast-food organizing all but failed, Kelleher's most satisfying success came in 1983. After the Greyhound Burger King challenged ULU's election victory, using delaying tactics for three years, the first fast-food union finally signed a collective-bargaining contract with an employer. ULU also eventually organized several light industrial plants. From 1978 through 1984, ULU started locals in five cities and organized thousands of workers. Though ULU was technically separate from ACORN, its Constitution and By-Laws make clear that the union shared ACORN's goal of "economic justice for low and moderate income people in the neighborhoods and in the workplace." The documents specifically stated that the two groups would "work together in any way that will benefit our members and all low and moderate income people."

Several organizers who cut their teeth with ULU would become prominent in the labor movement: Mark Splain became an AFL organizing director, Kirk Adams became chief of staff to SEIU president Andy Stern, and Myra Glassman became field director of SEIU Local 880.

ULU's work caught the attention of a few international unions, who saw a group with gutsy determination and ability to organize workers that many traditional unions neglected. ACORN's tactics—door knocking, listening to people's concerns, and building neighborhood-based organizing committees—were quite effective. From 1978 to 1984, a variety of international unions approached ULU with feelers about affiliating; ULU by then had about twenty organizers nationally, not enough to become a self-sufficient national union. ACORN turned down the offers until the SEIU offered organizing subsidies for the local operations, legal assistance, political assistance, and, most important, an agreement to preserve ULU's independence. In 1984, with SEIU's newly elected national president John Sweeney committed to organizing the unorganized, Rathke, Cantor, Kelleher and the other ACORN organizers agreed to affiliate.

In combining union and community organizing and politics into one entity that fought to reduce poverty, Rathke's ACORN was operating far outside the U.S. norm, especially because the union organizing would soon include the South. Even in big cities where unions were more widespread, the working class perceived workplace politics and community politics as separate spheres. Working-class politics in the community focused on issues of family, neighborhood, ethnicity, government contracts and jobs, and the distribution of local services, as Ira Katznelson explains in *City Trenches*.[8] Workplace politics revolved around issues of wages and conditions. Mobilized by trade unions at work and urban political machines in their neighborhoods, U.S. workers never developed a language of class that combined their concerns about both work and community life. (When Keith Kelleher and Madeline Talbott married, their union symbolized the uniting of labor organizing and community organizing that ACORN hoped to achieve in one association.)

What had ACORN morphed into? It was partly a group with "a militant style and a radical program" and those who could not accept this gradually dropped out of its ranks, as Madeleine Adamson and Seth Borgos concluded in *This Mighty Dream*, published in 1984.[9] But ACORN was not just a protest organization, although members protested. It was not just a community organization, although it built neighborhood chapters. It was not a liberal lobby, although ACORN's members lobbied for liberal causes. It's staff were not just organizers, they were also entrepreneurial. They founded a business that sold paper to nonprofit organizations in three cities and was exploring a residential heating oil cooperative. At a time when foundation money was drying up for community-organizing projects, ACORN was unique in not relying on philanthropy. Membership dues and grassroots fund-raising represented 85 percent of ACORN's income. And now it was starting a union. For Rathke, ACORN was not only effective, but bigger, and therefore better.

People who encountered ACORN had a difficult time comprehending it. Even union leaders and other close allies of ACORN, such as the head of Arkansas's AFL-CIO, couldn't quite understand what Rathke was doing. He had produced an admixture of organizing group, national political party, community, and workplace union.

Most ACORN organizers, who worked long hours for low pay, felt they were part of a powerful force. They rose in the morning went to work, excited about the issues they would tackle that day. The next looming problem they would face had plagued nearly every inner city where ACORN organized. The practice causing this problem was not easy to pin down, yet it was widespread and the evildoers were upstanding members of the community.

The loss of manufacturing industries—and the jobs and tax base that went with them—was changing the face of cities like St. Louis. White middle-class residents were fleeing to the suburbs in the wake of the movement of jobs to these areas driven by government policy such as federal outlays for highways, and defense spending in suburban areas like Orange County, California. Economic disparity between suburbs and cities widened, accompanied by deepening fiscal crises in the nation's older cities. Most policy makers viewed these changes as a kind of natural law they called "market forces"—the inevitable rise and fall of older cities. But ACORN's organizers in cities like Boston and St. Louis began to discern a red pen in the invisible hand of the market—especially in the pattern of banks' lending decisions.

Chapter 6

Partnering with the Enemy

In 1976, Missouri ACORN's head organizer, Mary Lassen, one of the Harvard graduates, was engaged in a statewide tax reform campaign and at the same time searching for a local St. Louis issue that could produce a victory, build neighborhood chapters, and lead to new recruits.[1]

In the mid-'70s, as ACORN began expanding from three states to twenty, Lassen's organizers going door to door had begun to see a pattern—the routine rejection by local banks and savings and loans of inner city families' requests for loans to fix up a home, purchase a house, or expand a business.[2] The families had accepted the banks' explanations that they did not meet the lenders' standards until organizers began helping them discover that many other families and entrepreneurs in their community, who clearly earned enough money to pay back a loan, had met with the same treatment. ACORN members would deposit their savings in these banks, who then refused to make loans in their communities. Other community groups across the country, especially in black neighborhoods, were discovering the same discrimination. Activists in Chicago called these lending practices "redlining." Even officials of banks with inner city branch offices literally drew a red line on a map to delineate black neighborhoods where they would not make loans, instead targeting their money lending to home buyers and businesses in the suburbs.

As one Chicago organizer said, "They're like vacuum cleaners, sucking up the money from the neighborhoods and investing in the suburbs with loans to developers." By siphoning money out of these inner city communities, banks helped promote urban blight.

In the early 1970s, ACORN joined community activists in various cities to forge a loosely coordinated national campaign, led by National Peoples Action (NPA), to change federal banking regulations to end this kind of discrimination. (Unlike ACORN, NPA is a loose network of neighborhood organizations, but it came out of the same Alinsky organizing tradition.) NPA's extraordinary leader, Gail Cincotta, a Greek American housewife and mother of six sons, came to personify the battle between working-class neighborhoods and the banking industry. NPA had a major ally in Sen. William Proxmire, a liberal Democrat from Wisconsin who was a strong advocate for antiredlining legislation in Congress. The first major victory came with the passage of the Home Mortgage Disclosure Act (HMDA) by Congress in 1975, which required banks to disclose their approvals and denials of mortgage applications, by address and census tract.

ACORN Missouri's organizer Mary Lassen used the HMDA data to tell a dramatic story. With a reputation within ACORN as a smart strategist, Lassen had grown up in Groton, Connecticut, and graduated Harvard summa cum laude; she was twenty-three. She had written a thesis on the United Mine Workers reform movement and been active in the United Farm Workers boycott campaign and the campus antiwar movement. Now, using multicolored maps and charts, she showed which minority neighborhoods were being starved for credit and which banks were the culprits.

On September 30, 1976, the day the HMDA went into effect, Lassen and other organizers, working closely with Richard Ratcliff, Washington University sociologist, launched a campaign in St. Louis against downtown banks. The research team documented loans rejected by banks simply because people lived in an inner city black neighborhood. On November 16, St. Louis newspapers and TV stations sent reporters to ACORN's press conference to document Ratcliff's dramatic and newsworthy findings; bank discrimination became a public issue.

Ratcliff's study showed that banks were making lending decisions based on the racial make-up of neighborhoods rather than the credit worthiness of would-be borrowers, a clear case of racial bias. Ratcliff proved that the redlining practices were widespread across St. Louis's entire banking sector. Clearly, these banks' top executives as well as the front-line loan agents needed to change the way they did business. Lassen organized community leaders to convince bankers—suburban residents with stereotyped images of city neighborhoods—that redlining was wrong and they should revise their perceptions and lending practices.

ACORN soon discovered that moral persuasion was not enough. Lassen and her green, young staff helped the members organize themselves into small groups and select banks with poor lending records based on Ratcliff's findings. Unannounced, they descended on the banks, carrying picket signs and flyers. As more and more members visited the banks, officers pleaded with Lassen to help them meet with these folks, hoping to quiet the protests, which were galvanizing news coverage and creating bad publicity for the banks. To make sure the maximum number of people could attend the meetings with the bankers, Lassen scheduled them at night. ACORN brought props such as a large poster listing demands with a space to check off each bank's response. That way the bankers could not simply make vague promises to reform their practices. For each demand, ACORN expected the bankers to respond yes or no.

At the initial meetings, only a few banks agreed to change their lending practices. ACORN needed more leverage. Lassen had learned that many banks did business with the city government; for example, the city deposited its accounts in a number of banks and used banks to issue checks. This gave the city some leverage over the banks, even though it had no legal authority in terms of regulating lenders, which were under state and federal jurisdiction. So ACORN leaders decided to lobby city officials to adopt a new and unprecedented policy called "linked deposits" that would require the city government to deposit its funds in banks that did not discriminate in lending. To be eligible for city deposits, a bank had to sign an ACORN-drafted anti-redlining pledge and post the pledge in its lobby.

Although the city government's funds accounted for only a small part of the banks' business, the bankers worried that other customers—individual depositors, unions, churches, social agencies, and so on—might follow the city's lead and stop doing business with offending banks. The linked-deposit policy, in short, could lead to a boycott of the banks that failed to meet ACORN's anti-redlining test. Several of St. Louis's largest banks began to change their practices, reaching out to community groups in black inner city neighborhoods to promote affordable mortgage loans to residents so they could buy a new home or fix up one they owned.

Lassen and ACORN staffer Madeline Adamson describe the growth of the St. Louis ACORN chapter due to its anti-redlining campaign: "The campaign was a great success in organizational terms. It established ACORN as an effective community organization and as a technical expert on this issue. It built good relationships for the organization with other local groups, St. Louis Aldermen and state legislators. It helped develop new groups in previously unorganized parts of the city, and more sophisticated leadership. No other campaign elicited as many phone calls from people wanting to get involved."[3] Activists in other cities had similar experiences.

If they really wanted to end redlining, activists across the country realized, they needed a bigger stick—a federal law that would make racial redlining illegal and that would penalize discriminating banks. In 1977, a coalition led by the NPA's Cincotta pressured Congress to enact the Community Reinvestment Act (CRA), a law that would revolutionize banking practices in the United States. Gail Cincotta would come to personify the battle between working-class neighborhoods and the U.S. banking industry. The new act would put teeth in the HMDA law.

Since the New Deal, federal regulatory agencies, through deposit insurance and access to central bank credit, had ensured that banks were safe and profitable; the CRA would extend the regulations to require banks to invest in neighborhoods where they took deposits, which would give Lassen more leverage. The banks opposed the CRA, but Proxmire and other congressional supporters minimized its visibility by tucking it into a large bill that included changing city grant formulas. (The CRA's supporters also had the good fortune to lobby the government before the election of Ronald Reagan and the nation's turn against government regulation.)

Under the CRA, if the banks excluded low-income minority neighborhoods from their loans, investments, and financial services, agencies such as the Federal Reserve and the Federal Deposit Insurance Corporation (FDIC) could deny the bank approval for lucrative mergers or acquisitions. The CRA was unique because it encouraged citizen groups to enforce it; since nearly all banks that had branches in minority neighborhoods were practicing redlining, the CRA gave community groups the chance to lodge a complaint against banks and savings and loans, alleging suspect lending practices based on the banks' own HMDA data. If the regulators found discrimination, it could hold up a profitable deal.

The CRA would also be a boon to civil rights organizations that for years had tried to end housing discrimination; fair housing laws were difficult to enforce because they depended on realtors and landlords identifying individual victims of housing discrimination. The only redress for a victim was on an individual basis through legal settlements. But the CRA provided groups with the necessary ingredients for a good organizing campaign.[4] It affected many people (bank redlining practices impacted not just individual residents, but whole neighborhoods), there was a clear problem (redlining), a clear target (banks), and a clear solution (reinvestment).

Change did not come overnight. Bankers held national conventions to concoct ways to avoid the CRA. At one American Bankers Association convention in the early 1980s, howls of laughter erupted from one of the meeting rooms as the speaker, an expert on the CRA, wrapped up his presentation by pointing to the boldly printed word projected on a screen behind him. "In conclusion," he shouted above the laughter and applause, "you can have your Community Reinvestment Act Programs, you can have your Community Reinvestment Act Policies, you can have your Community Reinvestment Act Personnel. But as you can see it's all just . . . CRAP!" The bankers were laughing because federal bank regulators ignored the law and community groups lacked the clout to enforce the CRA.[5]

In the mid 1980s, a revolution in inner city investment lending would commence. The groundwork for the change came from the organizing efforts by groups like NPA and Lassen's ACORN chapter. Activists in different cities met at conferences, corresponded by phone and mail, and read about each other's efforts through the media. Ironically, a remarkable anti-poverty success story would be aided by the wave of deregulation—reducing government restrictions on business—that began sweeping the country by the late 1970s.

The efforts of politicians like segregationist George Wallace and Richard Nixon, who since the late 1960s had wooed the vote of white working class with antigovernment rhetoric, dovetailed with the big business agenda to reduce government oversight of their practices. Even some liberals endorsed deregulation, claiming it would increase market competition and protect consumers against legally sanctioned monopolies, such as AT&T, the telephone monolith. Business's first victories came under Jimmy Carter's administration, which reduced government regulations over airlines, trucking, railroads, and interest rates. But with Ronald Reagan's election in 1980, big business had an ally and ideological soul mate. Under Reagan, deregulation accelerated.

Chase Manhattan, Citicorp, and other large commercial banks lobbied the Reagan administration and Congress hard to deregulate banks. They wanted to revise Depression-era regulations that restricted monopoly ownership of banks and that required one sector of the banking industry—savings and loans institutions—to focus its business on providing home mortgage loans. The banking lobbyists wanted to ease the way for profitable interstate bank mergers. They argued that banks needed to buy up smaller banks and merge with other large commercial banks to stay internationally competitive. Under Reagan, federal regulatory agencies relaxed merger restrictions, which gave large banks the green light to buy smaller banks and S&Ls. This move brought unintended consequences that would dramatically change the future of ACORN.

When banking industry lobbyists convinced Reagan and Congress to loosen the rules to allow banks to merge and S&Ls to engage in commercial lending, the Community Reinvestment Act was still the law of the land, although largely dormant until 1989. That year a bank in Chicago became the first big bank to have a merger application denied on CRA grounds, sending shivers up the spine of the banking industry. Mergers are high-stakes events. Delays in regulatory approval can mean changes in the agreed-upon sale price if stock values go up or down. From then on, to avoid adverse publicity and regulatory challenges that could delay and even scuttle their lucrative merger plans, Chase Manhattan and other large commercial banks began negotiating agreements with protesting community groups. Banks agreed to conduct outreach and educational programs, as well as provide below-market home repair and mortgage loans.

Individual homeowners were not the only beneficiaries of the CRA. Banks began reaching out to Community Development Corporations, nonprofit housing groups that sponsored affordable housing and job-creating businesses. These groups had emerged in the late 1960s, aided by small federal programs and the Ford Foundation. By the late 1980s, their number had grown to more then two thousand, mostly in older urban neighborhoods. Successful CDCs provided effective and workable solutions to the housing problem; among them were Mid-Bronx Desperados, Tacolcy Economic Development Corporation in Miami, Hispanic Housing in Chicago, several CDCs in Pittsburgh and Boston, and New Community Corporation in Newark.

Under pressure to channel credit into redlined neighborhoods, banks created community reinvestment divisions and forged partnerships with these community-based organizations to increase mortgage loans in urban areas. Bank managers in those divisions began providing community groups—many of them church connected—with low-cost credit to build affordable housing. To encourage the church and other groups' support, the banks also gave them philanthropic grants to underwrite their organizational operating expenses. In this way, and by avoiding aggressive, confrontational inner city community groups like Lassen's ACORN, banks could minimize the cost of their CRA commitments while satisfying the concerns of politicians and federal bank regulators. With the federal commitment to the working poor shrinking, millions of lower income families were forced to remain in unaffordable apartments, struggling to choose between paying the rent or purchasing food.

But ACORN wouldn't go away. Responding to the housing crisis the number of ACORN chapters grew, and more of them organized anti-redlining campaigns. Since Lassen's first campaign in St. Louis, ACORN's staff had become adroit in conducting research, using the media, and negotiating with banks, and they spread this expertise around the country. ACORN's activism was shaking the money tree.

A National, Hierarchical Organization

Banks continued to invest in community development in response to ACORN's protests, however, the money was going not to ACORN, but to local nonprofit development groups. ACORN staffers watched in frustration as such groups not only signed agreements but also entered into ongoing partnerships with banks to build affordable housing and obtain grants for their operating expenses. These groups were reaping the fruits of ACORN's organizing victories.

ACORN wanted a piece of the action for its own national organization and local chapters, and toward this end, it had one advantage over other community groups: it was a hierarchical, fairly disciplined, nationally federated organization. It could act simultaneously on the local and national level, waging campaigns against local banks while lobbying Congress to change banking regulations and targeting big national banking corporations with headquarters in California, New York, North Carolina, and elsewhere.

To get more than crumbs from the banks' CRA table and earn the same benefits as the less feisty CDCs, ACORN had to overcome two barriers. It would have to enter into partnerships with its targets, the banks, and it would have to find members within its ranks willing to lead its campaigns. For some of ACORN's left-leaning organizers, who viewed the banks as part of the capitalistic system responsible for racism, poverty, and inequality, the idea of partnering with banks was hard to swallow. Furthermore, throughout its history, ACORN had protested against many big corporations, but it had never forged an ongoing business partnership.

How would such an operation be set up? ACORN would have to create a separate nonprofit tax-exempt corporation to receive government and private grants so that it could build affordable housing and counsel prospective home buyers. If ACORN took that step, it would have to confront the dilemmas that befell activist groups that branched out into building affordable housing. ACORN would be forced to view the world through the lens of a profit-making entrepreneur. ACORN would become a business, albeit a nonprofit one, and thus a landlord, a contractor, a developer, and a social service agency. ACORN 's organizers and leaders were concerned that if they become homeowners' counselors, they would lose the momentum required for effective community organizing and movement building. A host of ACORN organizers believed that providing individuals a specific service and building housing would lead to being co-opted by government and business elites. How could ACORN continue to organize tenants against landlords, the symbols of private greed? ACORN organizers might be reluctant to mobilize tenants in their own buildings or fearful that their own tenants would organize against ACORN. A pair of Rathke's old mentors, Richard Cloward and Frances Fox Piven, had warned against doing anything that would discourage the mobilization of the poor.

On the other hand, ACORN faced a changing political landscape. During the 1970s and early 1980s, most cities were losing their tax base with the exodus of low-skilled manufacturing firms. Carter, Reagan, and Bush cut federal funds for urban programs. Tax cuts, vastly increased defense spending, and dramatic reductions in social spending, especially housing aid, to local governments meant that city officials had fewer resources for programs to help the poor. Banks couldn't replace the government as a source of antipoverty funding, but they could provide ACORN with funds so working-class families could buy homes.

Even when ACORN won battles, it could face enforcement problems. The CRA presented ACORN with an opportunity to maneuver private banks into financing the building and rehabilitation of slum apartments and obtain philanthropic grants to hire more organizers, who would recruit more dues-paying members, and help ACORN grow, which in turn would help enforce its victories with more oversight of corporations.

Mike Shea, who had joined ACORN as an organizer in Arkansas in 1976, proposed at a national staff meeting that ACORN create a nonprofit housing corporation and go into the housing counseling business. Shea saw an opportunity and he had the support of Rathke. Surprisingly, there was almost no serious internal debate about this proposal. In the mid 1980s, ACORN created a housing division and then spun it off into a separate corporation, ACORN Housing Corporation (AHC) of Illinois. Chapters in New York, Philadelphia, Phoenix, St. Louis, and Little Rock followed suit.

ACORN had entered the complex business of low-income housing development. Local chapters needed housing developers and managers to navigate the complex deals required to develop low-income housing. There was no simple standard approach, for every housing project was different. Each involved multiple subsidies from federal, state, and local government agencies, arcane accounting, brokered tax abatements, negotiations with construction firms and lenders, and other creative scrounging. Shea and other ACORN staff had to cope with government bureaucrats, mortgage bankers, and shakedown racketeers vying for control of local construction projects.

ACORN's housing business got off to a rocky start in 1986 with the renovation of a house at 1015 Schiller Street in the middle of an empty neighborhood in Little Rock. Lacy and Daniel Williams bought it, looking forward to living in their first house. But soon after they moved in, gang members began to loiter on the lawn. Flasks of vodka and broken bottles riddled the street gutters. In less than a year, the Williams family was forced to move, unable to carve out a small safe place to live. One nearby resident called the area Vietnam, a neighborhood of empty lots, forgotten houses, and gang turf. A few years later, the city tore the house down.

In rundown neighborhoods, developers' chances of success are higher if they rebuild an entire area rather than a single dwelling, an opportunity rare for an activist community group. Since ACORN did not have enough capital in Arkansas to purchase an entire block, it fixed up houses where it could find them, spreading its energy thinly over hundreds of blocks.

The Dudley Street Neighborhood Initiative in Boston, the first nonprofit community group to be given powers of eminent domain, and IAF's Nehemiah project in Brooklyn are two exceptional success stories for resuscitating an inner city neighborhood.

After some initial trial and error and largely because of Mike Shea's almost fanatical dedication, ACORN figured out the complicated affordable housing business. The CRA allowed ACORN to deliver housing and home ownership counseling services to its existing members, identify potential new recruits, and increase its staff. Lucrative deals for ACORN began to accumulate.

Also, like the earlier squatting campaigns, ACORN's CRA campaigns demonstrated to Rathke and ACORN's other leaders that they could learn from successful campaigns conducted by other groups, creatively adopt them to their local situation, and then nationalize them—that is, carry out similar campaigns in cities across the country at the same time, thus building a national movement for reform. ACORN's CRA effort was a major turning point for the organization. It vindicated Rathke's strategy to build a cohesive national organization and highlighted another ACORN asset—its ability to adopt its tactics to a changing political climate. It also vindicated Rathke's emphasis on raising money. If ACORN were to compete against large corporations and mainstream political parties, it would need funds. As Rathke would later say when emphasizing the importance of raising money to improve ACORN's tech capacity: "There is no reason for us to be proud of pea shooters, when all of our enemies are using machine guns."

A New Leader

As the 1990 national ACORN convention approached, the media broke the savings-and-loan crisis, which the national staff at ACORN decided was yet another opportunity for ACORN to demonstrate its muscle against the country's financial powers. At the convention, the group elected a new president, Maude Hurd, forty-six, who would help mount and direct this new phase in ACORN's national CRA campaign.

As a young African American woman raising five children in Dorchester, a working-class Boston neighborhood, Hurd got involved in ACORN the way most members do. In 1982 an organizer knocked on her door and asked, "What are your concerns about your neighborhood?"

She had never been asked that before. "At first I didn't want to be bothered," she recalls. Her experience with other community groups was that they didn't accomplish much and didn't last long. "One of the differences with ACORN was the organizer asked me what *I* thought," she explained. The trash-filled vacant lot next door to her house, was Hurd's answer to the organizer.

She had tried for years to get that lot cleaned up. Frustrated by her failure, she agreed to attend an ACORN community meeting about the many garbage-strewn vacant lots in her neighborhood. At the meeting the group decided to try a get a appointment with Mayor Ray Flynn, who called himself the "neighborhood mayor," ACORN members sent letters to Flynn's office but received no response. Phone calls didn't work either. Encouraged by ACORN organizers, the group decided to try a direct action, a protest. Hurd and a few other ACORN members went door to door in their neighborhood, recruiting others who were also upset by the unsightly vacant lots that pockmarked their community. She then led more than a hundred ACORN members on a march into City Hall. In the lobby outside Mayor Flynn's office, they piled bags full of debris from the abandoned vacant lots. This action launched a monthlong campaign that eventuated in a program that cleaned up more than seven hundred lots.

"It was a scary experience for me and a lot of folks," Hurd would recall, "but it got results, got news coverage, and got some vacant lots cleaned up. At that point, I was convinced that people working together like that can work." She realized that ordinary people could successfully demand a say in policies that affected their lives. "Before that experience with ACORN," she says, "I never thought of myself as a leader. At work, singing in the choir, or whatever it was, I saw myself as a background person." Now she was inspired to overcome her fear of public speaking.

Hurd came to Boston in the early 1960s, after high school, from the small town of Blakely, Georgia, married, and began a family. When her husband died from brain cancer, to support their five small children she worked in an alcoholism treatment program for women at the housing project and trained as a counselor. In 1983, after joining ACORN, Hurd attended the ACORN Leadership School, held that summer at Loyola University in Chicago. As part of the training, ACORN members learned they would participate in a confrontation with the Peoples Gas Company because it was shutting off people's services, leaving them with no heat and hot water. Hurd was anxious about this proposal because she was not comfortable with conflict. She was brought up to "not make waves" and was proud that her kids were "well behaved and obedient."

Yet ACORN's training sessions teach potential leaders the creative use of conflict to bring about the results members want. Trainers rehearse and re-rehearse what it takes to succeed in a combative, fractious public encounter.

When Hurd arrived at the gas company's offices with the other leaders, she was quite nervous, thinking, "I've never been part of an action this large and that vocal." Then the police came, and she became very scared, imagining, Oh, my God, people might get put in jail. She had never been in a situation like that. Yet as she watched the ACORN leaders take charge of the situation and make their point, she thought, Gee, I think I could do that. She began overcoming her discomfort with conflict, a critical trait for a living democracy and for an ACORN leader.

Hurd learned that low- and moderate-income people don't have the power to solve many of their problems alone, and that conflict is an essential byproduct of making change happen. Frances Moore Lappé would later write about ACORN: "Living Democracy means ongoing change, and change implies, minimally, that somebody thinks we can improve on the status quo. No big shock, then, that somebody else feels criticized. So change entails conflict."[6]

Soon after she finished her training, Hurd was elected to chair the Dorchester chapter of ACORN; she later served as the Massachusetts delegate to the ACORN national board. Eight years after she joined ACORN, she became the national president, a nonpaying post, while maintaining a full-time job with a medical foundation helping at-risk youth with substance-abuse problems. Her leadership skills would be repeatedly tested.

More Mergers, More Growth

As bank mergers accelerated in the 1990s, ACORN used the provision in the CRA to file challenges against banks seeking regulatory approvals who had not met CRA requirements, forcing the banks to the bargaining table. Some banks preferred a settlement with ACORN to either being pilloried in the media by community protests or enduring a full-scale review by one of the federal supervising agencies. Hurd, whose folksy, down-home disposition masked a sharp, focused mind, found herself across the negotiating table from the presidents of some of nation's biggest banks. Initially, she was intimidated, because "they seemed to have all the knowledge and all the power." Over time, though, she discovered that "they don't know it all, and I often know more about the issues than they do."

A woman with a stern face and soft eyes, Hurd was becoming a shrewd negotiator against adversaries that included corporations that often preyed upon low-income consumers. She frequently went toe-to-toe with government officials in Boston, as well as in Washington, D.C., to pressure them to enforce the law. Business executives and elected officials often underestimated Hurd, as they did ACORN, which often worked to her advantage. She could turn on the charm, but she also knew when to threaten her opponents with lawsuits and direct action.

When ACORN decided to pursue a challenge, it would schedule meetings with elected officials or bank regulators to voice its demands. Hurd chaired these meetings, where ACORN members would press federal and state regulators to make sure that as a quid pro quo for receiving a merger approval, the bigger bank agreed to specific programs and practices to benefit residents of poor neighborhoods. At dozens of negotiating sessions representing ACORN, Hurd helped secure these commitments, called "community reinvestment agreements"; they totaled about a billion dollars in loans for low-interest home mortgages.

Soon after Hurd became president in 1990, Mike Shea, the head of ACORN Housing, learned that North Carolina National Bank planned to merge with C&S/Sovran to create NationsBank, the fourth-largest financial institution in the country. Shea and Hurd saw the potential of negotiating with a bank that had branches in dozens of southern cities where ACORN had local chapters. ACORN's researchers discovered that North Carolina National denied black and Latino loan applications two to four times as often as white loan applications. The banks even discriminated against applicants of different races who had the same income: middle-income black applicants were seven times as likely to have their loans denied as middle-income white applicants.

Having conducted the research, ACORN enlisted elected officials, including House Banking Committee chair Henry Gonzalez and Senate Banking Committee chair Donald Riegle, to call for public hearings by the Federal Reserve Board. Demonstrations gained publicity and embarrassed NationsBank into submitting a plan for community investment to the Federal Reserve as part of its merger agreement. The bank agreed to fund the ACORN Housing Corporation; in exchange, AHC agreed to find, screen, and counsel low-income and minority applicants for a new low-cost mortgage product with interest at 1 percent below market rate, a product worth hundreds of millions of dollars to AHC borrowers. NationsBank agreed to underwrite $1 billion per year in these mortgages, benefiting six thousand first-time home buyers. The agreement established the first multistate agreement, covering Texas, Georgia, Washington, D.C., and Maryland.

Hurd, Shea, and Bruce Dorpalen, ACORN Housing's director of counseling, helped negotiate for alternative borrowing eligibility requirements that would count welfare, Social Security, and food-stamp benefits as income and substitute records of regular rent and utility payments for a credit record for people who had none.

These new standards allowed thousands of families to become homeowners through ACORN's mortgage-counseling program.

At its annual convention in New York in 1992, ACORN organized a bank summit to display its community investment agreements with several major banks, including First Fidelity, Mellon, PriMerit, and Chemical. The banks sent representatives to the summit to establish programs for low- and moderate-income people to qualify for mortgages in their communities. Citibank, the nation's largest bank, refused to participate, and in response, Hurd led ACORN conventioneers to a lively protest in front of Citibank's Manhattan headquarters. Chastened by the media attention, Citibank agreed to schedule a negotiating session with ACORN, which led to a three-way deal among ACORN, Citibank, and the Federal National Mortgage Association (Fannie Mae)—a $55 million, eleven-city lending program financed by Citibank and thirteen other major banks eager to avoid CRA blockages.

During the Reagan and Bush years, ACORN worked with its allies in Congress to pressure bank regulators to enforce the CRA on behalf of the poor. ACORN resorted to protests, demonstrations, sit-ins, and other tactics to draw public attention to the issue of persistent bank redlining. Its friends in Congress forced reluctant regulators to do their jobs—regulate banks.

ACORN hoped that with Bill Clinton in the White House, it would finally have a president who took the CRA seriously. His appointments to the four major federal bank regulatory agencies, HUD, and the Justice Department's Civil Rights Division were significant improvements over those who filled these posts under Reagan and Bush, and ACORN soon developed a close relationship with HUD secretary Henry Cisneros. HUD, under Clinton, gave ACORN and other grassroots community groups funds to "test" banks and landlords to uncover redlining and racial discrimination.

Hurd never imagined that she would meet with the president of the United States, but in 1993, she and twenty other ACORN members met Bill Clinton in the White House. She noticed the opulence of the Oval Office and the high shine on the president's expensive shoes. What made the biggest impression was that, like many of the organizers she knew in ACORN, Clinton neither patronized, intimidated, nor erased her. When he spoke to her, he looked at her as if she was the only person in the room.

Being charmed by the president did not divert Hurd from her goal. Clinton had met with ACORN because they were gaining a reputation as a political force to be reckoned with, a small but valuable part of the Democratic Party base. Ultimately, ACORN wanted Clinton to spend his political capital on public policies to help lift people out of poverty, improve conditions in inner city neighborhoods, and provide resources and validation to ACORN and other grassroots groups.

Clinton made significant changes in both government personnel and policy that ACORN wanted. Yet while CRA enforcement improved under Clinton's Justice Department and bank regulators, and ACORN received funds from HUD for housing, counseling, and racial testing, in November 1994, under the leadership of conservative GOP Speaker Newt Gingrich, the Republicans won a majority of seats in the

House for the first time in forty years. With the takeover, Clinton was forced to forge compromises that alienated some of his key supporters, including ACORN.

ACORN would not retreat from the national stage, and Hurd faced a new test of her leadership. In 1995 Hurd and five hundred ACORN protesters barged into a luncheon at the Washington Hilton to confront House Speaker Newt Gingrich over cuts in federal programs for the poor. The protestors waved trays and chanted, "Nuke Newt!" forcing the cancellation of Gingrich's appearance.

Hurd's most chilling experience came during House of Representative Banking Committee hearings on the Community Reinvestment Act. The banking industry resented the growing scrutiny of banks' performance by the CRA. Bank lobbyists convinced hard-line Republicans to eliminate some of the law's key provisions, which would weaken the government's ability to monitor and punish redlining in big cities. Confident Republicans on the committee, working behind closed doors, offered a series of innocuous-sounding reforms that, in effect, would have repealed the CRA.

ACORN brought its members to attend the House of Representative Banking Committee hearings. Dozens of ACORN members stood in line the night before the hearings (displaying the persistence important in ACORN's successes) to squeeze out paid banking lobbyists for seats in the hearing room. At the hearing, Hurd insisted on speaking. When she tried to testify, police grabbed her, slapped handcuffs on her, and locked her up. "It was the most frightening thing," she recalls. To cope, she and the four others who were arrested sang freedom songs. After a call from Massachusetts representative Joe Kennedy and a rainy day visit to the jailhouse by California representative Maxine Waters, the protestors were finally released. As they left, a guard told Hurd, "I don't know who you are, but you must know somebody important." Hurd's later comment: "We are up there rubbing elbows with some very powerful people. We are a force to be reckoned with. We're ordinary people doing some extraordinary things."

The CRA activists rallied congressional Democrats to unanimously oppose every Republican proposal to weaken the CRA. Clinton, who always supported the CRA, never wavered from an early pledge to veto any bill containing enfeebling provisions. At the end of 1996, the CRA emerged intact.

ACORN Housing

For the next fifteen years, the ACORN Housing Corporation expanded, entering into new agreements with banks that balanced financial needs of the community and the banks' need to make a reasonable profit. Typical was the deal with J. P. Morgan & Company. "Thus we have J. P. Morgan & Company, the legatee of the man who once symbolized for many all that was supposedly evil about American capitalism, suddenly donating hundreds of thousands of dollars to ACORN," wrote ACORN critic Sol Stern. "This act of generosity and civic-mindedness came, interestingly, just as Morgan was asking bank regulators for approval of a merger with Chase Manhattan. Not to be outdone, Chase also decided to grant more than $200,000 to ACORN."[7]

Since 1985, AHC had entered into memorandums of understanding (MOUs) and partnerships with two dozen financial institutions, offering bank products to new customers in thirty-eight offices nationwide. At first the banks resented negotiating with ACORN. As one community reinvestment banker put it, "The banks know they are being held up, but they are not going to fight over this. They look at it as a cost of doing business." Once banks took off their racist blinders, they discovered new markets and came up with profitable products that met the needs of ACORN's constituents.

ACORN's practice was controversial, even outside the banking industry. Conservative critics such as Robert L. Woodson, president of the National Center for Neighborhood Enterprise, accused corporate America of capitulating to ACORN to "buy peace from groups that agitate against them." In his opinion, according to Sol Stern of the conservative Manhattan Institute, "the same corporations that pay ransom to Jesse Jackson and Al Sharpton pay ransom to ACORN." Reflecting an ideology held by business publications such as the *Wall Street Journal* and *Investors Business Daily*, Stern claimed that ACORN's continued use of the CRA was crass opportunism and bad public policy; in the *City Journal*, just before the subprime mortgage crisis struck, Stern wrote:

> The discrimination that the CRA sought to cure no longer exists today. . . . Lenders can adjust the interest rates they charge borrowers according to the riskiness of the loan, so that they can make a profit by lending in the inner city. Today too, hundreds of individual mortgages are packaged together and sold to investors as "mortgage-backed securities," whose overall default rate is much easier to predict than the default probability of any individual mortgage. Thanks to these innovations, the capital available to inner city borrowers is now plentiful.[8]

Stern's opinion on mortgage-back securities would be refuted by the subprime crisis and several studies that demonstrated that landlords, real estate agents, and lenders treated whites more favorably than blacks and Latinos, even with income factored in.[9]

Liberals also criticized ACORN's methods. For thirteen years Paul Grogan was president of the Local Initiatives Support Corporation (LISC), a Ford Foundation–backed intermediary that raises funds for CDCs. Under his stewardship, LISC passed on to communities billions of dollars of loans, grants, and equity. Grogan and Tony Proscio observed in *Comeback Cities* that "millions of individual borrowers and home buyers have found credit where for decades there had been only rejections," a change Grogan, who earned a comfortable six-figure salary, attributed to the CRA. In their analysis, the authors mocked those like ACORN for their "in-your-face style of protest that Tom Wolfe famously dubbed 'mau-mauing' and their preference for confrontation over visible results."[10]

Like many liberals, Grogan wanted to believe that people without conventional access to money and power could make their voices heard without using tools like direct action and in-your-face tactics. Brad Lander, the head of the Pratt Institute and the former executive director of one of the most successful community development corporations in the United States, corrected Grogan: "This caricature has little to do with the actual direct action, grassroots organizing that has grown out of the civil rights movement and the work of Saul Alinsky. While often 'in-your-face,' this organizing is driven by a quest for concrete results—an end to predatory lending, the establishment of living-wage laws, fair employment and housing practices. . . . It is often the only way that people without conventional access to money and power can make their voices heard, even if there is a CDC with a fabulous track record in their community."[11]

While a few self-styled leaders without a base shook down the banks under the CRA's umbrella, the innovative law in fact encouraged citizen engagement for its enforcement, including the organizing power of groups like New Jersey Citizen Action, NPA, and ACORN. Despite some failures, such as the one in Little Rock and a short-lived experiment with land trusts in Chicago, ACORN Housing Corporation has built hundreds of affordable housing units in Dallas, Little Rock, Phoenix, and Chicago.[12] In New York City, the New York ACORN Housing Company owns and manages seven hundred apartments, providing low-income residents with quality, stable housing at below-market rates. For these tenants, the average monetary benefit of living in an ACORN apartment rather than finding, renting, and maintaining a rental apartment on the open market is $2,400 per year or $200 per month. This represents an average savings of $1,680,000 per year for ACORN tenants and $16.8 million over the last decade. ACORN housing development and management programs have benefited communities with $33.6 million in investments and rental savings.[13]

ACORN the outsider was becoming ACORN the insider.[14] Citigroup's website would highlight in a marketing brochure its partnership with ACORN along with other more established groups like Habitat for Humanity International and the National Urban League. In the mid 1990s, when NationsBank wanted to merge with Bank of America, based in California, its executives reached out to Shea, the president of ACORN Housing, to testify on behalf of NationsBank at public hearings held by the Federal Reserve Bank in San Francisco. ACORN was the only community group to testify in favor of the merger, which the Federal Reserve approved, and not surprisingly, as Shea said to his staff, NationsBank was "eternally grateful" for AHC's testimony.

By leveraging money from corporations as a result of its organizing campaigns, ACORN thought it was bringing new meaning to its historical goal of financial self-sufficiency. In the 1970s and 1980s, internal fund-raising consisted of membership dues, canvassing, and various local and national fund-raisers such as raffles and ad books. For the next ten years, raising money directly from corporate campaigns provided a new stream of financial support.[15] But would the partnerships continue if ACORN became too controversial? That would depend on many circumstances, including whether ACORN had powerful political alliances.

Discrimination in the 1980s wasn't the only housing problem facing the poor and working class, though, and using the CRA wasn't the only strategy in ACORN's arsenal. In every city where it set up shop, poor and working-class families faced an acute shortage of decent, affordable housing. Unemployment was rising, rents were skyrocketing, and the first signs of an epidemic of homelessness were visible in the nation's cities. As more and more houses were abandoned in America's cities, people desperately seeking housing began the illegal practice of squatting in them. Some ACORN organizers thought this could be an opportunity to make an impact on local and national policy. Philadelphia, where home abandonment was widespread, became a testing ground for ACORN's next foray: urban homesteading.

Chapter 7

Urban Homesteading

Housing had once been a political issue that mobilized large numbers of Americans.[1] In the late 1940s, with an enormous pent-up demand for housing after World War II, labor unions, veterans groups, and even PTAs spearheaded campaigns for local public housing (temporary housing for working-class families and veterans) and subsidized mortgages (to help working-class families and veterans buy their first homes). In the 1960s, civil rights groups mobilized to enact "fair housing" laws and ban racial discrimination by landlords and realtors, while tenant groups began fighting against the urban renewal bulldozer and for renters' rights, and unions continued their commitment to expand government-subsidized apartments. By the late 1970s, however, the political constituency for affordable housing had declined.[2]

In the early days of ACORN, Steve Kest had recruited his younger and taller brother Jon, who left Oberlin College for a year to organize for ACORN in Arkansas. Jon transferred to the University of Pennsylvania to finish college, and in 1977, Rathke tapped him to open the Philadelphia ACORN office. Jon's next-door neighbor, Francine Streich, was earning a bachelor's degree in occupational therapy in the university's School of Allied Medical Professions and led a campaign to keep that school from being shut down in favor of expanding the university's veterinary school. Jon was attracted to her campaign and even more to Fran. Five foot five, blond, adventuresome, brave, she was simultaneously sweet and intense. Kest offered to help her with her campaign. They worked together in what would be a losing cause—the school closed down, but the campaign brought them closer. In June, immediately after graduating from Penn, now a couple, they opened an ACORN office, where Jon worked full time. With insufficient money to pay both Jon and Fran, even at ACORN's very low salaries, Streich worked part-time.

Jon Kest's limited organizing experience in Arkansas provided him with the key tenets for mobilizing the poor in inner city Philadelphia: sign up dues-paying members and win victories by relying on their participation. Philadelphia's new membership would range from welfare recipients to a few middle-class professionals, but its heart was the working poor. For decades, modest single-family brick rowhouses in North Philadelphia had provided many of ACORN's working-class families with affordable housing in a livable working-class neighborhood. Over the same years, speculators and absentee landlords were purchasing buildings, renting them to poor families, keeping the rent money rather than investing it in repairs, and eventually walking away, leaving the buildings abandoned. They also stopped paying property taxes, forcing the city government to foreclose on the buildings and assume ownership.

With no plan to repair the vacant buildings, the city allowed them to deteriorate. Eventually, neighbors complained that the vacant slum buildings were eyesores and magnets for drug dealers, so the city government started to demolish them, leaving what one commentator called "gaps like missing teeth in formerly solid blocks." City officials estimated that twenty thousand houses were abandoned, with the densest concentration in North Philadelphia.

For the first two years, Kest and Streich fought to clean up vacant lots, put up stop signs at dangerous intersections, and help members avoid utility shutoffs. Rathke would say that, like Keith Kelleher and Madeline Talbott, Kest and Streich epitomized the adage, "In for a penny, in for a pound." They lived in the Kensington section of Philadelphia in an apartment house with broken mailboxes, dark corridors, and rats. As Kest and other ACORN organizers knocked on doors in the neighborhood, they kept hearing the same complaint: people wanted action to fix up the abandoned buildings. To build the chapter and recruit members, ACORN needed a strategy to help people solve this housing problem.

Although housing remained a serious problem not only in Philadelphia, but also in most U.S. cities, it wasn't a hot political issue among Washington's powerbrokers. The prohousing lobby was composed primarily of those with a direct financial or political stake in housing the poor: big-city mayors and local government housing bureaucrats; private housing developers, landlords, and speculators who scooped up federal housing subsidies; and groups concerned about the plight of the poor. These groups were politically weak, fragmented, and generally viewed unfavorably by members of an increasingly suburban Congress and white middle-class homeowners.

The urban lobby was losing clout as cities came to represent a smaller portion of the overall electorate and as national political action committees replaced city-based political machines as the key to winning urban seats in Congress. The prohousing coalition agreed that Washington should provide more funding for affordable housing, but they disagreed on many other things, like rent control, enforcement of antidiscrimination laws, and where federal funds should go—directly to developers or through city halls.

The National Low Income Housing Coalition (NLIHC) served as the key lobbyist for the antipoverty agencies and community groups. Founded in 1974 by Cushing Dolbeare, a liberal Quaker activist from Philadelphia, in response to the Nixon administration's moratorium on federal housing programs, the NLIHC issued reports on the housing crisis, testified on Capitol Hill on behalf of increased funding for low-income housing, and produced a newsletter informing its local members about legislation. Dolbeare even encouraged people to contact their representatives in Congress to support or oppose particular bills. But NLIHC, like many other single-issue groups based in Washington, lacked the capacity to mobilize people at the grassroots level. It was what political scientists call an "advocacy" group, not an "organizing" group. Lobbyists and researchers, not organizers, comprised its small and underpaid staff. Its methods were polite and nonconfrontational.

Ideas from the Street

Kest and Streich knew they would not get help from Washington. While they were getting ACORN off the ground, they came upon a ubiquitous theatrical character, Milton Street. Inspired by the civil rights movement, Street believed that civil disobedience could fix up abandoned buildings. With his scraggly beard and big Afro, he made a tenuous living selling hot dogs from a cart outside Temple University and became the leader of a black street vendors organization. He became a controversial figure when he charged Mayor Frank Rizzo with wasting federal funds awarded to the city for urban improvement. Street also criticized Rizzo for doing nothing about the thousands of homes foreclosed by HUD as a result of unpaid federal loans. A master of the art of public confrontation, he mobilized the poor to take over the vacant federally owned houses and fix them up. Clad in an old army jacket, screaming and shouting, he settled two hundred squatters into those single-family houses in an effort he called the Walk-in Urban Homesteading Program.[3]

President Carter's HUD secretary, Pat Harris, who thought of herself as a champion of the poor, attacked the squatters as "no better than shoplifters," and the president of the Philadelphia City Council warned of the "beginning of anarchy." But the public supported Street, and the press was sympathetic. A *Philadelphia Daily News* editorial on August 8, 1977, declared that Street "is putting people who need homes into houses that have stood vacant far too long. . . . Rather than doing battle with Street, the Rizzo administration and HUD should get behind the man and help him."[4] The city allowed the squatters to remain and even granted some of them title to their houses at nominal cost.

ACORN leaders like Reba Brown, who was involved in her church, and Grover Wright, who had been a civil rights activist, were deeply attached to their North Philadelphia neighborhood and desperate for the city to do something about the abandoned homes that blighted the area. They worried that the vacant buildings undermined property values and threatened neighborhood safety. Inspired by Street's limited success, Fran Streich urged them to try squatting. She had no idea this inspiration would lead to a dramatic change in federal law.

Despite its dangers, they enthusiastically agreed. ACORN's squatting efforts were intended to persuade the federal government (which owned the properties) and Philadelphia officials, including Mayor Bill Green, a reformer who succeeded Rizzo, to help support their effort and to subsidize the costs of rehabbing these vacant buildings.

Streich had good reason to believe a local squatting campaign was winnable. It could mobilize two large constituencies: families that needed housing, and residents of neighborhoods with countless abandoned houses. The campaign appealed to the self-interest of this widespread group of people who believed that what ACORN was pitching—a house for their family—filled an immediate need. In most housing reform programs, the benefits are too diffuse and remote to attract widespread grassroots engagement. In the squatting campaign, the benefit was immediate: if you squatted, you got the house.

Squatting was also an economically efficient government housing program. Squatters got generous rehabilitation loans, a relatively inexpensive way to rescue low-income housing that promised to restore abandoned property to the tax rolls. ACORN's national network took the local campaign and turned it into a countrywide effort, a sequence of events that would become a hallmark of ACORN's modus operandi. Also, ACORN was able to mobilize local squatters for a citywide and even a national campaign because the crusade emerged from the bottom up. Not all the squatters, but a critical mass, comprehended the policy issues and embraced the detailed programs for reform that ACORN's professional staff developed. They understood the issues and demands because they took shape from their individual and collective experience.

Although squatting was illegal, the press and clergy, as well as the public and many housing officials, saw the cause as just and moral. Framing actions in moral terms foreshadowed some of ACORN's future campaigns against poverty, especially its campaigns for moral minimum wages and a "living wage."

ACORN attracted squatters by placing flyers in neighborhoods asking: "Need a house? Call ACORN." The audacious tactic drew hundreds of previously unorganized individuals into ACORN offices and caught the attention of the local media. Moving poor and working-class families needing shelter into empty houses offered TV cameras and news photographers what they like—visually dramatic events. When ACORN's squatting efforts met with resistance from HUD and Mayor Green, ACORN just kept up the pressure. Streich kept the campaign simple to understand—the public confrontations bonded the goal of sheltering the homeless with the abandoned houses caused by government negligence.

Streich knew from discussions with her members that neighbors preferred a squatter next door rather than an abandoned shelter for junkies. Thus, the squatting campaign forged allies between the squatters, their neighbors, and neighborhood-based institutions, the churches as well as politicians. Streich could count on enthusiastic neighbors and community-based institutions to help sustain homesteading, since they had an interest in monitoring and enforcing it.

Scores of ACORN members took the risk of illegally squatting. The movement was well publicized to draw attention to the problem of vacant buildings and to underscore the squatters' pride in their neighborhoods. ACORN relied on the media coverage to generate pressure for change. The risk takers became transformed from passive observers to courageous political activists fighting to improve ghetto neighborhoods and to assert their right to decent housing. Sympathetic ministers and local officials participated at meetings and rallies, generating favorable media coverage.

Unlike most antipoverty and progressive groups, ACORN expressed its support for government activism in value-laden tones that rang true to most of the middle class. ACORN couched its radical ideas in everyday language that most Americans could understand and support. Its squatting campaign appealed to American traditions of self-help and hard work: the squatters weren't demanding something for nothing; they were willing to work hard to repair homes that had been left abandoned by unscrupulous and neglectful landlords and owners. The squatters claimed that they were looking for an opportunity, not a handout.

Eventually, ACORN embarrassed both HUD and Mayor Green into providing financing for the squatters and the transfer of the deeds. Consequently, ACORN's squatting and homesteading program in Philadelphia turned hundreds of abandoned buildings into decent affordable homes for the squatters.

ACORN's Nationwide Campaign

At ACORN's 1979 annual convention in St. Louis, Streich held conversations with ACORN organizers in other cities about Philadelphia's success. The word spread. Abandoned housing was abundant in Atlanta, Detroit, St. Louis, Dallas, Columbus, Tulsa, Pittsburgh, and Phoenix, but no mayor or other political leader had a plan for addressing it. Streich and leaders from Philadelphia ACORN traveled to each of these cities to teach their counterparts how to mount a squatting campaign. By April 1982, there were hundreds of ACORN squatters in thirteen cities. In St. Louis, Dallas, and Pittsburgh the official response was swift and harsh. Squatters were arrested and found themselves defendants in a civil suit for $500,000 in damages. Many officials denounced the squatters and refused to negotiate with them.

In other cities, local officials were more sympathetic. Madeline Talbott's ACORN chapter helped push the Detroit City Council to pass a resolution setting up a large-scale urban homesteading program and clemency for the squatters. In Atlanta, favorable stories and editorials encouraged Mayor Andrew Young, a former aide to Martin Luther King, to negotiate with the squatters.

Through these campaigns ACORN gained national exposure on housing issues. It enhanced its reputation not only as a feisty protest group but also as an effective practitioner of community development in low-income neighborhoods. Although ACORN organizers realized the squatting campaigns would not solve the nation's housing crisis, its leaders and staff hoped their symbolic power would challenge the national complacency about housing and that the simultaneous squatting campaigns in different cities would lay the groundwork for a large federally funded homesteading program.

On June 5, 1982, ACORN members in seven cities squatted in HUD-owned houses despite HUD officials' threats to evict and arrest squatters. These actions were intended to generate media interest in ACORN's plan to sponsor a squatters' Tent City in Washington, D.C., later that month, just a few hundred yards from the back porch of the White House. For two days in late June, the National Parks Service tried repeatedly to remove ACORN's two hundred Tent City squatters, who had gathered from ten cities. Despite harassment and intimidation, the protesters held their position, marched on the White House, and testified before a congressional committee about the housing crisis in America.

While public officials had warned ACORN that its confrontational tactics would backfire and sway public opinion and political influence against its goals, ACORN had learned repeatedly that such protest tactics worked. The squatting campaign, including the Tent City protest, led Congress in 1982 to enact the National Homesteading Act, which reformed federal policies and procedures to make it easier for low- and moderate-income people to purchase properties owned by the HUD.[5]

New funds for homestead acquisition and rehabilitation aid were appropriated for Phoenix, Columbus, and Brooklyn. Mayor Coleman Young of Detroit, once an implacable opponent of the squatters, was pressured by ACORN to set up a program to give away five hundred government-owned properties and approved a city plan that would permit homesteading in privately owned, tax-delinquent houses.

ACORN organizers smartly cast the squatting demands within traditional American values of individual initiative, self-reliance, and the importance of homeownership. Yet basing programs for the poor on self-reliance could play into the hands of those who wished to absolve the government of responsibility for housing and other antipoverty programs, a criticism the Left leveled at the Reagan and Bush administrations' approach to reducing poverty by relying on churches and volunteer associations. Using the language of self-help could prop up the kind of Reagan rhetoric that claimed: "Government is the problem and not the solution." While Reagan praised neighborhoods as "arenas for civic action and creative self-help" and lauded the "renaissance of the American community, a rebirth of the neighborhood," as the heart and soul of rebuilding America, his idea of community inspired a movement more in the tradition of the Know-nothings, nativist societies of the nineteenth century, and the neighborhood protection associations of 1950s suburbia.

Despite the work of ACORN and numerous other organizations, the fight against poverty dropped well under America's radar. Most of the civil rights organizations focused more on issues such as busing and affirmative action, which often had little relevance to the economic concerns in poor black communities. Poverty is, above all, about the distribution of wealth and power; ending poverty requires removing the barriers to a better education and jobs opportunities, which can only occur when the poor and their allies wrest some of the power and wealth away from those who have it.

"Without a struggle, there can be no progress," Frederick Douglass said. "Those who profess to favor freedom, and deprecate agitation, are men who want crops without plowing up the ground, they want rain without thunder and lightning." Yet most well-meaning antipoverty groups and people concerned about equality became more cautious and developed innocuous policy groups, public interest law firms, and service organizations. They stayed out of the fray, remained silent about politics and power, and became less effective. ACORN would take another tack entirely.

A New Road

The decision by Kest, Streich, and other ACORN organizers to embark on a squatting campaign in Philadelphia would for several reasons turn out to be a major turning point for ACORN. In fact, one cannot comprehend ACORN's success and growth, especially in New York, without appreciating the fateful decisions Kest, Streich, and the leaders made when they decided to address the abandonment problem with a squatting campaign.

The homesteading campaign, together with ACORN's CRA organizing, would lead to a complete break from anything ACORN had done before. ACORN would create a new spin-off institution, ACORN Housing, that would raise significant funds for ACORN, help enforce and monitor its housing victories, and become a vehicle for ACORN's role in the redevelopment of the cities of New Orleans and New York. Further, while ACORN would continue to attract white members, a result of the squatting campaigns was to weight the membership toward mostly African American, making ACORN less the multiracial group Rathke hoped for.[6] It was easier to be multiracial in rural Arkansas than in a segregated city like Philadelphia. To the foundation officers, other community activists, and government officials, ACORN was looking more like a black, militant, poor people's association, organizing in the cities and willing to engage in civil disobedience. Curiously, the national leadership in ACORN never had an in-depth discussion about escalating the squatting campaigns. The growth flowered within ACORN's decentralized decision-making structure.

By 1982, headquartered in New Orleans and operating in twenty states, with a national budget of $2.3 million (up from $250,000 in 1975), ACORN had 50,000 dues-paying members. With ACORN's solid base at the local level, Rathke had grown confident that the group could support itself without relying on the government or foundations.[7] ACORN's national board authorized new issues in a range of areas, from cutbacks in community development funds to housing, health care, and welfare.

The rapid expansion had not come without a price. Eight of ACORN's most experienced staff left, demoralizing some who remained. Some staff thought expansion had stretched ACORN too thin and advised Rathke to spend scarce money on strengthening the existing local and state chapters; Rathke opted for more expansion. Georgia and New Jersey, among other states, witnessed the opening and closing of offices several times.

Organizers burned out and quit. Mary Lassen left in 1980; she and her husband wanted children and Lassen didn't think ACORN's employment policies and culture were family friendly. Other good organizers left, feeling that as ACORN got larger, it had become lethargic. New organizers reflected a wide disparity in talent and commitment, as well as in local accomplishments.

ACORN barely had enough money in the treasury to pay its staff. Personnel and bills were paid late. There were big communications gaps among members from local chapters. Except for those who attended national meetings, most of the members in one state had no idea what members in other states were doing. Unless addressed, these issues could undermine ACORN's future.

While ACORN continued to help enhance the lives of the poor, the improvements represented less than what Rathke and his followers had envisioned. Beyond helping thousands of families obtain decent housing, lower utility rates, and more, Rathke foresaw his group helping to influence federal government policy so it would provide economic opportunities for everyone left behind by the private market. By the mid and late 1990s, ACORN's success would begin to attract the attention of America's national media. But in the early 1980s, because of changing economic and political forces, ACORN was swimming not only against the growth of corporate power and values and a new conservative grassroots movement, but also against the changing strategies and agenda of the Left.

Chapter 8

Political Ground Shifts

> You must now speak Sir John Falstaff fair,
> which swims against your stream.
> —Shakespeare, *Henry IV*

Rathke and ACORN's other workers were reminiscent of those feisty organizers for local farmers' groups who in the late nineteenth century toured the country giving lectures, organizing chapters, and creating a populist movement that developed an alternative agenda to the emerging corporate values of the Gilded Age.[1] Despite its limitations, ACORN won local victories and even some national battles, building on the positive achievements of the New Deal, the civil rights movement, and the Great Society's antipoverty crusade.

For three decades after World War II, the income gap between rich and the lower classes had steadily closed. By the 1980s though, no matter how hard ACORN's people worked, the country was becoming more unequal and poverty was growing. And like the populists of a century earlier, Rathke and ACORN were swimming against the tide created by a change in corporate values and power.

Not only did the percentage of poor increase, but also the gap between the rich and the poor. The number of poor swelled by 2.2 million in 1981, giving the nation its highest rate of poverty since 1967. By 1984, poverty had risen to nearly 34 million, a level not seen since the 1960s, before the Great Society program. Census data revealed that the gap between upper- and lower-income U.S. families was wider in 1984 than at any time in decades. The poorest 40 percent of all families received 15.7 percent of national income, and the top 40 percent, 67.3 percent. Throughout the 1980s, these trends would accelerate.

Their day-to-day impact was particularly harsh in the places ACORN was organizing—the nation's big-city ghettos. Whites constituted a majority of the nation's poor, but they were not concentrated in the poorest neighborhoods. In contrast, nearly half of the black poor lived in a ghetto neighborhood. Thanks to the civil rights movement and fair housing laws, many black middle-class families had escaped the ghettos, but the black poor were stuck in the nation's worst neighborhoods, with the highest crime rates, slum housing, and lack of public services.

Social scientists called this group the underclass, the ghetto poor—in sociologist William Julius Wilson's phrase, the "truly disadvantaged."[2] The persistence of the black ghetto was due to the flight of high-paying blue-collar industrial jobs out of big cities, cuts in job training and other programs, the sad state of urban public schools, and the ongoing discrimination against blacks by employers, landlords, and banks.

Reasons for these economic and demographic trends included the changing economy—international competition, new transportation, and communications technologies. The deterioration of the quality of U.S. democracy was another big factor; as Princeton economist Paul Krugman pointed out in *The Conscience of a Liberal*, small groups of the rich and powerful were dictating public policy.[3] A third factor was a remarkable political power shift toward an alliance of big business (ACORN's major political obstacle), the religious Right, the Republican Party, the moderate wing of the Democratic Party, and corporate-funded conservative think tanks. The weak, the poor, and those who lacked the advantages of wealth were losing political power. In addition, by the mid 1980s what sociologists call mediating institutions, such as organized labor, big city political parties, fraternal groups, and civil rights associations, who had formerly organized and spoken up for the poor and powerless in policy and political matters were losing members.[4]

In the midst of these trends, the growth of ACORN was an anomaly. ACORN had few collaborators capable of contending with the muscle of big business and their allies among movement conservatives. For instance, the union movement, which had lifted millions of American workers into the middle class, had lost considerable clout. Under the leadership of AFL-CIO presidents George Meany and Lane Kirkland, the union movement not only lost members, but much of its vitality as well. The AFL-CIO failed to bring new workers into unions. It made little headway, outside the public sector, in organizing employees in the growing service sectors of the economy. It had lost touch with many union members and done little to educate and mobilize them during election campaigns.

In the 1970s, Meany and his generation of union leaders expressed little interest in organizing unorganized workers outside heavy industry, comprised disproportionately of women, immigrants, and African Americans. In 1972, Meany said to these workers: "Why should we worry about organizing groups of people who do not want to be organized? . . . I used to worry about the membership, about the size of the membership. But quite a few years ago, I just stopped worrying about it, because to me it doesn't make any difference."

A few unions, such as the SEIU and the UAW, still viewed themselves as part of broader movements for social justice and allied with ACORN, as the UAW did in ACORN's Detroit union drives. But as early as the 1970s, many unions had lost the activist spirit that had ignited their earlier crusades for workers' rights and struggles for better housing and health care for all Americans. That loss of vitality led to a decline in numbers. In the mid-1950s, unions had represented 35 percent of the workforce; by the 1980s, it represented less than 25 percent.

The New Liberalism, Identity Politics, and Professional Organizations

Besides bucking economic and demographic changes in the second half of the twentieth century, ACORN faced a new generation of public interest activists heading new organizations whose structure and direction looked nothing like those of ACORN.

Unlike these post 1960s groups, ACORN resembled associations that had successfully mobilized poor and working-class Americans during the first half of the twentieth century. These included several national associations with local lodges or chapters that encouraged lower-income people and the middle class to socialize and engage in community service. The groups helped bridge the nation's class and social divide by identifying common concerns.

For example, in the 1920s, the Fraternal Order of Eagles led successful campaigns for old-age pensions; the General Federation of Women's Clubs successfully organized campaigns for mother's pensions; and the American Farm Bureau Federation and the Grange played a critical role in generating political pressure for land-grant colleges and other government aid to farmers. After World War II, veterans' organizations such as the American Legion and the Veterans of Foreign Wars had waged successful campaigns for pensions and educational assistance. The G.I. Bill, which brought a college education to millions of returning veterans, was possible only because the American Legion—with a membership that ranged from poor to upper middle class—demanded that the program become a universal entitlement.[5]

Although ACORN's founders and leaders did not model their group on the civic associations of the pre-1960s, the organizational model Rathke developed for ACORN resembled that of groups like the American Legion; like ACORN, such groups provided a vehicle through which the middle, working, and lower classes spoke with one voice. These pre-1960s civic groups also lobbied on the local and national levels and had a good track record of promoting national legislation that helped the less affluent. One cannot emphasize enough that these groups cared about the poor because, like ACORN, they had members who were poor and working class.

American popular culture, such as the *Honeymooners* TV show with Jackie Gleason, has trivialized and stereotyped these fraternal groups as silly clubs where men wear childish hats and swig beer. In reality, these groups had a good track record of promoting national legislation that helped the less affluent.

As was true of ACORN, the organizers of civic groups like the Fraternal Order of Eagles made sure that poorer members and less well-educated Americans had opportunities to develop civic skills of self-government and to attain positions of responsibility and trust. "Members and officers of voluntary federations . . . were tutored in the organizational skills they would need to participate effectively in democratic politics," according to sociologist Theda Skocpol. "Of necessity, rotating leaders learned how to run meetings, keep record books, make speeches, and organize events." The groups taught "countless numbers of Americans what it meant to be a presiding officer, a secretary, a treasurer, an elected chaplain, a representative of a local group to a higher representative body, and so forth."[6]

The leaders of these civic groups knew that to have any leverage over public officials, a voluntary federation had to be able to shape public opinion through newspapers and other media, and develop a network of members who could lobby and influence legislators at every level of government and across many legislative districts. To maintain their own organizations, and to wield financial and political clout, they had to continuously recruit new members and develop new leaders through social networks and person-to-person contacts.

Each of these groups had ambitious citizen-organizers who understood that the associations they built needed to put down strong local roots. They were, in Skocpol's phrase, "federated organizations, with a national structure and deep local roots." They represented a truly democratic way of engaging ordinary people, across class lines, in public life. Dominating our civil society and helping to shape our politics until the early 1960s, these groups provided a place where the working poor could effectively engage in public life. Jews, blacks, and women, often excluded, built parallel organizations, benevolent societies, social clubs, and issue groups that played a role in training a generation of leaders and activists. Many middle- and working-class and poor blacks who were involved in the civil rights movement had learned their skills in churches, Negro women's clubs, and black men's fraternal orders.

With the 1960s, everything suddenly changed. The activists of the women's, antiwar and civil rights movements of the 1960s found the reactionary positions of these older civic groups unacceptable and stigmatized them as exclusionary, open to either men or women (but not both), barring blacks from membership, or blindly patriotic and militaristic.

The kind of organizations the new generation of activists built hardly resembled what ACORN was building. After the successes gained by the civil rights movement, the politics of the Left took civic groups in a new direction. Liberal public interest groups like Common Cause, the National Abortion and Reproductive Rights Action League (NARAL), and the Environmental Defense Fund emerged. Hundreds of new public interest organizations were organized top-down and inside the Washington, D.C. Beltway, and all neglected organizing the poor. (Even the Children's Defense Fund, which advocated for the poor and was linked to several social service agencies, failed to build local activist membership chapters that included the poor.) Headquartered in Washington, staffed by lawyers, lobbyists, and policy experts, these groups sought to influence the government by relying on the courts, regulatory agencies, and congressional subcommittees, rather than by mobilizing followers. While the professionals related well to congressional staffs and other elites, many group members donated money but were not involved in local chapters. Most groups had no members at all. Except for a few other national networks such as Citizen Action, Alinsky's IAF, and National Peoples Action (NPA), few civic groups were even attempting to mobilize the poor and working class.

Instead of developing state and local chapters in the ACORN mode, groups like these sought support from foundations and from direct-mail fund-raising and emphasized single issues. For example, NARAL's call for members was chiefly a fund-raising tactic to encourage donations; the group became best known for its professional spokespeople, who debated groups like the National Right to Life Committee. Liberal activists relying on foundations and mass-produced fund-raising letters or narrow issues that often polarized a shrinking electorate ran to the courts and staff members of congressional committees. The good that liberal activists accomplished, starting in the 1970s, would be offset by the outlook of the middle- and upper-middle-class elites who had cut their ties to the interests of the lower-middle class and the working poor.

None of these groups had a Wade Rathke traveling the country, putting together a network of organizers and leaders state after state, and encouraging them to build local chapters of poor and working-class people with their own elected leadership and support from the national office. The new groups devoted little if any staff time to mobilizing their membership in direct action or even elections. They paid much higher salaries than ACORN; rarely brought individuals together across lines of income, education, and social status; and siphoned donor money away from groups that mobilized the poor, like ACORN, IAF and the Gamaliel network of faith-based community organizations.

Closely related to this new direction in civic groups was a trend that Skocpol points out made it harder for ACORN to achieve its goals. Liberal college graduates who might have joined ACORN in the 1960s or 1970s instead went to graduate school, then joined professional trade associations such as the American Bar Association or the National Association of Social Workers. Within their professions they would support progressive causes, and when they wanted to support a cause outside their professional associations, they sent checks to their favorite national advocacy groups. To help the poor, they might work in soup kitchens or donate money to a nonprofit focused on their chosen social woe. ACORN made no effort to reach out to these people. In fact, ACORN didn't want them, fearing that professionals would undermine the power of the low-income members.

In another trend that worked against ACORN, many teachers and welfare-state workers (social workers, psychologists, and other human service workers) who served their communities in educational and in nonprofit social agencies saw no need for a cross-class civic association like ACORN to improve the plight of the poor. They saw their own work—much of it funded through government and foundations—as the epitome of community responsibility. (A group called HumanServe tried to counter this trend by mobilizing the poor through voter registration, with some limited success.)

All these professional and human services organizations and public interest groups practiced class-based politics: moderately liberal on social issues, moderately conservative in economics. In short, this top-down advocacy created in 1970s and 1980s by professional, service, and public interest leaders spoke with an upper-middle-class voice. The new focus brought about some good results, for example, an increase in legal status for gay couples and more rights for the disabled, but it neglected the concerns of the poor.

ACORN's program and majoritarian strategic vision were also at odds with the growth of the identity politics movement and the rights revolution that fueled many of the new public interest groups and began dominating liberal and left-wing politics. The rights revolution demanded statutory and constitutional protections not only for women and for black and brown ethnic minorities, but also for criminal defendants, students, homosexuals, prisoners, and the handicapped. Even though a majority of ACORN members were black and women, the issues ACORN chose—redlining, school closings, taxes, utility rates, housing, and welfare—were economic class concerns, not issues of race and gender.

ACORN had fallen prey to what Bill Fletcher Jr., a longtime labor activist, has called the "white populist error." Rathke thought he could build a cross-class association, with support from labor unions, by attacking poverty caused by corporate abuse; his populist error was ignoring cultural issues of race and gender. ACORN's economic agenda emphasis on shared economic injustices, Rathke thought, would inoculate it against the divisions that arise when a group confronts racism and sexism. He was wrong, and in terms of organizational growth, his error kept large numbers of Americans away from ACORN. Its big tent was too small.

ACORN Mind-Set on Gender and Race

Rathke dismissed the priority issues of progressive woman's groups such as day care, equal wages, and abortion as unimportant. When confronted with this potential problem by ex-ACORN organizer Gary Delgado, Rathke said: "It's never come up. If a local group wants to take up the issue of abortion, that's its prerogative. We have had a group in Memphis address the question of rape—in a public school situation where a young women was raped, we went after the principal on how he dealt with her." He also referred to ACORN's antirape campaigns in Boston, New Orleans, and Detroit. But ACORN rarely supported women's issues. It endorsed the Equal Rights Amendment only when its failure to do so would lose the Texas Women's Political Caucus support for ACORN's platform at the 1980 Democratic Convention.

Although by the mid 1980s, 70 percent of ACORN's rank and file were women, most of them black, and the majority of its leaders were women, Rathke and other white middle-class males like the Kest brothers dominated staff decisions. Not only did this discrimination contribute to the organization's neglect of women's concerns, it began to affect staff morale.

Even committed ACORN organizers like Fran Streich and Madeline Talbott complained that the atmosphere within ACORN was not sufficiently supportive for women and families. Many women legitimately felt they had little to say about policy. According to former ACORN staffer Madeleine Adamson: "The turnover rate for all organizers is high. For women, it appears to be even higher. The reasons are varied, but a few stand out. They have to do with lifestyle—the difficulty of integrating any other interests in life with organizing, particularly having a family, and with the difficulty of competing in what is still a male-dominated field." Delgado in his book on ACORN, *Organizing the Movement*, concluded: "While women do have power within the organization, they do not in fact have power on the staff: on a staff of over 150, fewer than five women have access to major decision-making." In short, ACORN's reliance on Rathke and sometimes on the old boys' network to make the key staff decisions would endanger its future growth and effectiveness.

That ACORN also avoided framing its issues racially hampered its work with local community black power organizations. Delgado concluded that this avoidance limited, for example, ACORN's ability "to form linkages with single issue minority groups organized around desegregation, police brutality, or saving vital services."

ACORN's choice of issues and its staff culture also undermined its ability to recruit and retain a staff that included women and people of color, a change Rathke and others claimed they wanted. Yet they appeared clueless about how to accomplish this goal without sacrificing the existing staff hierarchy, ACORN's class-based politics, and perhaps their old boys' network. The ACORN mind-set needed to change.

ACORN and the Democratic Left

ACORN's strategy of uniting a large coalition of the poor and working class around their shared economic interests was also out of step in the 1980s with the liberal politics of the Democratic Party. The few organizations on the Democratic Left that, like ACORN, emphasized class-based politics, economic issues, and the importance of unions were on the wane. Groups such as Michael Harrington's Democratic Agenda, which had strong support from the UAW and the machinists union, and Tom Hayden's Campaign for Economic Democracy in California played a meaningful but ephemeral role in U.S. politics. By the end of the 1980s, they would disappear.[7]

At the same time the Left was deemphasizing class concerns, an economically conservative brand of liberalism antagonistic to the New Deal and economic populism was emerging within the Democratic Party that limited any potential party influence by ACORN. Politicians such as 1984 presidential candidate Gary Hart and Paul Tsongas were representative of this conservative brand of liberalism, sometimes called "neoliberalism." It emphasized social issues like abortion rights, civil liberties, and civil rights but was suspicious of unions and deemphasized government intervention in the economy, promoting instead the idea that social progress could be achieved by encouraging free-market methods, fiscal responsibility, and fewer restrictions on business, that is, implementing business-friendly policies would assure economic growth, create jobs, and improve the welfare of the entire community. The neoliberals accurately accused the "more liberal" wing of the Democratic Party of failing to recognize that the public sector had gotten too bureaucratic and unresponsive to the citizens it served, who resented paying increased taxes for programs for the poor that didn't work.[8] Except for a few issues, such as the Community Reinvestment Act and the Earned Income Tax Credit, this new agenda resulted in policies that hurt the poor. A new politics emerged causing a backlash against liberalism, as millions of working and middle-class Americans abandoned the Democratic Party and became Reagan Democrats or Independents. Edsall and Edsall persuasively argued, "Working-class whites and corporate CEOs, once adversaries at the bargaining table, found common ideological ground in their shared hostility to expanding government intervention." Since the New Deal, the Democrats had forged a "bottom-up" coalition that united the interests of the poor and the middle classes. In the 1980s, Republicans outmaneuvered the Democrats by exploiting race and taxes and value-laden issues like abortion, school prayer and gay rights, often in coded language and fashioned their own "top-down" coalition, pitting the rich and the middle classes against the poor.

Meanwhile, a large multi-issue grassroots movement was penetrating establishment politics. It was also cross-class—middle and upper. Conservatives were succeeding on the right the way Rathke had hoped he would succeed on the left. Suburban warriors, as Lisa McGirr calls them, including middle-class mothers, hosted coffee klatches for Barry Goldwater in their tract houses. Conservative doctors, dentists, housewives, and engineers agitated against sex education, abortion, busing, affirmative action, the weakening of the family, and the loss of religion in national life.[9] Conservative millionaires, corporations, and foundations funded and endowed think tanks and professorships to help shape the intellectual climate and policy agenda. The Republican Party recruited socially conservative Christian pastors to lead a new religious-political movement that combined its traditional social conservatism with the libertarian or free-market movement that organized after the defeat of Barry Goldwater. There was nothing inherently compatible about social and free-market conservatism—indeed, historically they have been at odds—but the intentional creation of the modern religious Right and its ideology is one of the great right-wing organizing successes. Reagan, with the support of an energized rank-and-file right-wing movement, set about changing the shape of U.S. politics with tax cuts, vastly increased defense spending, and dramatic cuts in social spending. It was the beginning of an era in which the Right would try to dismantle all the institutions created by the New Deal to make America a more equal society through unions, progressive taxation, and Social Security.[10]

ACORN's class-based organizing dropped out of fashion with nearly everyone on the left. Rathke, like Alinsky, had believed that the key political tug-of-war was whether the middle class would align with the rich or the poor; by the end of the 1980s, the pattern was clear. And the harvest for the poor promised by the Reagan supply-siders and neoliberals would never trickle down.

Amid the shifting U.S. political tides, ACORN organizers kept their eye on a smaller target: the next campaign. In fact, when it came to defining success, Rathke, other ACORN organizers, and its leaders had something in common with movement conservatives like the powerful Grover Norquist, founder of Americans for Tax Reform in 1985. Norquist, in a *New Yorker* interview, compared politics to warfare. So did ACORN. Todd Gitlin, in *The Bulldozer and the Big Tent*, called movement conservatives "ruthless about winning." So was ACORN.[11]

To counter the policy trends emerging out of Washington in the early 1980s, ACORN's national board authorized campaigns that would fight the cutbacks in community development funds, housing, health care, and welfare. Rathke understood that ACORN didn't have the power to make a national difference without expanding the organization geographically. To be a truly national organization, ACORN had to target New York.

Chapter 9

New York: A New Model

One of Rathke's first contacts in New York was Ron Shiffman, the eminent director of the Pratt Institute's Center for Community and Environmental Development. A brilliant planner with a long history of dealing with the city as well as community groups, Shiffman sported a long, fuzzy red beard. The two men looked more like bohemian artists than radical political activists.

According to Shiffman, New York had many nonprofit community and church groups involved in community development. The first in the country, the Bedford Stuyvesant Restoration Corporation, had been started in Brooklyn in 1967. The concept originated with Robert Kennedy after his famous walk through the area's neighborhoods. These groups, however, heavily dependent on foundations and federal funds, were reluctant to bite the hands that fed them, Shiffman said. But the city had no group committed to skilled community organizing, particularly in low-income areas like East New York. Shiffman encouraged Rathke to focus on areas that lacked community-base activity.

Later in 1982, Rathke asked Jon Kest and Fran Streich, just married, to move to New York. They were experienced, having built up Philly ACORN, and Jon was from the New York area and anxious to return. They set up shop in the Reverend David Dyson's Lafayette Avenue Presbyterian Church in Fort Greene, Brooklyn, a hotbed of inner city activism. Dyson had worked with César Chávez and the United Farm Workers and as an organizer in the labor movement. Jon and Fran spent a year and a half becoming familiar with the city and its leaders and by 1984 had recruited more than four thousand dues-paying members.

It was not the best time to be fighting poverty. New York City was in the midst of a public safety panic fueled by its tabloid newspapers. "What unnerved most city dwellers," writes historian Fred Siegel, was "the sense of menace and disorder that pervaded day-to-day life."[1] New York's gestalt in 1984 was symbolized by Bernard Goetz, the "subway vigilante," who on December 22 shot four young black men in a Manhattan subway car after, he said, the men threatened him and tried to rob him. Many white residents sympathized with him, especially descendants of Italian, Irish, and Jewish immigrants who had moved to the outer boroughs of Queens and Staten Island. Many unable to move out to suburbs felt trapped in neighborhoods undergoing racial and economic change.

Less visible to the press was a breakdown of another sort—the collapse of the low-income housing market. Like several other large U.S. cities, New York seized vacant buildings in the inner city when landlords and speculators abandoned their properties and failed to pay their delinquent taxes. As the number of New Yorkers needing affordable housing mounted, so did the inventory of abandoned vacant housing owned by the city, reaching some six thousand units by 1985. Not surprisingly, thousands of low-income families occupied these properties, including a woman in the Bronx named Bertha Lewis, who would soon join ACORN.

Some of these squatters had moved in when landlords walked away from their properties, others after the city took possession. Either way, they were occupying the buildings illegally. The question for city officials was whether to evict them, look the other way and let them remain in these deteriorating and dangerous slums, or target city funds to fix up the properties to make them safe and habitable. Kest saw in this situation a real organizing opportunity for ACORN. In 1985, New York ACORN embarked on its first major campaign, modeled on Kest and Streich's successful squatters' crusade in Philadelphia.

New York ACORN's Squatter Campaign

Many of ACORN's members lived in Brooklyn's East New York, a predominantly black and Puerto Rican 5.6-square-mile tract, home to some of the poorest people in the city, a community full of graffiti-covered bodegas and auto-body shops where gunfire resonated in the streets. Hundreds of solid working-class families lived near abandoned neighborhoods of drug addicts, empty lots, and empty homes. In 1968 a visiting mayor, Kevin White of Boston, called it "the beginning of the end of our civilization."[2]

Several community groups throughout New York had supported squatters before ACORN came on the scene. On the Lower East Side, long an entry point for immigrants and the poor, more than three dozen buildings had housed squatters since the 1970s. Other groups sprang up about the same time as ACORN, supporting squatting in Harlem, Chelsea, and the Upper West Side. Some of these groups failed in their goal to permanently house the squatters because they lacked the complex technical know-how required to finance and manage safe, affordable housing. A few however, such as the Banana Kelly Community Improvement Association in the South Bronx, preserved and rehabilitated the buildings for the squatters. The East Brooklyn Congregations, an IAF affiliate, confronted public officials, bureaucrats, bankers, and real-estate operators in order to build hundreds of affordable homes in East New York in the 1980s. Its members were low- and moderate-income black and Hispanic residents, not squatters. As was true of all IAF groups, members often came from strong families who had a bit of financial wealth, an enormous amount of spiritual wealth, and a commitment to community.

But these neighborhood organizations had no plan to join or build a citywide, multi-issue political force. The mostly black and Hispanic squatters and families participated in these activities without a political agenda beyond wanting a legal place to live. What was unusual about ACORN was its vision. Kest and Streich viewed the squatting campaigns as part of a process of building a powerful multi-issue, cross-class, city organization capable of linking with other grassroots groups across the country.

On January 1985, ACORN's New York chapter, led by Louise Stanley, a fifty-one-year-old postal supervisor, began pleading with the city to renovate two thousand abandoned, rotting East New York buildings—to no avail. Frustrated by the municipal government's intransigence, Kest and Streich organized a sit-in at the office of Brooklyn borough president Howard Golden, demanding that the city turn over vacant buildings to the poor. The meeting unnerved Golden's assistant, Marilyn Gelber, even though she had visited some of these slum buildings and sympathized with the plight of the families raising their children in such squalid conditions. After several other attempts to get the city to take action, ACORN's people took matters into their own hands.

Kest and Streich, having organized squatters in Philadelphia, thought they could win a similar campaign in New York. Since organizers could not go door to door to recruit homeless people, Streich repeated her Philadelphia strategy. In search of folks willing to fix up and move into vacant properties, organizers distributed flyers to families at bus stops, grocery stores, and homeless shelters reading, "Do you need a home? Call ACORN." Hundreds of potential squatters responded. From a list of buildings Shiffman had surveyed to make sure they were structurally sound, these would-be squatters selected ones they thought were appropriate. Federally funded legal aid lawyers gave them an orientation that included a briefing about the risks they were taking, since squatters had almost no rights. All squatters signed statements to the effect that they knew this move was illegal, that it involved the risk of arrest, and that they could lose whatever they put into the house.

As in the Philadelphia campaign, ACORN argued that squatting was morally right, even though it was illegal. Moreover, it made political sense—it could help mobilize people in desperate need of housing and residents of surrounding neighborhoods, frustrated by the city's neglect of their communities, who wanted responsible people to inhabit these buildings. Vacant houses were invitations to rape, drug dealing, and arson.

ACORN's organizers met with the volunteer squatters to explain the political, legal, and logistical aspects of the campaign. They made sure that the potential squatters met with the homeowners and renters already living on these blocks to put a face on the idea of "squatter." They had these neighbors sign petitions stating that they supported ACORN's plan to occupy and then repair the vacant buildings on their blocks.

On June 15, 1985, ACORN families, using hammers and crowbars, began to pry the metal seals off abandoned city-owned buildings and started moving in. With ACORN's help, Ernestine Ross, a fifty-seven-year-old grandmother who worked part-time as a custodian's assistant for the Board of Education, moved into a house at 461 Essex Avenue along with her son, daughter, and three grandchildren. With no radiators or running water, the building had been a hangout for drug dealers and users. Ross and her family put in new walls, new ceilings, baseboard heating, and pipes for plumbing. To others in need of housing she would say, "We take a little money that we get every week from our paychecks and we put in a little sheetrock, a little window here and there, and we fix up a few rooms. You can do the same thing, and I'm ready to help."

Norma Jusino, thirty-nine years old, and her husband, Francisco, forty-five, an ambulance driver, took over a house on Blake Avenue with their six children and grandchildren. Like the other squatters, little by little they put much of the money they earned into the house. For the first time they no longer feared eviction by a private landlord, but like the other squatters, they were afraid that someday the city might evict them.

Kest and Streich believed that, to succeed, the squatters needed the support of elected officials and churches. They attracted the sympathy of Howard Brandstein, director of Catholic Charities Home Ownership Project on the Lower East Side, who commented: "When we see people squatting, we recognize it is not a romantic solution but rather a response out of desperation given the housing crisis, the level of gentrification and displacement." Rev. John Kennington, the regional coordinator of the Roman Catholic Archdiocese of New York's substance-abuse ministry on the Lower East Side, helped organize the taking of several buildings; he believed such action would stem the "displacement" of residents by private developments in the area.

State senator Thomas J. Bartosiewicz, a liberal Democrat whose district included East New York, supported ACORN's taking the buildings even though the actions were illegal. "This is just the beginning," he told the press. "There are 2,500 other buildings like this in East New York, and we're going to be back here time and time again. Sometimes this is the only way to dramatize the plight of the residents and to prod the city to take action."

Opposition from City Officials

City officials had a legitimate complaint with the squatters. Charles Perkins, speaking for the city's Department of Housing Preservation and Development, asked: "Why should we allow the person with the greatest muscle, who breaks down the door first, to have the unit rather than other people who may be on a waiting list?" The city's Public Housing Authority had thousands of families awaiting housing. Perkins claimed the squatters were stealing buildings that would otherwise be used to house the homeless and the poor. He also said the buildings were sealed because the city deemed them unsafe and uninhabitable. "People think that if they do the work, they can pressure the city into giving in," Perkins added. "We never, or virtually never, negotiate with someone."

Although Mayor Ed Koch wanted to crack down on the squatting, his deputy commissioner in the Department of Housing Preservation and Development, Joseph Shuldiner, was unsure whether to support or oppose ACORN. Shuldiner, who would become an assistant secretary of HUD during the Clinton administration, understood that ACORN was gaining political support for the squatters among a growing number of New Yorkers who were concerned about gentrification. He commented to the press: "Homesteading has become part of a larger, different kind of struggle. I think in some communities, many people are very concerned with the issue of gentrification. They feel they are being pushed out, and that rather than let these buildings go, they seize them and insure their long-term use."

ACORN understood that only people who had run out of options would engage in a dangerous, illegal, and time-consuming action like squatting. The private housing market and government housing policy had both failed. The private market has never supplied enough housing for the poor and working class, and Koch presided over a city that owned thousands of vacant buildings and had more than 175,000 families waiting for public housing. The city government owned about two-thirds of the real estate in Harlem but had no plan to repair neglected buildings. To make matters worse, President Reagan dismantled the federal role in housing and cut back aid to the cities.

ACORN was looking for tools to fix what the market and the city had broken. The housing shortage was especially severe in East New York. Typical was a family with five children who lived in an apartment with no heat or hot water and a hole in the roof. Their property owner, to whom they paid $350 a month, was the city. A growing number of families couldn't afford to pay rents that allowed landlords to make a profit. Tax laws that encouraged property owners to milk properties and then walk away exacerbated the problem. Only a well-organized poor people's campaign backed by a sympathetic middle class could put enough pressure on elected officials to help.

Streich and Kest discovered to their advantage that, first, city officials couldn't keep track of their six thousand abandoned buildings and, second, once city officials learned that squatters had moved in, the process of evicting them would be long and expensive. If squatters had occupied a building for more than ten days, for example, the city couldn't just call the police to evict them but had to take them to court. As a result, the city had not taken action against many of the squatters, and in a few cases, sympathetic officials gave assurances that squatters would not be prosecuted. So far the city had not taken any action at any of ACORN's twenty-five buildings. That was about to change.

In the spring of 1985, with the mayoral election approaching in the fall, city officials decided to crack down on the squatters. No one knows for sure why, but an abandoned three-story building at 412 Vermont Avenue became the focal point of the bitter struggle. Clive Dougal, a thirty-three-year-old immigrant from Belize who lived with his parents, two brothers, and six sisters, was determined to move into the house. He had already carried out rotten boards and garbage bags filled with debris, replaced shattered windows, and repaired holes in the walls. With a hammer in his hand, Dougal vowed, "Before the end of August, I'm going to be in there."

ACORN leaders had pledged to "take" as many abandoned buildings as they could for squatters until the city's housing crisis was solved, but they wanted to avoid a violent confrontation. On August 2, ACORN warned the police of its intended action at 412 Vermont Avenue, where state senator Thomas J. Bartosiewicz would help lead the charge. As dozens rallied outside the abandoned city-owned building, police moved in and arrested fifteen people, including Bartosiewicz, for breaking into the building. Tom Kelly, spokesperson for Mayor Ed Koch, called the move "illegal and unsafe." He told reporters that the city was already in the process of trying to renovate the building and that the squatters were hampering that effort. In reality, ACORN had been trying to get the city to renovate the building for months; city officials had done nothing.

Those arrested were released with summonses for trespassing, disorderly conduct, or both, violations that carried maximum penalties of fifteen days in jail and $250 fines. A trial was set for October. They all vowed to reoccupy the building.

A few days later, on a warm summer night, ACORN leader Louise Stanley barked through a bullhorn to the cheering crowd outside 412 Vermont Avenue: "We're entitled to decent housing and we're going to have decent housing, even if we have to take it." That night ACORN celebrated its occupation of the twenty-fifth building in the squatting campaign. As promised, Dougal and his family finally moved in. "We at ACORN," shouted Stanley, who lived in a nearby house she had fixed up, "plan to take over as many buildings as we can to solve our housing crisis." She said she hoped the squatters' movement would help turn her neighborhood around. Rev. Eugene Wright, another ACORN leader, told the crowd: "While squatting is illegal, we think what the city is doing is immoral."

Mayor Koch and his top housing officials were determined to remove Dougal and the neighbors who came to support him from city property. Neighborhood families—many living on less than $7,900 a year, well below the poverty level, were just as determined to fight for decent affordable shelter. ACORN set up block watchers to keep an eye out for police and city officials. One Sunday afternoon when block watchers were unavailable, Dougal and his family returned from a day's visit to family members in another neighborhood. They found the building gone. He later learned that the city, under orders from Mayor Koch, had called a private company under contract with the city that had sent several men with a wrecking ball and bulldozer to 412 Vermont Avenue. Within a half hour, the two-story building was history.

In October, at the request of District Attorney Elizabeth Holtzman of Brooklyn, all charges filed against the state senator and the fourteen other demonstrators were dropped. Mayor Koch immediately denounced Holtzman for being "soft on crime" and suggested that she had a political motive for dropping the charges. "If I had to guess," Koch said, "it is because she may be running for something." Holtzman, who had been mentioned as a possible candidate for the U.S. Senate, said she had followed the same policy and standards that had been used for arrests at peaceful protests in front of the South African Consulate and elsewhere.

Leaving the courthouse, Senator Bartosiewicz said the dismissal of the charges was a "major victory, the first of what we hope are many victories. The people who should be standing before the court are the mayor and all of those who have turned an icy shoulder to the most desperate among us, while leaving more than 6,000 buildings vacant." The mayor said he was "incensed" by the decision to drop the charges, which he said would encourage people "to take the law into their own hands." In his opinion, he said: "It is not nonviolent. It is violent. They break down doors. What is now to stop other people in Brooklyn from simply saying, 'There is no law, the D.A. has said you can take law into your own hands.'"

Janet Swingle, an organizer for ACORN, viewed the district attorney's action as a victory: "It's like the city is saying we did nothing wrong. It encourages us to think that we will succeed." The controversy became an issue in the 1985 Democratic mayoral primary between the incumbent, Ed Koch, who opposed the squatting, and city council president Carol Bellamy, who spoke out in favor of the squatters, as did a *New York Times* editorial. Koch won the primary and went on to win the general election. ACORN had lost the battle for 412 Vermont, and their enemy was still mayor. But the war was not over.

The ACORN squatters were an intrepid bunch. In October 1986, about a year after the trespassing charges against the squatters were dropped, Jacinto Camacho moved into a rundown three-story house at 925 Glenmore Avenue as an ACORN squatter and started fixing it up. A sixty-seven-year-old retired electrical mechanic, Camacho had come to the United States from Ecuador in 1967 and for fourteen years lived alone, doing carpentry, painting, and plastering seventy hours a week, two shifts a day. In 1981, he had brought his wife and three of his children to America and they lived in overcrowded quarters.

While trying to fix up the house, Camacho endured some frightening experiences, for a hundred drug addicts were used to shooting up there. Working from six in the morning until eight at night, he would sometimes bump into the addicts as they ran up and down the stairways. Patiently he removed them, sometimes by talking pleasantly and sometimes by calling the police. When police asked him if the house was his, Camacho always said yes. He looked like a responsible home owner, and he had the courage to walk a legal tightrope—breaking the law himself while asking the cops to evict illegal squatters who happened to be drug addicts.

At first Camacho spent most of his time cleaning up debris. He paid for repairs with his Social Security check of $387 a month. He repaired the house by hooking up to a quarter-horsepower motor and securing the doors with material he salvaged from the street. He bought $1,400 worth of ornamental iron grilles at payments of $100 a month to protect the ground-floor windows and doors and slept in the house for two winters without heat, electricity, or a weapon to protect him. His daughter, who worked part-time, helped with the bills. Four times the city housing agency tried to evict Camacho, and each time ACORN arranged for a volunteer attorney or government-funded legal aid lawyer to defend him.

ACORN was maneuvering in the netherworld of city politics. Koch's political coalition, built on white, ethnic, middle-class voters, pursued policies designed to promote private investment and jail criminals. While his administration gave tax breaks to real estate investors and developers like Donald Trump, Koch mostly ignored the poor except when they protested or when a newspaper published a story about the tragedy of poor people in Brooklyn and the Bronx living in conditions reminiscent of those in impoverished Calcutta.[3]

Camacho was an immigrant, illegally squatting and resisting legitimate efforts by city officials to evict him for trespassing, an act he and his neighbors thought was morally correct—similar to the civil rights movement's moral high ground for civil disobedience. Meanwhile, the mayor was under pressure to provide more housing but felt compelled to evict squatters to demonstrate that he was tough on crime.

Though the city had a huge bureaucracy devoted to housing issues, even after Koch's 1986 reelection his administration had no realistic plan for addressing the city's deepening housing crisis.

Kest and Streich knew that the squatters campaign would succeed only if they ultimately could bring Koch and his top aides to the negotiating table. Meanwhile, they doggedly continued to use a dependable variety of tactics to force him to turn over the abandoned buildings to ACORN. Streich negotiated with foundations, banks, and city officials she knew were eager to show their commitment to low-income housing, although they were ambivalent about supporting squatting. She also knew that Brooklyn borough president Golden was feeling pressured about what his borough would do. Marilyn Gelber, his assistant, told the *New York Times*: "We are the largest borough in population and have the largest number of city-owned buildings, and we felt it wrong for city policy to focus so exclusively on Manhattan."

Gelber's first meeting with ACORN was a sit-in—"quite an introduction," she recalled. Still, ACORN had done its work in the community and Gelber was impressed. ACORN's demand for more housing for low-income residents in vacant buildings resonated with her. "We had been pressing Housing Preservation and Development to get these buildings to local people," Gelber told the press. "But the city's policy was to sell them, at auction."

ACORN opposed the city's plan to auction these properties off to the highest bidder or as part of a lottery, viewing this as a haphazard way to rebuild neighborhoods, for there was no guarantee that the highest bidders or lottery winners would repair the buildings they purchased. Indeed, ACORN feared that by auctioning off these buildings, the city might be putting them into the hands of speculators who had no interest in repairing the buildings, especially for the poor. Kest and Streich talked with ACORN leaders and decided to turn the city's auction and lottery into a public controversy. They demanded to meet with city officials to get them to end the lottery and to develop a plan for disposing of these properties that would guarantee that community groups like ACORN could help poor people repair and occupy the buildings.

To facilitate the negotiations, ACORN brought in a key ally, the widely respected planning professor Ron Shiffman, who four years earlier had urged Rathke to bring ACORN to New York. For a year and a half, Shiffman negotiated with the city, expediting the deal with ACORN's promise to forgo squatting in the future.

A New Model

On October 2, 1987, two years after ACORN's first squatting action, city officials capitulated. For ACORN, this was an extraordinary victory. In the heart of Brooklyn's East New York section, in front of an empty lot covered with tall grass and on which sat the upside-down chassis of an old Ford Falcon, ACORN organized a rally, complete with banners, speeches, and a man waving a big American flag. The address of the empty lot was 412 Vermont Avenue. On this sunny day several ACORN leaders, including Louise Stanley, took members, city officials, and reporters on an unhurried walk to ACORN's newly rehabilitated houses ten blocks away. "We brought all this into focus—and the city didn't like us for that," said Stanley. "But they had to deal with us, because we were persistent."

Camacho, the retired mechanic from Ecuador, showed reporters one of the rooms he had painted at 925 Glenmore Avenue. "In the same way, I've tried to train my sons to be serious, to do serious work and take care of their families." Five of his fourteen grandchildren were now in the United States, along with his three of his seven children. "The whole family is coming," said Camacho. "What I did was illegal. But if you don't try, you don't get anything. I never had any weapons—just my own hands and the help of God." Pointing to family members with him, he added, "The house is for them."

The Koch administration agreed to turn over fifty-eight city-owned buildings to the ACORN squatters, whom ACORN organized as the Mutual Housing Association of New York (MHANY). The city appointed MHANY to run the buildings and gave it title to the land on which the buildings stood. The city also awarded grants for technical and architectural aid and $2.7 million in city loans for renovation, which would provide housing for 180 families. The squatters were allowed to keep their houses.

ACORN's creative community organizing was essential to this victory. Shiffman, the expert, helped give legitimacy to ACORN, a group whose confrontational and illegal tactics angered city officials. The New York Foundation, a philanthropic organization, and the Consumer-Farmer Foundation, which agreed to serve as the project's banker, managing the revolving loan fund, aided the negotiations. It also helped that the vice president of Consumer-Farmer was Harold DeRienzo, who in the mid-1970s had founded Banana Kelly, a nonprofit housing group that had organized protests in the South Bronx, confronted city authorities, and negotiated deals to build affordable housing. With Shiffman and Pratt's architectural and technical expertise and Consumer-Farmer providing financial services, ACORN transformed the squatters into a legitimate nonprofit group. The squatters who joined ACORN desperate for any housing at all were now working with planners, architects, and organizers, receiving city funds, and getting positive media attention—an incredible transformation in only a few years.

The deal had potentially important policy implications. For the first time New York would test out a new model—mutual housing—for low-income housing development. In a mutual housing association, neighborhood residents form a collective, contributing some money and a lot of sweat equity to rehabilitate buildings for their own use in return for public support and limited ownership. The city gave ACORN money and technical help in return for restricted rights of resale. The collective—in this case the MHANY—retained title to the land. When an owner chooses to sell, the association has the right to repurchase for a price reflecting only individual investment, not market value.

This form of ownership is an accepted practice in Western Europe and Canada, where housing is viewed more as a social program than a private commodity. Versions of this approach had been tried in a few U.S. cities, including Philadelphia, St. Louis, and Phoenix. Felice Michetti of the city's Department of Housing Preservation and Development touted the idea as an attractive model for neighborhood groups across the city.

To ACORN, mutual housing represented a new form of social contract between the city and its poorer residents, who obtained buildings at a nominal fee while giving up their right to speculate and maximize profits. ACORN favored the mutual housing setup, since it would keep the housing for low-income residents in perpetuity, and the large number of units would provide economies of scale in purchasing goods and services.

For the leaders of ACORN this was a big triumph. Not everyone agreed it was a victory—many officials thought a plan that gave its imprimatur to squatting was wrong. "I don't think you could ever make squatting legal," said one New York City Council member. "Can you imagine what that would do to a city like this?" (This reasoning was similar to the arguments put forth by white moderates who labeled as anarchy Martin Luther King's civil disobedience tactics. In "Letter from Birmingham Jail," King retorted that some laws have to be broken to improve social conditions and human rights.)

But some sympathetic affordable housing experts were skeptical, as well. They suggested that mutual housing requires a level of community organization and sustained commitment that will be hard to duplicate widely. To make a significant impact, the city would have to commit money and property on a large and ongoing basis. They didn't believe this would happen.

Conservative critics accused the city of turning over property to nonprofit groups just when New York real estate was the hottest business in town. Why should ACORN, unlike other property owners, enjoy government protection against the uncertainties of the marketplace? Further, no matter how high the market rose, the law under the mutual housing form of ownership forbade ACORN's owners to sell their apartments at a profit—in other words, it's a poor investment. Occupants could never hope to do more than break even on their investment of time, money, and labor; they were poor when they moved in, and they would be poor when they moved out. If they decided to sell, they had to sell back to the MHANY collective at cost. The collective could thus amass renovated apartments at a fraction of their market rate.

The squatters, as well as many city officials, disagreed with the critics. ACORN opted to trade the right to accumulate market-rate equity in their homes that former squatters had enjoyed for the assurance that the housing units would remain affordable. Whether occupants remained poor would depend on educational and job opportunities. For Jacinto Camacho, Norma and Francisco Jusino, Ernestine Ross, Clive Dougal, and the other squatters, the experience reconfirmed their faith in government and in justice, but most of all, in themselves and their organization, ACORN. (Nineteen years later, Comacho's daughter, Cecilia, would go to work for ACORN.)

The squatters' mutual housing victory would prove temporary. When Republican Rudolph Giuliani was elected mayor of New York City in 1993, homesteading policy would change. As part of his Quality of Life campaign, Giuliani instructed his new staff at the Department of Housing Preservation and Development not to tolerate squatters. After Giuliani's reelection in November 1997, HPD served the residents of 672 East 136th Street with an order to vacate on the grounds that certain devices used by some of the residents were deemed a fire hazard. Approximately ten days later, HPD arrived to carry out the order to vacate, accompanied by an army of police officers clad in riot gear, with helicopter support. The approximately seventy residents were forcibly evicted and their possessions removed. Under the Giuliani administration the building remained unoccupied and began to deteriorate. Soon, a small group of former residents reoccupied the building as squatters.[4] (Ironically, after Mayor Michael Bloomberg was elected in 2003, HPD turned over the property to ACORN Housing to halt the building's deterioration, redevelop the building, and put it back on the affordable housing market.)

Nevertheless, by the end of Giuliani's second term, a thousand low-income New Yorkers lived in homes owned or managed by MHANY. ACORN had partnered with banks it once criticized for redlining to negotiate lower mortgages and grants for affordable housing. ACORN and its Housing Here and Now coalition would next negotiate commitments with Mayor Bloomberg to set aside thousands of affordable housing units and would get the mayor to propose a $130 million Housing Trust Fund to create and preserve 4,500 units.[5]

And ACORN elsewhere? About the same time that Kest and Streich were establishing ACORN's presence in New York, Madeline Talbott and Keith Kelleher moved on to Chicago to do the same, only they would develop a new way to ensure a minimum wage for impoverished workers.

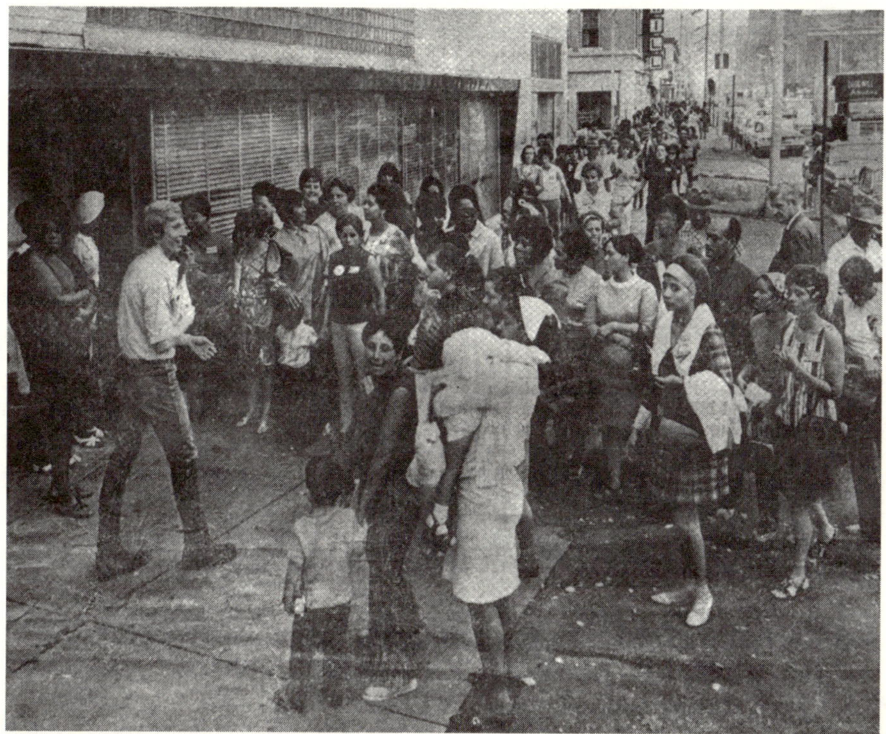

Figure 1. On September 3, 1969, Wade Rathke organized mothers on welfare to march on the welfare offices in Springfield demanding money for household supplies and clothing. Rathke talks with the marchers before trying to enter the building. (Photo by Steve Lemonis in *Springfield Daily News.* Photo courtesy of Wade Rathke)

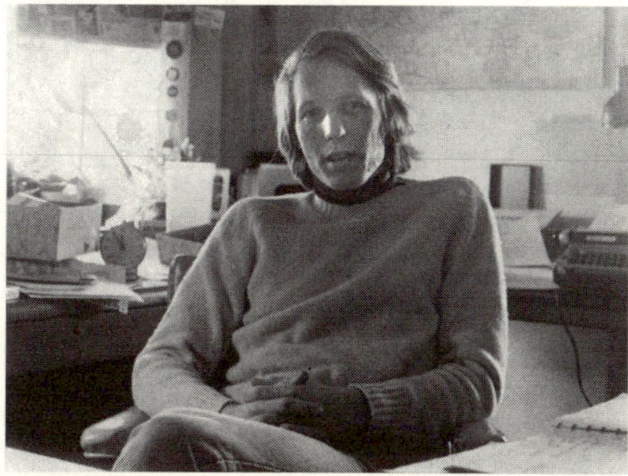

Figure 2. Wade Rathke in his Little Rock office, 1975. (Photo courtesy of Wade Rathke)

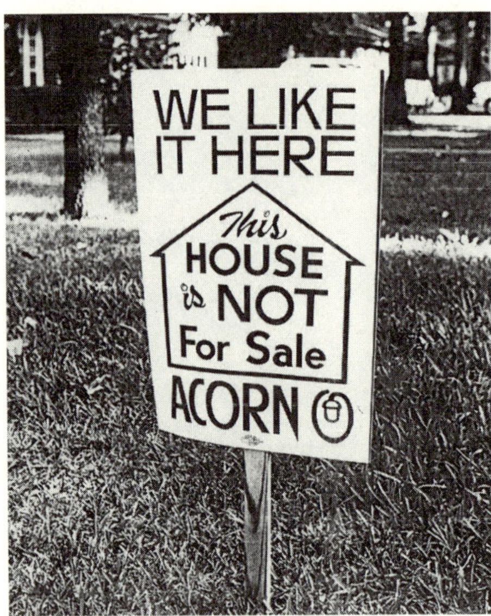

Figure 3. Anti-blockbusting campaign in Little Rock, Arkansas, 1972. (Photo courtesy of ACORN)

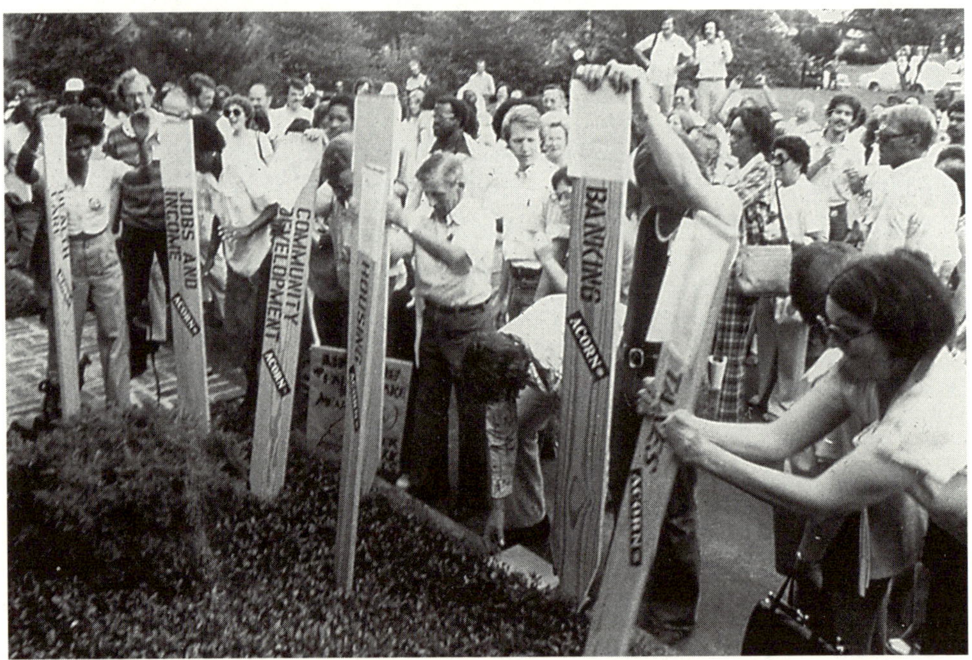

Figure 4. After ACORN's members overwhelmingly passed the People's Platform, 200 of the 1,500 ACORN delegates marched to the suburban home of S. Lee Kling, the chair of President Carter's campaign finance committee. Here, organizers and members plant nine boards in Kling's lawn with labels corresponding to the planks in the platform. Wade Rathke, *center*; Jon Kest, *rear left*. (Photo courtesy of ACORN)

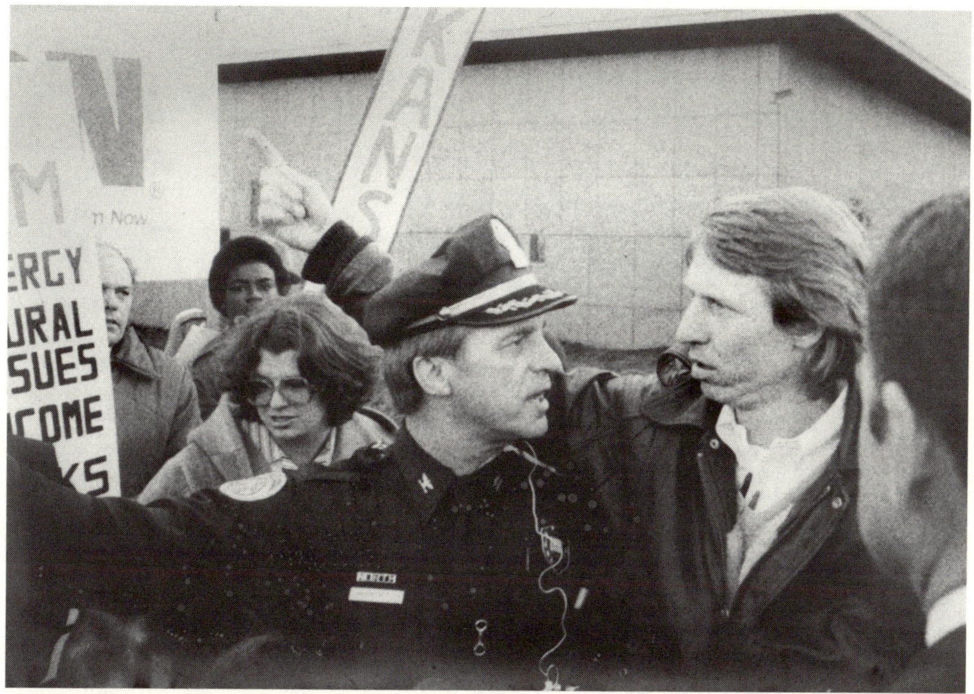

Figure 5. Hundreds of ACORN members marching to the Democratic Party's midterm convention in Memphis in 1978, as Rathke refuses to halt the march and signals marchers, around the police captain's back, to continue. ACORN held its first national convention nearby. Rathke regarded political participation as a way to expand ACORN's overall reach nationwide, as well as a tool to advance ACORN's issue work locally, and used this occasion and the 1980 Democratic Party's primaries and convention to open ACORN chapters in twenty states. At the convention center, ACORN members demanded platform changes reflecting their concerns about affordable housing, jobs, energy costs, and health care. (Photo courtesy of ACORN)

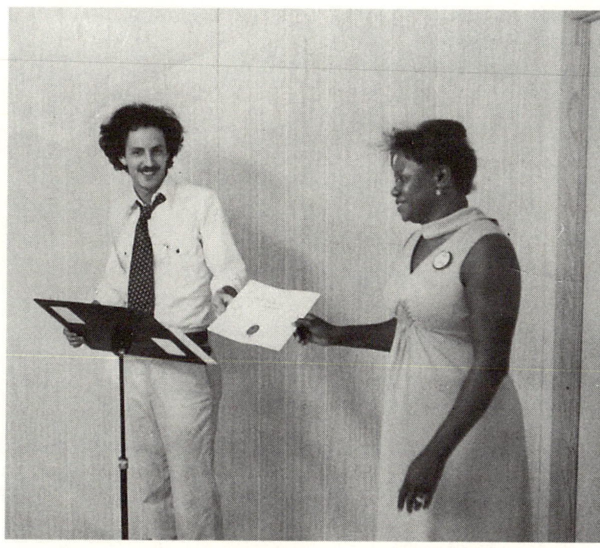

Figure 6. Steve Kest presents ACORN member L. V. Darrough an award for collecting signatures in the campaign to remove the sales tax from food and medicine. Little Rock, 1978. (Photo courtesy of ACORN)

THE
FASTFOOD
WORKER
ULU
FOR WORKERS ONLY!
MANAGERS-HANDS OFF!
AN OFFICIAL PUBLICATION OF DETROIT FASTFOOD WORKERS/UNITED LABOR UNIONS
UNION RIGHTS ARE HUMAN RIGHTS
SIGN THE PLEDGE!

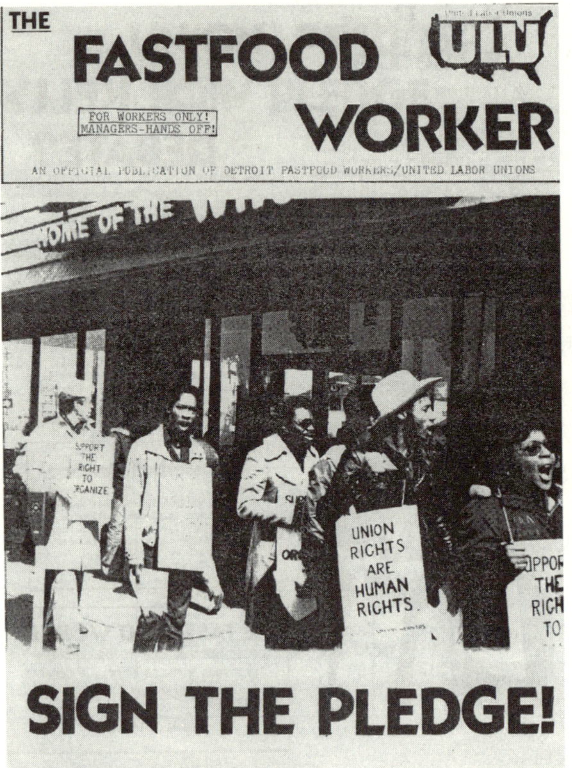

Figure 7. With an eye on the rapid increase in low-wage jobs for home care, janitorial, hotel, and restaurant workers, Rathke assigned Dan Cantor to lead ACORN's campaign to organize fast-food workers, and United Labor Unions published the weekly *Fast Food Worker* as part of its effort to organize Burger King and McDonald's employees. By combining union and community organizing and politics in one entity that fought to reduce poverty, ACORN was operating far outside the U.S. norm. (Photo courtesy of ACORN)

End Food + Medicine
TAX
Mo. Tax Reform Group - ACORN

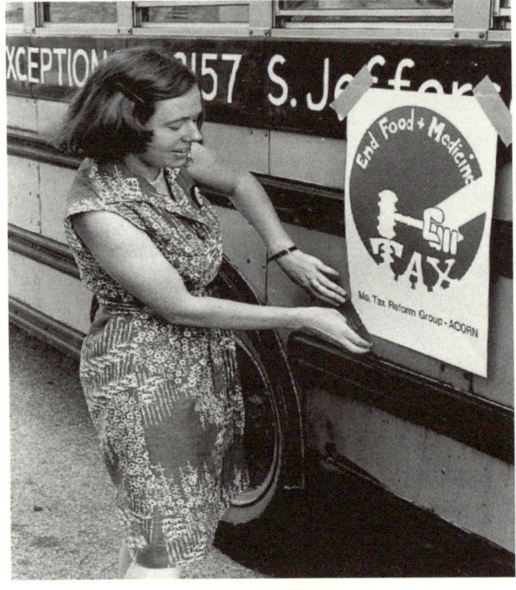

Figure 8. Mary Lassen, former ACORN head organizer in Missouri, prepares to board a bus with ACORN members in the summer of 1976 to deliver signed petitions to the secretary of state, part of a campaign to end the sales tax on food and medicine. Lassen and other organizers had begun to hear complaints from inner-city St. Louis families unfairly rejected by local banks and savings and loans when they sought loans to fix up or buy a home or expand a business. Lassen would soon be mobilizing anti-redlining campaigns, which would lead to agreements between ACORN and its enemies the banks. (Photo courtesy of Mary Lassen)

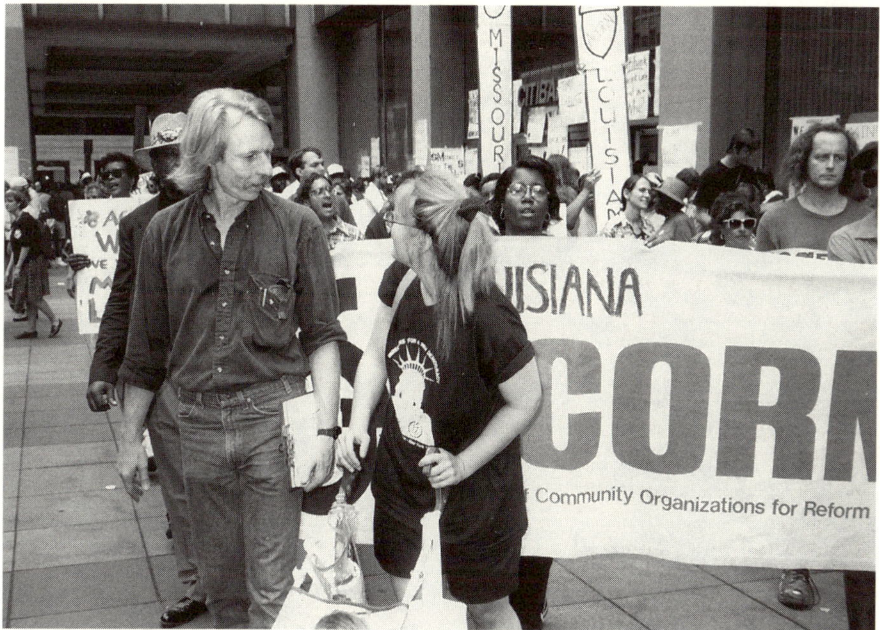

Figure 9. Wade Rathke leads a 1988 demonstration in New York at which 1,500 ACORN members took over the lobby of Citibank headquarters. Here, Rathke talks to longtime ACORN organizer Fran Streich (pushing her daughter, Jessie). With Madeleine Adamson from ACORN's D.C. office, *at right*, in front of the Louisiana standard; Philly ACORN staffer Steve Lucinski, *tall, far right*; Louisiana ACORN leader Lanny Roy, behind Rathke; Linda Roy, behind Streich, holding the sign. (Photo courtesy of ACORN)

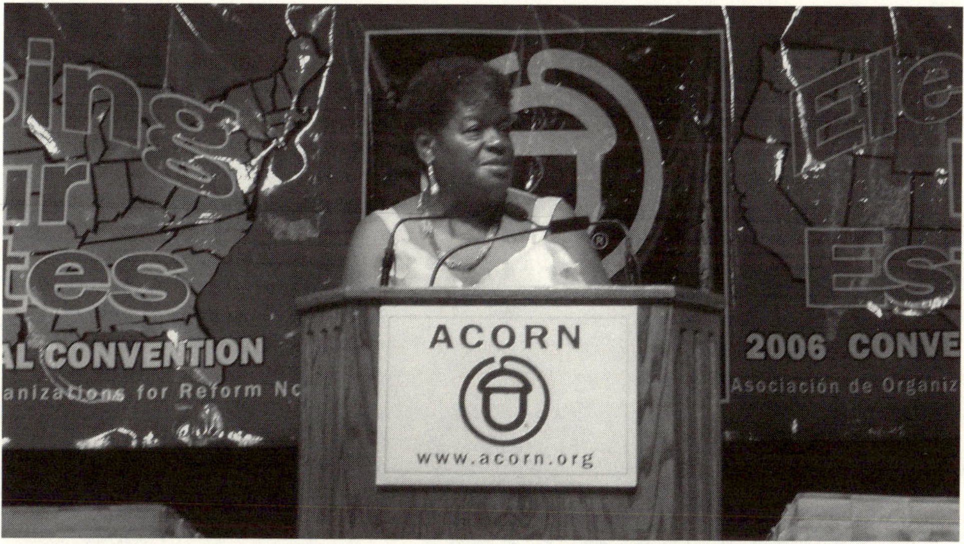

Figure 10. Maude Hurd, elected ACORN president in 1990, speaks at a national convention. Hurd got involved in ACORN, as do most members, when an organizer knocked on her door and asked, "What are your concerns about your neighborhood?" (Photo by Bonnie Friedman)

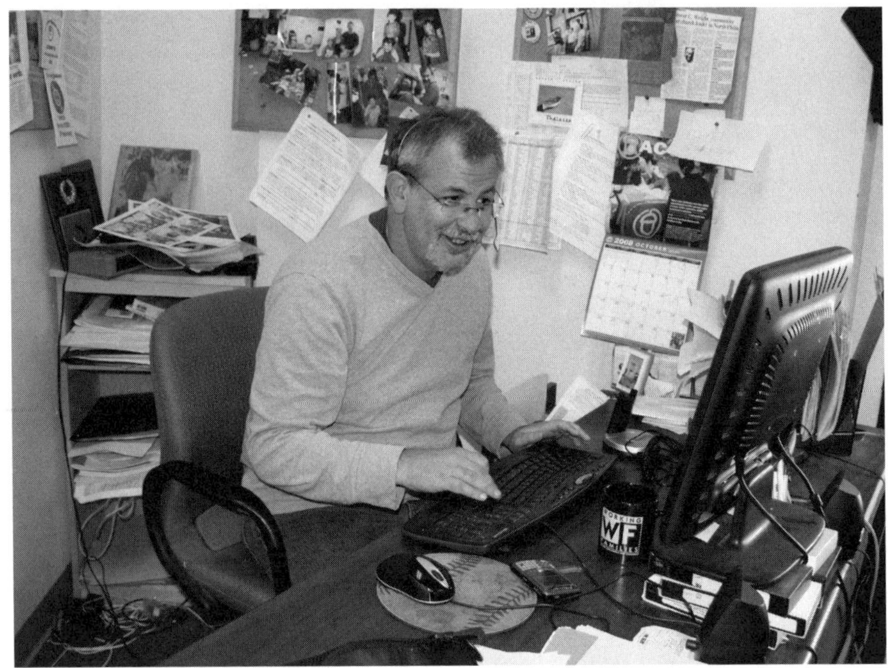

Figure 11. Jon Kest, New York's head organizer in his Brooklyn office at 2–4 Nevins Street in 2008. Recruited in 1977, Kest and his wife, Fran, organized chapters in Philadelphia and New York that focused on squatting and homesteading. The squatting campaign led Congress in 1982 to enact the National Homesteading Act, which reformed federal policies and procedures to make it easier for low- and moderate-income people to purchase HUD properties. (Photo by Bonnie Friedman)

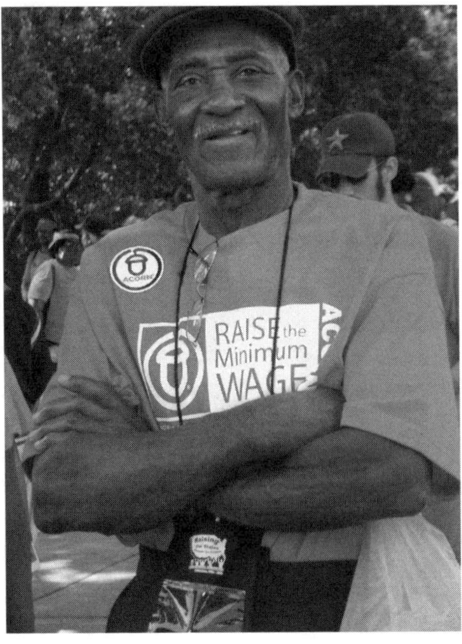

Figure 12. ACORN member active in ACORN's minimum-wage campaign, Columbus, Ohio, 2006. (Photo by Bonnie Friedman)

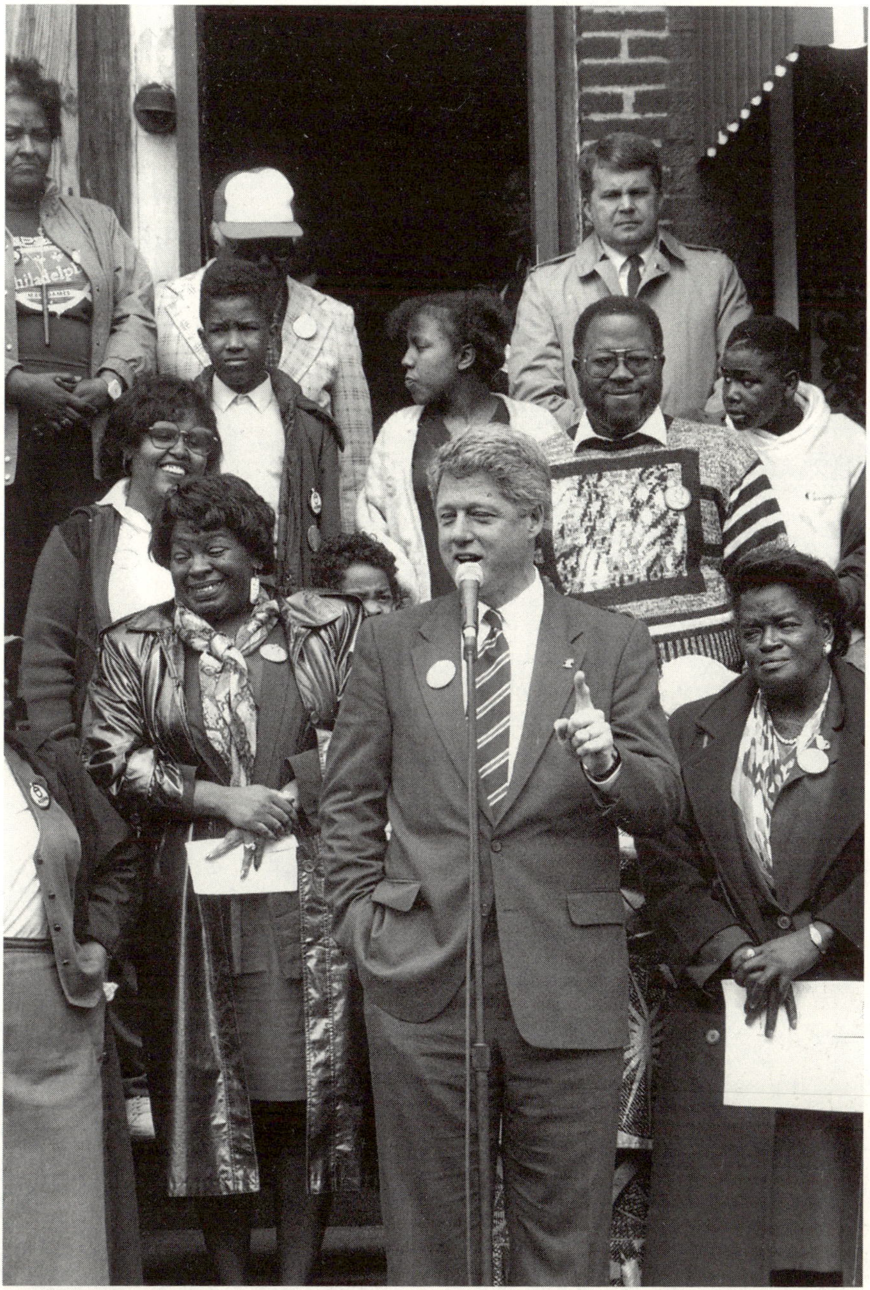

Figure 13. Bill Clinton, Maude Hurd, and ACORN members in Philadelphia (Photo by Scott Hamrick)

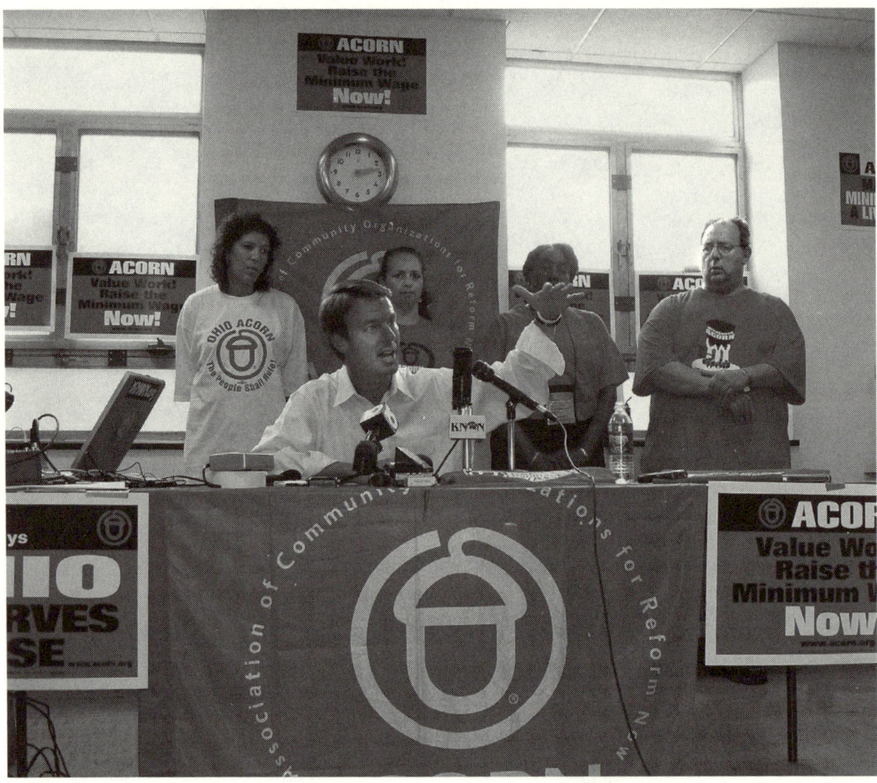

Figure 14. *Left to right*, ACORN leaders Julie Smith, Maria Polanco, Maxine Nelson, and Paul Satriano with John Edwards at a press conference calling for an increase in the national minimum wage, Columbus, Ohio, 2006. (Photo by Bonnie Friedman)

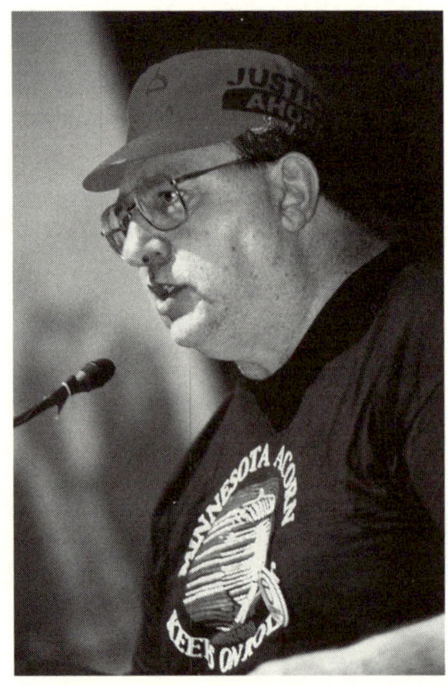

Figure 15. Minnesota ACORN leader Paul Satriano at a 2002 press conference condemning Household Finance Corporation's abusive home-lending practices. HFC would soon agree to distribute a record-breaking $484 million to abused borrowers and to set up a $150 million fund to provide additional relief for them. (Photo by ACORN)

Chapter 10

A Living Wage

> Liberty requires opportunity to make a living, a living decent according to the standards of the time, a living which gives man not only enough to live by, but something to live for.
>
> —Franklin D. Roosevelt, renomination speech,
> Democratic Convention, 1936

In 1983, Madeline Talbott, ensconced in Detroit, got a call from Wade Rathke, now a close friend and mentor, who told her: "Just like ACORN needed to be in New York, we need to be in the Second City. And you need to be the head organizer there. You know you're one of our best organizers. You've earned the opportunity."

"What about Keith?" Talbott asked. By now her husband was organizing health-care workers into the ACORN union, ULU.

"He's going to continue the labor stuff in Chicago," answered Rathke.

Keith and Madeline soon packed their bags and moved to Chicago, Madeline to build the Illinois chapter of ACORN and Keith to organize bus drivers, home nurses who cared for the sick and elderly, fast-food workers, and janitors into the local ULU.

Soon after they arrived in Chicago, Madeline and Keith began organizing the low-income home-care workforce and founded the Chicago Homecare Organizing Project, which affiliated with Local 880 of the Service Employees International Union (SEIU), the new name for ACORN's union local. ACORN began winning the kind of victories it had won in Michigan and more, as well as generating the same kind of opposition—not only from the business community, but also from rival community groups worried about their turf. A leader of a respected and successful faith-based Community Development Corporation resented "outsiders coming in and starting their own organization, instead of consulting and working with the existing community leadership." Although Talbott always reached out to other groups, ACORN would not shed its reputation among some community groups in Chicago, as elsewhere, as an organization that's hard to work with.

A year later, in 1985, Barack Obama moved to Chicago. While Talbott was building ACORN, the twenty-four-year-old Obama, just graduated from Columbia University, started his new job as a community organizer with the Gamaliel Foundation. Obama helped poor blacks on Chicago's far South Side, a neighborhood staggering from steel-mill closings, fight the city for jobs, playgrounds, after-school programs, school reforms, and asbestos removal. Like ACORN organizers, Obama worked in the tradition of Saul Alinsky. Unlike ACORN's, Gamaliel's base was not individual dues-paying members but a network of churches. Unlike ACORN's leaders, who wanted to build a movement for social justice, Gamaliel claimed it was only a neighborhood group empowering citizens. To those inside the community-organizing world, this is an important distinction.

Obama used one tactic common to ACORN's campaigns—he led groups of adamant citizens to confront officials, an approach markedly different from the tradition in Chicago, where most church leaders and antipoverty public interest groups, as well as most black Democrats, instead exploited personal connections. Talbott initially considered Obama a competitor when both were working to get asbestos insulation removed from a Chicago housing project, but his work impressed her so much that she invited him to conduct a few trainings for her staff. When Obama's asbestos-removal campaign in Chicago's public housing projects stalled, he began reassessing the potential of community organizing. Obama saw that community organizers needed allies in city government. Inspired by the election and accomplishments of Harold Washington, Chicago's first black mayor, Obama began to think about running for public office. Perhaps a charismatic elected official could make a bigger difference than a community organizer. He would soon decide to go to Harvard Law School, but he would return to Chicago and ACORN.

Talbott and Kelleher Dig In

In 1990, Madeline Talbott became ACORN's national field director, responsible for supervising all the state head organizers and for training new organizers. She had developed a strong statewide ACORN presence in Illinois and hosted the 1990 ACORN national convention, where the speakers included Rev. Jesse Jackson, Rep. Charles Hayes, and Rep. Joseph Kennedy. After their addresses, Kennedy led a march past City Hall to one of Chicago's premier commercial high-rises. Hundreds of marchers snuck past security guards to protest the actions of the Resolution Trust Corporation as part of ACORN's campaign to push pressure on the S&L bailout agency.

Meanwhile, after seven years of organizing, Keith Kelleher's Local 880 numbered barely a thousand members, mostly home-care workers. Other union organizers told him to forget about the home-care industry. They made some telling points: home-care workers were not real workers, but merely part-time babysitters; they can't be organized; it is a high-turnover industry. They also told Kelleher that "poor and moderate-income black, white, and Latino women just can't be organized," and that "most home-care business was not very profitable, so how can you win wage and benefit increases? And the profitable ones knew how to break unions."

Kelleher remembered that the history of the major industrial unions was replete with examples of skilled trade union leaders like those in the carpenters union who dismissed auto workers, steel workers, garment workers, and other industrial workers as "not real workers." So despite these obstacles, he and Local 880 pressed on.[1]

In 1992, Local 880 and ACORN saw a chance to flex their political muscle when Cook County's recorder of deeds, Carol Moseley Braun asked Talbott and Kelleher to play a major role in her voter registration and get-out-the-vote efforts in her run for the U.S. Senate. Barack Obama, who had recently graduated from Harvard Law School, returned to Chicago that year and took a job running Project Vote, a newly invigorated voter registration group, as well as an important place to make connections with progressive activists and philanthropists in Chicago and around the country. SEIU Local 880 and ACORN agreed to help Braun with a large-scale voter registration effort, joining forces with Project Vote (within a decade, Project Vote would join ACORN's family of organizations).

Working with ACORN and others, Project Vote approached dozens of community groups—sororities, churches, unions, motorcycle clubs—adding more than ten thousand voters to the rolls in the fall of 1992, mostly blacks, Latinos, and gays. The next step for Obama and ACORN was contacting new voters, then helping them file absentee ballots or driving, carrying, and chasing them to the polls on Election Day. Braun was elected, the first African American woman senator in U.S. history.[2] Three years later, in 1995, Talbott would work with a team of attorneys, including Obama, representing ACORN in a lawsuit against the State of Illinois for failing to implement a federal law designed to make it easier for the poor and others to register as voters.

As Obama thought about running for public office in 1995, talking with a Chicago newspaper reporter, he asked: "What if a politician were to see his job as that of an organizer, as part teacher and part advocate, one who does not sell voters short but who educates them about the real choices before them?"[3]

In his run for the presidency in 2007, Obama would apply the philosophical and practical lessons he learned on the streets of Chicago. He enlisted the help of Marshall Ganz, a Harvard lecturer and one of the country's most brilliant community organizers, to help train his get-out-the-vote volunteers. Sounding like an ACORN organizer, in his speeches he would often allude to his organizing history, urging followers to think of his campaign as a social movement in which he was just "an imperfect vessel of your hopes and dreams."[4]

A New Generation of Organizers

Senator Braun's was not the only victory that gave ACORN hope. Bill Clinton's win in 1992 put a Democrat in the White House for only the second time since the founding of ACORN. His election also gave ACORN some breathing room from the federal government's harassment. During the late 1980s and early 1990s, ACORN had endured years of an expensive and time-consuming federal grand jury investigation instigated by President George H. W. Bush's Department of Labor, alleging that ACORN was "too close" to a progressive labor union—SEIU's Local 100—and that it might be illegal for Local 100 to partner with ACORN's fights for social change. The DOL dropped the preposterous case a year into the Clinton administration. Rathke remembered how relieved he was when Clinton's DOL called ACORN's office and asked someone to come and pick up the truckload of records ACORN had meticulously numbered and given to the government. The incident left a deep imprint on Rathke and made him more cautious about ACORN's enemies looking into the organization's business.

In Chicago, a few years after Senator Braun's victory, Talbott was seeking young talented organizers to expand her operation—disciplined, prepared, and productive people that in ACORN lingo are "hard core." When Brian Kettenring walked into her office looking for a job, Madeline's eyebrows shot up and she thought, "Oh, my lord—how will I train this very white, very big, very awkward young man?" She found the twenty-three-year-old very intelligent, however, and despite some misgivings, hired him, trained him as a Chicago organizer, and sent him out onto the streets of Chicago.

Brian Kettenring, along with other young organizers such as Ginny Goldman in Texas, Matt Henderson in New Mexico, Kate Atkins in New Jersey, Bertha Lewis and Helene O'Brien in New York, Mitch Klein in Maryland, Kevin Whalen in Minnesota, and Darryl Durham in Georgia, was part of the new generation who would spearhead the next round of ACORN's civic engagement.

Kettenring was typical of some members of this new generation of young white organizers coming to work for ACORN. He had grown up in Summit, New Jersey, a comfortable, middle-class suburb whose claim to fame was a local rock group, the Velvet Underground, that had made its concert debut at the high school Brian would attend. His mother was an art professor who voted Democrat, his father a statistician for Bell Labs and a political Independent. The family attended Christ Church, whose members were mostly moderate Republicans. More liberal than most of his high school friends, Brian at sixteen favored Michael Dukakis in the 1988 presidential election, because he thought Jesse Jackson was too radical.

Brian attended Carleton, a small, top-ranked Midwest college where liberalism and political activism prevailed, partly because of the late U.S. senator Paul Wellstone, a professor of political science who taught there for twenty-one years. Brian's thinking began to change as the result of an incident in April 1992 in his sophomore year: Twelve jurors in the suburban community of Sylmar, California, rendered their verdicts in a case involving the 1991 beating of Rodney King by four LAPD officers. The case had received heavy media coverage before it went to trial, when a video of the beating was replayed constantly on national TV. Three of the four officers charged with the thrashing were acquitted, and inner-city Los Angeles erupted in flames.

Brian watched TV images of the burning city with horror, fear, and outrage. Harry Williams, who taught Brian's African American studies course, walked into class the next day and tossed copies of major newspapers on the floor in the middle of the circle of students. One headline blared, "LA Burning," with front-page photos of smoke billowing over the city. Professor Williams commanded the class, "Talk to the papers!"

Discussions about race with his working-class black and Hispanic classmates, who regarded the black professor as a mentor, intimidated Brian. He was uncertain about what caused poverty and injustice. When he asked in class, "Why would people destroy their own community?" he felt embarrassed. Feeling somewhat guilty, he wondered if he—a white liberal raised in an upscale suburb of New Jersey—was partly to blame for the plight of disadvantaged minorities.

Brian's work with ACORN Chicago was not very glamorous for a graduate of a prestigious college—low pay, fifty-five to sixty hours a week, mostly walking door-to-door at night in the unsafe neighborhood of Lawndale trying to recruit members to ACORN. At first, he was sure some gang member would kill him. Only after Madeline assured him it was safe (it wasn't) did he agree to amble around the neighborhood at night, his fear abated. He was like a midcentury door-to-door Fuller Brush salesman or a Jehovah's Witness hawking *The Watchtower*, only he was selling equality, democracy, and justice on $14,000 a year.

During his ACORN training, Brian learned that what ACORN needed most was new leaders, the ordinary folks who lived in the community and who, after joining ACORN, were supposed to emerge as speakers for and give direction to the organization. He had met several ACORN leaders and read about others—retired railroad blacksmiths and postal workers, home health-care aides and young welfare mothers. Now ACORN was trying to recruit more black and brown organizers, and Brian wasn't sure he was the right person for the job. In fact, when he knocked on Beatrice Jackson's door one evening in 1995, she wondered what a white boy was doing there on a cold winter night. Few people of any race walked around Lawndale at night, and the only whites who did were cops, drug buyers, and welfare caseworkers.

Jackson had been laid off from her job at Sears where she worked for thirty-seven years. She lived in North Lawndale, a once-bustling section where the original Sears Tower and businesses like Western Electric and International Harvester had provided thousands of middle-class jobs. Between 1950 and 1970 the area steeply declined as those businesses moved out and many of the middle-class Jewish residents followed. The high-wage jobs disappeared. The area became a collection of vacant lots, whose tall grass provided cover to drug dealers. Commercial strips were nearly dead, but violent crime flourished. The elderly residents remained in the neighborhood, while their friends and family died or moved away.

This was Brian's second night going door-to-door. He extended his hand and stiffly repeated the words he had memorized from ACORN's training manual on door knocking: "Hi, my name is Brian Kettenring and I'm with the ACORN community organization. A couple of the neighbors are getting together to fight for changes in this neighborhood. We want better schools, safer streets, and more good jobs. Are you concerned about some of these things or seeing your neighborhood improved?" Before she could answer, he continued: "A lot of your neighbors are concerned about speeding traffic, improving the schools, abandoned housing, better jobs, higher wages. Are you concerned about any of these things?"

Beatrice smiled. "I sure am."

"Do you have a minute to sit down and discuss these things and ways we might attempt to solve these problems?" Brian's low-key, rehearsed style masked his intensity. Beatrice invited him into her wood-frame duplex and led him to her cream-colored sofa in the living room. Brian had only fifteen to twenty minutes to make his pitch, with 5,000 households to visit in eight weeks, hoping to sign up 10 percent as dues-paying member families. (The typical number of households in an ACORN neighborhood ranged from 1,500 to 5,000.)

Bea Jackson became the first of hundreds of recruits for Brian. He also was responsible for identifying, encouraging and training people to become leaders, who would fight to improve the neighborhood and speak out in their community, while he stayed in the shadows. After several months, Brian discovered that Jackson had a special quality that trained organizers spot when seeking out new leaders. "We look for people who will work hard, who can lead and hold a base, and who can look you in the eye and hold their own," Rathke would say.

Brian wanted to devote whatever time was necessary to support Jackson, who showed an interest in developing her leadership skills. A new idea, however, was brewing in ACORN that would divert some of his attention. ACORN wanted to address the problem of a growing number of workers in Chicago earning poverty-level wages.

Building from BUILD

In 1994, an organizing campaign in Baltimore caught the attention of Steve Kest, Wade Rathke, and others at ACORN. A community group known as BUILD (Baltimoreans United in Leadership Development), part of the Alinsky-founded Industrial Areas Foundation, a local community organizing network, led a campaign that mobilized ordinary people to fight for higher wages for the working poor. One of those was Valerie Bell. She lived in a small rowhouse in Baltimore. With just a high school degree, she had secured a job with a private, nonunion custodial firm that contracted with the city to scrub floors and take out the garbage at Southern High School for $4.25 an hour with no health benefits. Like so many others, Bell struggled to pay the electricity bill, buy groceries, and pay the rent. It was not unusual for the head of a household to work forty hours a week, fifty-two weeks a year, but not make enough to keep his or her family out of poverty.

BUILD put together a coalition of churches and labor unions and lobbied the city to pass a "living wage" law that would increase wages above the national minimum. The law would apply to employees who worked for private firms that had contracts with the city—1,500 workers hired by private bus companies, security companies, and janitorial firms—raising their wages from $4.25 to $8.80 an hour over three years. At some risk to herself, Bell organized other custodians to join the living-wage campaign; when the custodial company discovered Bell's activities, it fired her. Undeterred, Bell stayed active with BUILD and helped gather petition signatures and organize demonstrations. BUILD recruited academics, who produced studies showing that it made no sense for the city government to save money in the short term by underpaying workers who then had to resort to a variety of government-supported homeless shelters and soup kitchens to supplement their low wages. Working with BUILD, Bell and others put so much pressure on the city that they convinced Mayor Kurt Schmoke to support them.

Because of this grassroots organizing effort, Baltimore passed the nation's first living-wage ordinance. Economists estimate that the law puts millions of dollars into the pockets of Baltimore's working poor each year and has had a ripple effect, pushing up wages for other low-paid jobs in the city.

Steve Kest realized that the living-wage issue had the kind of appeal that had helped earlier ACORN efforts succeed. Like the squatting campaigns and the CRA, providing living wages to working people was the ethically right thing to do; it carried the moral imperative that no one who works full time should have to live in poverty.

Lisa Donner, ACORN's Washington lobbyist, and Jen Kern, a new staffer, were sent to Baltimore to research what had happened there. Kern—twenty-four, a tall blond with large, intense eyes—had joined ACORN after graduating from Grinnell, a small, elite Midwest college where she played basketball and majored in anthropology and gender studies. At the Library of Congress, she pored over regulations, court decisions, and state constitutions from around the country to find out if ACORN could mount campaigns in other cities where it organized.

Kern was excited to discover several cities where ACORN could legally launch a campaign to raise the minimum wage above the federal standard. In many states the law allowed cities to include not just city contractors—as in Baltimore—but all local businesses that paid very low wages, such as privately owned restaurants. ACORN had tried unsuccessfully to raise the minimum wage at the state level in Missouri the next important question was, in which cities was this kind of campaign politically feasible?

The Chicago Jobs and Living-Wage Campaign

"I think *we* can do this," Madeline Talbott said to Keith Kelleher on one of the those gray Chicago mornings, when stinging winds off Lake Michigan defeat the will to get out of bed, much less change the world. It was late March 1995 and light snow surrounded their two-story yellow brick apartment building in Albany Park on the northwest side. This once predominantly middle-class Jewish neighborhood had become one of the most diverse in the Chicago area as waves of Latin Americans, Caribbeans, and Asians immigrated in the 1970s. Talbott and Kelleher bragged to friends that if you walked the whole neighborhood, you could hear sixteen different languages. Their comfortably spartan apartment was furnished with Goodwill items, hand-me-downs from relatives, and knick-knacks from garage sales. They shared the four-flat co-op with three other families. All the parents were community activists and organizers.

The morning conversation was typical of their discussions over the last two weeks. "We could win," said Talbott. When Keith raised his eyebrows in doubt, Talbott added, "Even if we don't, we'll still shake up Chicago politics." They had agreed that besides organizing unions, passing a wage ordinance was the only way ACORN could force the city government to create jobs that paid workers enough to escape poverty. They also agreed that the campaign couldn't be one of those legislative campaigns, where you approach some City Council members and simply *ask* for their support. Keith said with a sly smile, "It would be a great fight, the fight of our lives." Then he cut to the crux of the matter. "How will we deal with Daley?"

He was talking about Chicago mayor Richard M. Daley, son of the late Richard J. Daley, who had been one of the most powerful political bosses in U.S. history. Elected mayor of Chicago in 1955, he had held that post for twenty-one years, building his machine through patronage and racial politics, aligning himself with the business community, and promoting downtown office construction. From the early 1960s to the end of his reign, hotel, clerical, and other service-sector employment surged. But the new commercial and government-service jobs did not offset the loss of 232,000 higher paying manufacturing ones at firms like Bea Jackson's former employer. Displaced workers couldn't find jobs, and Daley neglected the older neighborhoods, especially minority ones, where the industrial decline took place.

In 1989, when Richard M. Daley was elected mayor, he began to rebuild his father's machine, partly by including some community groups from inner city black and Hispanic neighborhoods in his coalition. The core of his support, however, came from the Chamber of Commerce, the downtown commercial interests, the restaurant business, small entrepreneurs, and white ethnic voters. Like his father, Daley built the organization based on personal fealty: loyalty was more important than performance, policy, or political experience. Economic growth meant creating a positive climate for business.

A few weeks after Keith and Madeline first discussed the campaign, they finished breakfast and got their two daughters out the door and onto the school bus, then drove their Mazda minivan to their offices. They worked in downtown Chicago on Harrison Avenue in the south Loop—in the same building, on the same floor, only twenty feet apart, both their offices littered with mail and lists of board members, organizers, union leaders, and every Chicago bank and mortgage company and their phone numbers. They were a tight team.

At a staff meeting in the office kitchen about the campaign, one person was skeptical: "It can't be done, we'll be spinning our wheels, we'll never get enough votes on the City Council." Another said: "Daley controls the City Council. He's not like Baltimore's Schmoke. He's probusiness and he'll oppose us." Talbott admitted that such a high-profile loss would be scary, then spelled out how they might win. She later had little trouble convincing the ACORN leadership and members that this campaign would be good for the organization as a whole, and the Chicago Jobs and Living Wage Campaign was born. To join the steering committee, an organization had to have troops or money—its members would have to contribute a minimum of a thousand dollars, deliver a busload of people to coalition events, or both. Madeline had learned, as she often said, that you "can't depend on groups that can't move people."

By the summer of 1995, Talbott had put together a steering committee that consisted of ACORN; the Chicago Coalition for the Homeless; union locals, including Keith's SEIU local; the SEIU state council, as well as the Teamsters and the United Food and Commercial Workers (UFCW); several religious networks; and a few neighborhood groups. She convinced the unions that employees who were hard to organize at the workplace could benefit from a living-wage ordinance. The campaign and coalition would become a major ACORN innovation: the creation of an ongoing, permanent coalition.

In the kind of organizing ACORN does—sometimes referred to as "power organizing"—the point is not only justice; ACORN builds power by winning victories. The living-wage issue met the criteria. Talbott thought she had a winnable goal that was simple to understand and a pocketbook issue that brought constituents together. The first victory should build the organization and lead to other victories. With these rules in mind, the steering committee sat down to draft the ordinance.

The first item the committee had to resolve was how high to set the minimum living wage. They decided on $7.60 an hour, or $15,000 a year—the federal poverty level for a family of four. Then they had to decide whether to include all businesses or just businesses that received city contracts or subsidies to pay their workers. This was a tricky question. On one hand, the more businesses included, the larger the opposition. On the other hand, the more businesses included, the more beneficiaries of the increased wage, meaning more people power. The group decided that attaching strings to public moneys was a more politically acceptable first step than demanding that the ordinance cover all employees. They decided the ordinance would apply only to firms that received city contracts and subsidies. To avoid opposition from very small private companies that had city subsidies, they agreed that the subsidy had to be more than $50,000 and that the company must have at least twenty-five employees, with the exception of those that employed construction workers (virtually all of whom earned above $8 an hour). The ordinance would also apply to companies that held city contracts valued at a minimum of $5,000. The committee's research indicated that many of the affected employers were paying the national minimum wage of only $4.25 an hour and that the ordinance would affect one thousand businesses and ten thousand employees.

Madeline, Keith, and their new organizer, Brian Kettenring, would staff the campaign. "I am excited," the cerebral Kettenring told Talbott, "because it combines grassroots organizing with an explicit jobs and anticorporate strategy." Research by two professors of economics at the University of Illinois showed that money granted to companies by the city amounted to a half billion dollars a year, with few strings attached. Companies did not have to hire minority or city residents or pay a living wage. Increased wages required by the ordinance would cost such companies about $2 million.

By the fall of 1995, the Chicago Jobs and Living Wage Campaign had lobbied all fifty members of the Chicago Board of Aldermen and organized rallies, street demonstrations, and town hall meetings, attracting hundreds of supporters and public attention. Twenty-six aldermen agreed to cosponsor the legislation, a bare majority of the City Council. With such a start, Talbott thought they would win.

Mayor Daley and the Chamber of Commerce were opposed. If asked, Daley claimed that efforts to increase the minimum wage would devastate small businesses that were on financially fragile ground. Labor unions sent a letter to the mayor requesting a meeting; he ignored it. Cardinal Joseph Bernardin of Chicago wrote to Daley asking him to support the living wage. AFL-CIO president John Sweeney sat down with the mayor, but he did not budge. The mayor cited thick piles of studies from liberal as well as conservative economists showing that big hikes in the minimum wage ultimately kill low-wage jobs, as employers replace now-expensive receptionists with voice-mail systems, or pile more duties onto experienced employees instead of hiring additional staff. The mayor believed that increasing the costs of city contractors would require them to raise the prices they charged the city, eventually requiring tax hikes that would drive employers—and jobs—out of town to cheaper locales, isolating the poor who were left behind.

Talbott and Kettenring needed a symbolic target. They discovered the Farley Candy Company and its competitor, the Brach Candy Company of Chicago. Farley was a minimum wage, nonunion candymaker that received a $3 million tax abatement from the city. It operated in the Little Village area on Chicago's west side, with a growing Mexican American population. Farley was suspected of hiring undocumented workers. (When the Teamsters attempted to organize the company, it threatened to fire or deport all its workers.) At a comparable manufacturer, the Brach Candy Company, the workers earned fifteen to eighteen dollars per hour. Brach, lacking city subsidies, was in danger of shutting down its west side plant. "That was the issue," said Kettenring. "The city is subsidizing poverty-wage jobs with public money for private gain, while ignoring a living-wage company."

To draw the public's attention to the minimum-wage increase, members of ACORN and SEIU picketed the Farley factory. They wanted to make Farley, a "sweatshop" company using undocumented labor, the poster child for the living wage. Using a variety of tactics, the ACORN coalition was determined to make Farley the embodiment of a company that should not receive millions from city taxpayers unless it agreed to pay its workers a living wage. On one weekend, for example, ACORN coalition members went to a Farley discount store and did a shop-in. They went up and down the aisles, filled grocery carts with candy, brought them up to the checkout counter, stood in line to make the lines go slower, and left the carts when they reached the cashier.

In December 1995, the Living Wage Coalition planned an event at a Teamsters hall on the city's west side, where for the first time hundreds of grassroots members of the coalition would gather to see their aldermen sign on to the principles of the living-wage ordinance. Topping the goal of 500 attendees, 750 people came out to the event, and more than a dozen City Council members came up to sign the principles. The campaign gained momentum.[5]

In early January, Talbott read a news story about the Vienna Beef Company that gave her an idea. The story reported that Jim Bodman, chair of Vienna Beef's board of directors, was proud of his "family-oriented workplace." Approximately 70 percent of the people who worked there also had a relative working for the company, located on the south bank of the Chicago River just northwest of downtown, one of the hottest residential growth areas in the city. This prime real estate attracted the attention of a developer who planned to turn an empty parcel near the Vienna Beef factory into residential property. "We can't sit still and let residential units be built right near us. It will be the beginning of the end," Bodman told his associates. "We're a three-shift company. Our noises will become an uncomfortable presence for residents to be that close." Vienna Beef needed the city to zone the land as a commercial area. A public struggle began pitting the developer against Vienna Beef, with many politicians lining up against Vienna.

There are few cities in the world, thought Madeline, where the hot dog receives the kind of praise and respect it gets in Chicago. Saving Vienna Beef not only had the hallmarks of an indigenous Chicago campaign, but also could help discredit the antibusiness label some had attached to the Living Wage Campaign. Madeline called Bodman, they met and became partners, and the Living Wage Campaign took up the cause of Vienna Beef, which employed 430 people at wages of more than eight dollars an hour. The campaign highlighted the injustice of a city's funding poverty employers like Farley while driving decent employers out. In February 1996, five hundred supporters of the Living Wage Campaign stepped into ten buses and rode to the Vienna Beef factory, where Bodman, who had packed five hundred corned beef sandwiches for his guests, greeted them at noon. After lunch, the supporters canvassed the neighborhood, collecting more than two thousand signatures opposing the Vienna Beef zoning change from commercial to residential.

The next week Mayor Daley intervened on Vienna Beef's behalf. The Living Wage Campaign had won over a corporate supporter for their ordinance and proved that it could be pro-business as long as the business was willing to treat its workers well. But Daley still opposed the ordinance, and without his support the Living Wage law would not pass.

Daley and the Chamber of Commerce continued to argue that the ordinance would cost millions of dollars and require a property tax increase. Researchers from the University of Illinois at Chicago, Roosevelt University, the Chicago Institute on Urban Poverty, and the Center for Economic Policy Analysis disputed that claim. Their studies concluded that the cost to the city would be negligible—less than one-third of 1 percent of the city's budget. Chicago was scheduled to host the 1996 Democratic Party National Convention in late August, and the researchers estimated that the cost of the living wage would be in the area of $10–12 million, about the same amount the city had spent on cosmetic infrastructure projects in preparation for the convention.

On a Teamster building across from the convention site, the campaign unfurled a huge sign trumpeting the Living Wage. Activists successfully sued to gain access to the Navy Pier to picket the mayor as he welcomed the Democratic delegates to the city. The campaign organized a "tour of shame" for delegates to visit low-wage-paying recipients of local corporate welfare.

After the convention, Daley's representatives contacted coalition partners to explore the possibility of negotiations. Once ACORN saw that these talks were going nowhere, they decided in the summer of 1997 to push for a vote to avoid losing momentum. Talbott and most of the leaders of the campaign sometimes thought a win was a long shot, sometimes thought they could win—many City Council members did not want to be forced to go on the record against an idea as popular as the living wage.

The council scheduled a vote on the living-wage ordinance on June 30, 1997. The leaders of the campaign—including John Donahue, executive director of the Chicago Coalition for the Homeless, Maggie Laslo, an SEIU organizer, Diane Lovett, Jon Green and Mike Stewart—organized two hundred people to gather at City Hall to demand that the City Council act. By this time, through local lobbying by ACORN's members and organized labor, the coalition had signed commitments from thirty-six of the fifty aldermen supporting the living-wage ordinance. What the campaign leaders did not know was that nineteen of those aldermen were afraid that Daley would deny jobs, money, and services for their neighborhoods; they secretly hoped to pass a motion to table the ordinance.

As the coalition protesters gathered in the lobby and the hallway outside the council chambers, it might have seemed to those who usually conduct business at City Hall like the start of a revolution. Daley did not even resort to the more traditional tactic of packing the chamber with city employees; the chamber that day was nearly empty. He ordered the doors to the council room barred. The throng wasn't having it. "Open the dooooor, Richard!" the crowd sang, and they pounded on the doors and walls of the chamber in rhythm. The police, unamused, promptly arrested all the leaders. Reporters who had assumed the living-wage ordinance was dead on arrival scrambled to revise their stories.[6]

Daley won that day, for the ordinance did not come to a vote. A motion to table consideration of the living-wage ordinance passed, 31 to 17, with two abstentions.

Victory at Last

After Talbott's release from jail, she and Kelleher reflected on what had happened. Seventeen Aldermen had defied their mayor. ACORN had brought together sixty organizations with a combined membership of over 250,000 people. The living wage had become a popular public issue. If they kept working, it wouldn't go away.

ACORN's and the coalition's power extended beyond the living-wage battles. Their reputation helped pass school reforms and get people elected. When the ACORN-backed activist Willie Delgado first ran for the legislature in the 1996 Democratic primary, he received few union endorsements and lost. Two years later, Delgado ran again for the same post and beat his opponent, this time with the support of unions. Delgado correctly attributed his labor support to ACORN's fighting side by side with the unions in the Chicago Jobs and Living Wage campaign. During the summer of 1998, to build an electoral threat to the aldermen who had opposed the 1996 living-wage ordinance, Living Wage Campaign organizers went ward by ward, getting residents to sign petitions to put a nonbinding living-wage resolution on the ballot. When the mayor and aldermen prepared to enact a hefty salary increase for themselves that required council approval, the campaign hit the streets outside two consecutive council meetings at City Hall. Led by Ted Thomas, president of Illinois ACORN, the group said if the council approved the salary increase and not the living-wage ordinance, they would be targeted for political defeat in 1999. With victory in sight they chanted, "Payback time in '99." Almost immediately, city officials representing the mayor called Living Wage Campaign headquarters and agreed to a deal. On July 29, 1998, after nearly three years of intense organizing, the Chicago City Council unanimously passed a living-wage ordinance.

The victory had an immediate effect. Members of the campaign were invited onto the City's Living Wage Implementation Task Force to ensure the ordinance would be properly enforced. Because city-contracted home health-care workers fell under the ordinance, the city agreed to increase their wages from around $5.30 an hour to $7.60, including back pay to January 1999. Next came a living wage for Cook County, which passed easily. Capitalizing on their momentum, most of the living-wage collaborating groups tried to pull off another upset victory. With the February 1999 city election season approaching, Talbott convened the steering committee of the living-wage campaign in late 1998. The committee agreed to push for the living wage as part of a broader project to reshape Chicago politics and adopted the slogan, "Payback Time in '99!" In 1999 ACORN president Ted Thomas agreed to run for alderman from Chicago's Fifteenth Ward. A retired postal worker who had never held public office, Thomas won endorsements from the *Chicago Tribune*, the *Chicago Sun Times*, and the *Chicago Defender* based solely on his record as a community activist and a leader of ACORN.

With ACORN's coalition working hard, and with a slight change in the precincts' demographics, Thomas surprised everyone by taking three of the four precincts by substantial margins. After all the votes were tallied, a chant arose from the assembled volunteers from labor and community groups: "The people, united, will never be defeated!"[7]

In addition, several stalwart living-wage supporters were reelected to the City Council while touting their pro-living-wage stance. This triumph over Mayor Daley's machine candidate (and a field of twelve candidates in the primary) demonstrated the popular political strength of the living-wage message.

Although not running for elected office, Martha Jernegons, a fifty-six-year-old home health-care aide with a daughter and several grandchildren, also won. Jernegons worked for a private agency that was reimbursed by the city. She received a $2.15 per hour raise—a 40 percent increase—to $7.60 an hour. Though she still lived below the poverty line and still lacked health insurance, her salary increase allowed her to pay off an old medical bill for six hundred dollars. "The raise gave me a different outlook on life," she said. "I feel better about myself. Now I can go to Payless and buy a pair of shoes."[8]

In 2002, the campaign again successfully increased the living-wage amount, this time from $7.60 to $9.05 an hour and with the support of the mayor, and indexed it to inflation. As part of the effort, living-wage supporters released several reports documenting the positive effects of the law and the need for its expansion. The victory and the expanded work in education and housing reform were catalysts that built ACORN Illinois.

Chicago ACORN's work encouraged other ACORN chapters to engage in minimum-wage and living-wage campaigns. In 1998, ACORN had established the Living Wage Resource Center to inspire and provide technical assistance to a living-wage movement. It hoped to provide materials and strategies to living-wage organizers all over the country. For the next four years, using its federated structure and local chapters as a foundation, ACORN led living- and minimum-wage campaigns to victory in St. Louis, St. Paul, Minneapolis, Boston, Oakland, Denver, New Orleans, Detroit, New York City, Long Island, Sacramento, and San Francisco.

Floridians for All

In 2003, Rathke sent Kettenring to Florida in ACORN's boldest attempt to put the minimum wage on the national agenda. His job: to lead a voter registration project for the November 2004 election, mount a referendum to raise the state's minimum wage a dollar to $6.15 an hour, and index it yearly to inflation. Eight long years had passed since Congress had set the meager federal minimum at $5.15.

Although their primary concern was to help lift families out of poverty by increasing the minimum wage in Florida, ACORN's leaders also hoped to spark a national movement to increase the federal minimum and help jump-start Florida ACORN. Another goal was to register voters in black and Hispanic neighborhoods—likely Democratic voters—who could affect the outcome of the presidential race in the largest battleground state (twenty-seven electoral votes). If John Kerry loudly supported their effort and then beat George W. Bush in Florida, ACORN's leaders figured that its minimum-wage campaign would get much of the credit. ACORN would make history.

Before embarking on the campaign, ACORN, which now had 160,000 low-income dues-paying members in twenty-eight states, commissioned a statewide poll that found overwhelming support for increasing Florida's minimum wage, especially among low-income and minority residents. According to one study, the state's low-income workers would get a whopping $443 million salary increase, which would have positive ripple effects throughout Florida. Orlando, as well as Miami-Dade and Broward counties, had passed living-wage ordinances, mandating higher wages and health insurance for those who worked for those localities. The Republican-controlled legislature, ironically known for its support of local control, overturned those ordinances by banning municipalities from passing minimum-wage laws.

Kettenring deployed a field staff of forty organizers, sixty canvassers, and more than two thousand volunteers to gather the signatures to put the measure on the ballot, to register voters, and to mobilize an Election Day get-out-the-vote effort.

Floridians for All—a coalition that ACORN's staff initiated of labor unions, community organizations, churches, senior citizen groups, and others—registered 210,000 new voters in the state's largest urban areas. ACORN's top strategists assumed that many poor Floridians who might otherwise stay home on Election Day would go to the polls to raise their wages and, once there, cast a vote in the presidential race as well.[9]

In August 2004, Floridians for All kicked off its campaign in eleven cities, anticipating that Florida's business community—featuring a large restaurant and tourism industry, including Disney, that depends on low-wage employees—would mount an expensive opposition effort. The next month, business leaders unveiled a plan to fight the amendment. "We are not going to allow union bosses to come into the state of Florida and make decisions that are going to hamper the state of Florida without a fight," said Rick McAllister, the Florida Retail Federation's president and chief executive. On October 12, the *Tampa Tribune* blasted the minimum-wage amendment, echoing the business community's line that it was unnecessary because the majority of minimum-wage workers were under age twenty-five, undereducated, and worked only part-time.

In October, the business groups launched television ads equating the minimum-wage initiative with Florida's recent hurricanes, calling it a job killer. ACORN countered with an ad campaign of its own on cable TV, showing a working woman with grocery bags in one arm and one of her two children in the other, urging them to vote "Yes on 5" to help them meet the spiraling cost of "basic necessities like food, rent, and health care." The ad was designed to encourage people to vote for an increase in the minimum wage because it was the morally right thing to do.[10] At the same time, accusations of voter-registration fraud mounted, forcing Kettenring and other staff to devote time to rebutting these claims rather than to voter turnout.

The GOP and its business allies began to worry when an October poll revealed that fully 81 percent of voters favored raising the minimum wage, while just 12 percent opposed raising it. There was more good news for ACORN: the poll confirmed that the minimum-wage initiative would help increase voter participation; ACORN's key turnout targets—African Americans, younger voters, and unmarried women—had become more interested in the election. For example, the poll found that nearly three-quarters of African Americans who had not voted in the past said that the minimum-wage issue was "very important" and would motivate them to vote.

Many unions, environmental groups, and civil rights organizations worked in Florida for months to register new voters, and ACORN's strategy of mobilizing voters around the ballot initiative had won praise from many liberals. John Henley, the Florida campaign director for the Service Employees International Union (SEIU), said: "Anyone who understands how campaigns work understands that ACORN is doing an amazing job."

Still, Kettenring and other supporters were suspicious of the polls, since a vast majority of voters would not benefit from an increase in the minimum wage and ACORN's opponents would soon scare these voters into voting against the ballot initiative. He was also concerned because Democratic support for the measure was muted, including that of presidential candidate John Kerry, who knew that his active support would alienate the business community and believed that Florida was too conservative to increase the minimum wage. The night before the election, several organizers for ACORN complained that Kerry had scarcely mentioned it. "Kerry is failing to seize the opportunity to use the issue to connect with voters," said Kettenring. "It could hurt our effort and his." Like so many other Democratic Party leaders, Kerry couldn't quite comprehend the idea that his party could come up with issues that could appeal to both the poor and the middle class.

On November 4, as George W. Bush won Florida by 300,000 votes and conservative Republicans won seats in Congress, ACORN scored an astonishing triumph in the red state of Florida that would almost immediately help the poor, as well as facilitate a change in the direction of national politics.

To the surprise of even ACORN's leaders, the ballot measure won in a landslide 72 to 28 percent, nearly five million votes to two million. The victory was remarkable because most of the voters who supported the ballot initiative were middle-class workers making more than the minimum wage. The measure won in every county in the state, including conservative counties in the Panhandle, where military bases and retired military veterans dominate the political culture. In those counties, more than two-thirds of voters supported the wage boost—about the same margin given Bush. Ordinary people did not believe a dollar increase would wreck the economy. Kerry made the fatal mistake of not publicly embracing the minimum-wage ballot.

ACORN's precedent-setting achievement was overshadowed by the defeat of the Kerry campaign and downplayed by the media: it was the first time a minimum-wage increase passed in a southern state. Because of ACORN, 300,000 workers would gain directly from the increase and another 550,000 would receive increases from "ripple effect" wage increases—nonmandated raises that businesses voluntarily provide some of their workers after the higher minimum-wage rate is implemented. The victory would yield over $121 million in wage increases per year.[11]

As far as increasing ACORN's visibility, the campaign received sufficient press to give ACORN credibility among Democratic Party insiders and liberal fund-raisers, and it put a bit of fear into the heart of the Republican Party leadership. Because of a lack of money to hire more organizers, and since ACORN ran the campaign under the name Floridians for All, however, the victory did not boost the visibility of ACORN's Florida chapter. Further, charges of voter fraud by Republican Party operatives, which led to an investigation by the Florida Department of Law Enforcement, remained unsettled.

Going after Wal-Mart

The effort to increase the salaries of America's low-wage workers faced a formidable barrier. While most people after the turn of the twentieth century thought of high-tech companies as the symbols of the new economy, Wal-Mart and other service-sector corporations were the true faces of our changing economic system. Most new jobs were in such low-wage service industries. Wal-Mart's legions of low-paid, non-unionized workers (some 60 percent of whom lack company-provided health insurance) were part of the fastest-growing labor-market sector. Wal-Mart soon employed more Americans than did the entire U.S. auto industry.

The practice of U.S. corporations, high tech and low tech, hiring employees from lower-wage nations instead of from the United States, coupled with the low rate of private-sector unionization—under 9 percent of the workforce—led to the stunning collapse of the capacity of low-wage workers to claim their share of the nation's corporate earnings.

While wages stagnated and the ranks of the poor and uninsured increased, corporate pay and profits skyrocketed. In 2004, with millions of Americans trying to keep up and get ahead, corporations and CEOs enjoyed a banner year. The average CEO made an obscene 430 times the income of the average worker, up from a ratio of 301-to-1 in 2003. Nothing symbolized this trend more than the chasm between the pay of the CEO and of the average Wal-Mart worker. In 1969, when GM was America's largest employer, the average worker at General Motors made about $45,000 a year, adjusted for inflation; CEO James Roche was paid $4.2 million. Wal-Mart workers earned on average less—$18,000; the CEO of Wal-Mart, H. Lee Scott, filled his pocket with almost $23 million.

To build the living-wage movement, Rathke urged ACORN's national governing board to support a campaign against Wal-Mart's employment practices. He put together a coalition called the Wal-Mart Alliance for Reform Now (WARN). ACORN would show its muscle when WARN forced Wal-Mart's retreat from plans to build stores in Orlando, Sarasota, Plant City, and Temple Terrace, Florida. ACORN, however, did not want to just stop Wal-Mart from opening stores. The most dramatic fight with Wal-Mart happened in Chicago.

In 2003, while ACORN was planning its minimum-wage campaign in Florida, Wal-Mart's marketing research revealed that Chicago's inner city markets represented a cash cow—$5 billion in annual buying power. ACORN's research indicated that Wal-Mart not only paid poorly, but also destroyed local businesses, cost taxpayers in subsidies to pay for Wal-Mart's workers' health care, and engaged in unfair labor practices. Instead of creating jobs, the average Wal-Mart actually decreased employment by driving its local competition out of business.

When Wal-Mart proposed opening stores in Chicago, the old living-wage movement was ready. In Talbott they had a general; in Tim Drea, the Chicago United Food and Commercial Workers' political director, they had a strong lieutenant; in Toni Foulkes, from the neighborhood of Englewood, an inspired organizer; in the coalition, a network of dedicated activists, including those from two new labor groups, the Chicago Federation of Labor and Change to Win. They needed a respected member of the City Council. Alderwomen Toni Preckwinkle, an authoritative African American woman, stepped up.[12]

On a partly sunny spring day in 2006, scores of ACORN members and volunteers fanned out in Chicago's lower-income neighborhoods, gathering signatures in favor of a law that would require giant retailers like Wal-Mart to pay employees a "living wage"—$10 an hour plus benefits. Wal-Mart's starting wage was about $7.25 an hour; more than half its workers had no health insurance. In Chicago, according to the Economic Policy Institute, a single mom with one child needed to earn $34,351 to meet her family's most basic needs; a full-time, entry-level job at Wal-Mart would bring in approximately $15,000. Opponents of the law included civil rights leader, former Atlanta mayor, and former U.N. ambassador Andrew Young, who played the race card, warning that the living-wage proposal would drive jobs and desperately needed development out of some of the city's poorest African American neighborhoods and lead Wal-Mart to abandon the city. Mayor Daley vehemently opposed what ACORN and the coalition called the "Big Box Living Wage." Wal-Mart spread its money around to members of the City Council and financed an ad campaign warning, "Don't Box Us Out!" Its executives called on its vendors to lobby elected officials. Both major Chicago daily newspapers editorialized against the wage ordinance. The *Wall Street Journal* labeled it "the red-lining of Chicago." The giant retail chain Target, which would also be affected by the new law, threatened to cancel or delay stores planned for the city. "All we are trying to do is get the largest companies in America to pay decent wages," countered Alderwomen Preckwinkle at public forums and City Council meetings.

ACORN's Toni Foulkes, who made a living decorating cakes and training workers for the Jewel supermarket bakery, was confident of victory. She told her customers that there was a reason the cakes she sells at a South Side Jewel store cost more than cakes at Wal-Mart: "They don't put love in 'em like I do," she said. "And their employees don't make what I make." She earned about $35,000 last year at her $12.85 per hour job, including overtime.

Despite the opposition of Wal-Mart, the Chamber of Commerce, and the mayor, on July 26, 2006, after years of organizing and months of agitation, ACORN's coalition pressured the Chicago City Council into passing, 35–14, what the front page of the *New York Times* called a "groundbreaking ordinance." It was the first ordinance in the nation that required all big-box retailers to pay a "living wage." Retailers with more than $1 billion in annual sales and stores of at least 90,000 square feet, by mid-2010, would pay workers at least ten dollars an hour in wages plus three dollars an hour in fringe benefits.

ACORN mobilized its coalition to use an anticipated veto by the mayor as a rallying point to defeat Daley's allies in the upcoming February 2007 elections. Daley did veto the bill, ran for mayor, and easily won reelection because no serious contender emerged. But a number of the pro-Wal-Mart aldermen aligned with the mayor and targeted by the coalition lost their seats. The ACORN leader Foulkes, with strong financial support from SEIU, won a seat on the Chicago City Council with more than 60 percent of the vote, defeating the candidate backed by Daley. The campaign may have lost a battle to the mayor's veto, but the war on Wal-Mart continued to pressure it to change its workplace practices. Talbott's coalition went back to the drawing board to plan another push for the big-box ordinance.

Flushed with its success in Florida, ACORN and its labor partners plotted a multistate minimum-wage initiative for 2006, particularly where Democrats had a chance to compete for key offices. The strategy, developed in collaboration with former vice-presidential candidate John Edwards, was designed to increase voter turnout and to provide liberal candidates with a morally righteous economic issue. Organizers also hoped to reach out to white, churchgoing voters of both major parties who earned barely enough to stay above the poverty line. They sought to counter the right-wing initiatives opposing gay marriage and affirmative action. They also hoped this state-by-state strategy would create a groundswell for raising the federal minimum wage.

On March 5, 2005, ACORN president Maude Hurd and Edwards announced that they would be working together on initiatives in targeted states to raise the minimum wage. "I am strongly committed to moving people out of poverty and into the middle class, and one of the most important things we can do is help families earn more money at work," Edwards said. "We desperately need to raise the minimum wage—its low level today is a disgrace."

As the midterm congressional elections approached, most political analysts assumed the GOP's ability to outspend the Democrats and its superior capacity to get out the vote of its enthusiastic supporters almost guaranteed a Republican victory. They were wrong. Democrats took back control of the House and Senate, with the help of ACORN's smart strategy that combined voter registration with the minimum-wage issue. Voters in six states in the South, Midwest, and far West—Arizona, Colorado, Missouri, Montana, Nevada, and Ohio—approved measures to raise state minimum-wage levels by $1 to $1.70 an hour and index them to inflation. These initiatives not only put more money into the pockets of low-income workers, but also, as ACORN's organizers predicted, increased voter turnout among urban and working-class voters in key states, especially Missouri and Montana, where Democratic candidates for U.S. Senate won narrow victories that put the Democrats in control of both houses of Congress.[13]

In addition, the legislatures in another four states—California, Arkansas, Michigan, and North Carolina—raised their state minimum wages early that year. As a result, twenty-eight states and the District of Columbia had passed legislation or approved ballot initiatives raising their state minimums above the federal minimum. Several of them—including all six that passed on November 7, as well as Washington, Vermont, Florida, and Oregon—included cost-of-living adjustments, which required the state minimum wages to rise with inflation.

One cannot underestimate what ACORN had done. Until 2006, the living wage was a radical idea. John Kerry was afraid to promote it in 2004. The transfer of income from employers to workers in eleven states that passed minimum-wage increases in 2006 equaled some $16 billion.[14] Moreover, with such allies as the AFL-CIO and SEIU, ACORN had used its local minimum-wage and living-wage victories as stepping-stones to propel the new Democratic-controlled Congress to support a significant increase in the federal minimum wage. After the 2006 elections the Democratic Party leadership embraced ACORN and agreed to look more closely at its issues. Democrats ranging from John Edwards to the more conservative Joe Lieberman sought to arouse voters by focusing on income inequality and the need to raise the minimum wage. Incoming House Speaker Nancy Pelosi promised to "give Americans a raise" by increasing the federal minimum wage from $5.15 to $7.25 over a two-year period. Bush opposed the idea and threatened to veto any congressional mandate.

Yet on July 24, 2007, ACORN president Maude Hurd addressed a rally in Washington, D.C., standing alongside Pelosi, Senate Majority Leader Harry Reid, Rep. George Miller, and Sen. Edward Kennedy—all there to celebrate the long-overdue increase in the federal minimum wage signed into law by George Bush. ACORN members in twenty states across the country rejoiced with rallies and press conferences. While ACORN lost its lengthy battle to increase welfare grants, it had begun to succeed in the ideological battle to make work pay.

Even as ACORN was helping workers receive a living wage, however, the banking and finance industry during the 1990s had begun selling a mortgage product to people who didn't qualify for traditional, conventional credit. It was called a "subprime loan." Families started defaulting on these mortgages, and some rushed to ACORN's offices worried about foreclosure. Mike Shea labeled the loans predatory. Shea, Rathke, and other ACORN organizers had an idea to help these folks. Their plan would send them on a collision course against one of the nation's most powerful financial institutions.

Chapter 11

Never Borrow Money Needlessly: ACORN and the Subprime Crisis

On the predatory lending side, some people have done unethical things. We don't do that.
—Bill F. Aldinger III, CEO, Household International

The faults of the burglar are the qualities of the financier.
—George Bernard Shaw

Mike Shea had been ACORN's home ownership man since the 1980s. He had worked on the squatting and community reinvestment battles, encouraged banks to make below-market homeowner loans to the poor and working class, and participated in ACORN's high-pressure negotiations that led to specially modified underwriting, low interest rates, and expert one-to-one counseling that taught new homeowners how to avoid default. Under Shea's supervision as the head of ACORN Housing, thousands of families had become first-time homeowners.

In search of work at the intersection of poverty and the environment, Shea had started with ACORN in June 1976, a new University of Michigan graduate lured by the group's triumphant action that halted Arkansas Power and Light's huge polluting power plant. Twenty years later, he had a string of accomplishments behind him, among them a successful ballot initiative campaign in Arkansas that increased the cost of power for businesses and decreased rates for low-income homeowners and tenants. A young associate lawyer, Hillary Clinton, had crafted the brief for the utility company's challenge, and in the end the law was not implemented. (Hillary Clinton would be the keynote speaker at ACORN's 2006 annual convention, and Bill Clinton would give the keynote speech at New York's twenty-fifth anniversary gala in 2007.)

Across the country an increasing number of the ACORN Housing Corporation's (AHC) clients were returning to AHC in danger of foreclosure, agonizing about the difficulties they faced paying their mortgages. They claimed to have been pressured, misled, and tricked by high-pressure salesmen to refinance the low-cost loans they secured with ACORN's help into new high-cost arrangements. Organizers who went door to door were hearing similar complaints; people were falling behind in their mortgages, and others had lost their homes in foreclosures. This was a disaster, since what little wealth existed in low-income minority neighborhoods survived in home equity. Homes make up over 70 percent of the net wealth of Hispanics and African Americans.

ACORN members who were not in danger of foreclosure complained to ACORN's staff about the growing number of foreclosures in their neighborhoods, which meant more vacant houses and lower property values. These ACORN members were experiencing the American dream of homeownership turning into a nightmare.

Savings and commercial banks had fled from ACORN's neighborhoods, leaving behind the poor and elderly, who became easy prey for a scheme peddled by a new breed of unscrupulous moneylenders beginning around 1993. They were marketing subprime, predatory loans. "Subprime," a fancy financial term, described loans for credit-risky, modest-income people, including middle-class families who had accumulated too much debt. To cover their risk, lenders charged such borrowers higher-than-conventional interest rates or sold them "adjustable rate" loans, which offered low initial interest rates that jumped sharply after a few years. Subprime loans typically had higher application, appraisal, and other fees, as well higher mortgage insurance payments, principle and interest payments, late fees, and fines for delinquent payments to protect the lender against increased risk.

Between 1993 and 1999, subprime loans went from 1 percent of home-purchase mortgage loans to over 10 percent, increasing foreclosure rates. During this period in Chicago, Shea's home base, subprime lending grew from just over three thousand to almost fifty-one thousand, while foreclosures doubled. "Subprime" would become a household word in a later wave of home foreclosures, declining housing prices, and bank failures that was entirely preventable.

The loans that Mike Shea was concerned about—as was Lisa Donner, ACORN's Washington, D.C.–based legislative director—were not just those given to credit-risky people. Shea and Donner were hearing story after story of salesmen lying to homeowners about the terms and costs of the mortgages they were offered. The homeowners were not merely victims of subprime loans; they were targets of an insidious version of the subprime loan that ACORN called "predatory."

Donner decided to see what ACORN could do about the foreclosure problem. A history and political theory major at Harvard, she had graduated in 1991, worked as an organizer for SEIU, and then as a lobbyist and organizer for ACORN. "People who work in ACORN come from lots of different backgrounds," she would say, appearing slightly embarrassed about her elite education.

Yet as smart as Donner was, she had difficulty understanding the subprime mortgage loan features because the language in the contracts was indecipherable legalese. Verifying the terms of a loan was extremely difficult, since many borrowers no longer had or never had the loan papers. When she requested new copies from loan companies, they stonewalled her. To pin down the lender-borrower exchanges, Donner had to find out what the lender said to the borrower, where and when these conversations took place, the borrower's financial situation before the loan, the reasons for refinancing, and so on. Donner was unsure how widespread the problem was because she had only anecdotal data based on the numerous complaints that came to ACORN. Slowly, doggedly, she accumulated evidence implicating several financial institutions in abusive lending schemes, including Advanta, Ameriquest, and Wells Fargo/Norwest Bank.

ACORN contemplated a lawsuit and, of course, demonstrations. On Saturday, June 26, 1999, chanting "Predatory Lender—Criminal Offender," more than two thousand ACORN members marched through Center City, Philadelphia, to a rally at the Federal Reserve Bank, where they demanded that the Federal Reserve use its authority to end unscrupulous and abusive mortgage practices. The group stopped along the route to demonstrate at the offices of financial institutions they believed engaged in predatory mortgage lending. The next day, three hundred ACORN members marched on the suburban home of Advanta Corporation president William Rosoff and staged a symbolic foreclosure in protest of Advanta's alleged predatory lending. The next day more than a thousand members canvassed North Philadelphia neighborhoods in a grassroots effort to make the community a "predator-free zone."

Donner and ACORN's organizers mobilized scores of demonstrations around the country, trying to attract attention to this growing problem. They met with limited success—a few news stories tucked away in the business pages—and only one concerned person with political influence, Federal Reserve member Edward Gramlich, who repeatedly warned other public officials, including Alan Greenspan, that the federal government needed to tighten its regulation of these high-cost home loans. (Gramlich privately urged Greenspan to send examiners into the mortgage-lending affiliates of nationally chartered banks and crack down on the increase in subprime lending, but Greenspan and most of the Federal Reserve were ideologically opposed to government interference, preferring industry self-regulation.)[1]

The ACORN leadership agreed it would take a lot more than a lawsuit and a few demonstrations by ACORN to dramatize the issues and get some relief for the victims of subprime loans and foreclosures. Donner needed a symbolic enemy, and she knew just who it should be: Household Finance Corporation. ACORN was getting numerous complaints concerning this company, headed by a hotshot new CEO, William F. Aldinger, a pioneer in mortgage financing.[2]

Household Finance and William Aldinger

In the late 1870s, in a small room in a Minneapolis jewelry store, Household Finance Corporation (HFC) founder Frank J. Mackey made his first small, unsecured, personal loan to a working-class family. He continued to make ten- to two-hundred-dollar loans with low interest rates to families who temporarily couldn't afford to purchase furniture, for example, or pay medical costs. In the 1890s, he opened offices throughout the midwestern and eastern United States. HFC became the first consumer finance company to go public. To boost sales it solicited customers with a new innovation: loans by mail. After the 1929 depression, HFC's new executives believed people needed to learn how to break their cycles of debt and published materials to educate customers about spending and budgeting. From the mid-1930s to the 1950s, people seeking loans were enticed by HFC's ubiquitous radio ad jingle that began, "Never borrow money needlessly, unless you must . . . " In a 1935 marketing film, the company congratulated itself for treating its customers with courtesy and respect, and throughout the rest of the twentieth century, HFC filled a void in the marketplace as a fair and decent company for people who lacked the credit history to qualify for conventional home loans. HFC compensated for its more risky subprime mortgages by charging borrowers higher interest rates than it charged their prime mortgage counterparts.[3]

Enter William F. Aldinger. In 1994, Aldinger took over as president and chief executive officer. America was experiencing a new Gilded Age—a frenzy of corporate mergers, widening economic disparities, and the biggest concentration of income and wealth since 1928. Economists at the Federal Reserve claimed that deregulation of the financial services industry was essential to the efficient running of the free-market system. Debt was good. Greed was great. Aldinger was a man of his time. From 1994 to 2000, he turned Household Finance into one of the largest subprime lenders in the country. At first he increased Household's profits through acquisitions. In 1998, for example, he bought Beneficial Finance, a rival consumer finance firm. When he ran out of companies to buy, he began promoting the sale of more mortgages. To beat the competition, Aldinger changed HFC's corporate culture, pressing his loan officers to aggressively seek customers. He encouraged high-pressure sales practices, relaxed standards, increased fees, and encouraged HFC sales personnel to make loans that left customers owing more than the value of their house.

HFC's staff scoured tax records around the country looking for first-home purchases. Using that information, HFC's salespeople hounded the homeowners for months, encouraging them to refinance. Household's agents hid the high fees from borrowers and confused homeowners with terms like "discount points," suggesting that the fees and points lowered the interest rate, which they should have but didn't. States had repealed usury laws and Household took advantage, charging rates that soared to over 20 percent.

Using bait-and-switch tactics, HFC touted low interest rates in teaser ads in low-income, working-class, and minority neighborhoods, often without explaining the "adjustable rate mortgages" (ARMs) tied to these interest rates. ARM interest rates go up after a few years and can cause a family's monthly payment to bounce 25 percent or higher.

Former and even current Household employees began confessing to ACORN what they did and how they did it. If a borrower could pay little or nothing down, was recently bankrupt, or didn't have the income to keep up the payments, it didn't matter. "Just bring us the customers, we'll make the loan," said one loan officer. *Forbes* magazine cited former agents who said HFC engaged in deceptive practices and quoted Seth Callen, a form branch manager: "It was a pressure cooker."

HFC made no effort to document applicants' ability to pay back a loan, sometimes just accepting their word that they could meet the monthly payments. "You could be dead and get a loan," recalled one loan officer. Household turned the usual logic of lending upside down. Instead of cautiously lending to those who could repay a loan, they made their money by making loans that people were unable to repay. The truth was, the loans were structured in a way that guaranteed failure.

Household had a banner year in 2000, making $15.3 billion in mortgage loans. Aldinger was paid handsomely—$32 million in total compensation.

A Battle in the Twin Cities

Lisa Donner was turning up a raft of sordid tales. She worked with dozens of ACORN organizers who were in the field, knocking on doors and asking people to detail their mortgage complaints. Seeking to identify as many victims as possible, she adopted some methods used by the lenders, including buying mailing lists of borrowers from companies like Household that ACORN suspected of predatory practices. She searched county property records for mortgages prepared by subprime lenders and put them on a mailing list. If ACORN was to win the war against predatory lending, it needed to find and organize some of the victims—the potential ground troops—as well as look for the few who would emerge as campaign leaders.

Jordan Ash, the regional supervisor of the ACORN Housing Corporation, working in Minnesota, had also become immersed in ACORN's campaign and was working closely with Donner. Ash, using various lists, sent a mass mailing to everyone in the Minneapolis–St. Paul area he suspected had been duped by a predatory loan.

Paul Satriano was on one of Ash's lists. He and his wife, Mary Lee, lived in St. Paul, not far from where HFC made its first loan. Their modest redbrick home, built in 1947 by Mary Lee's father, was located in a working-class section on the city's east side. The Satrianos bought the house from Mary Lee's siblings with a $105,000 mortgage from Beneficial, then a new HFC subsidiary. Paul, fifty-seven and thickly built, was a former steel worker and a transplant from Brooklyn's Italian ethnic neighborhoods, with an accent to prove it. He kept the books for a nearby Holiday Inn. Mary, also fifty-seven, worked as a dispatcher for a courier service.

Shortly after they bought the house in 1998, Paul was surprised to start receiving letters from Beneficial asking if he would like "an extra $20,000 to pay bills, take a vacation . . . " Once he received a check for $2,500 with a letter saying he could spend the money as he pleased, as long as he agreed to come to the Beneficial office and consider a loan. (The letter was what the finance business calls a "live check," used to bait customers into taking out high-cost mortgage loans.) Every letter from Beneficial said, "You are one of our best customers."

At first, Paul and Mary ignored the letters. In spring 2000, though, after traveling to New Jersey for Paul's sister's funeral, they decided to call Beneficial. They visited Beneficial's office and met a smiling, friendly loan officer and manager who made it sound easy to consolidate all their loans—car, credit cards, mortgage—into one mortgage and save money with a lower monthly payment. The loan manager told them, "You're special to me because you've kept up with your payments. I can help you because of that." The loan officer left Paul and Mary with the impression that they didn't have good credit and Beneficial was doing them a favor.

At 4:10 PM on the day of the new loan's closing, Paul received a call from his loan manager. "Come down soon; we close at five." Paul and Mary rushed to the office and arrived just before five. The manager and loan officer shoved more than twenty papers in front of them. Paul squinted through his glasses, trying to pierce the fog of legalese in small print, blind to the potential risks of his new loan. Mary asked if there was a prepayment penalty. There was, but the loan officer said no, and quickly diverted her attention by focusing on the rest of the paperwork, reminding her of the tax deduction of a home loan. The agent kept telling them what a break they were getting.

Beneficial ended up rolling the Satrianos' existing 8 percent, $105,000 mortgage and $4,000 auto loan into a $119,726 home-refinancing loan. The manager explained that under the new loan the Satrianos would make twenty-six biweekly payments a year instead of one a month, and the interest rate would be less than 8 percent. Although the paperwork and the representations were confusing, Paul assumed the loan officer was looking out for his best interest. He walked out of the office believing he had done a smart thing. In fact, he had just been hit with a cleverly hidden 13 percent interest rate and $8,860 for points.

In February 2001, Paul Satriano received a letter from ACORN's Ash, saying the Satrianos might have been the victim of a predatory loan. Paul and Mary Lee talked about the letter but did nothing. They had never heard of ACORN and didn't think of themselves as victims, although they suspected that something was wrong after they added up the new mortgage payments. Realizing that he might have been duped, Paul thought maybe he should meet with ACORN, but he was too embarrassed. Paul and Mary were not ready to say anything to anyone. Still, money was tight, and now they owed more money than before the new loan. Even so, five weeks passed after they received Ash's letter before Paul and Mary Lee agreed it would be crazy to do nothing. If they didn't take action, they might lose their home. Paul made an appointment with Ash.

Typical of people preyed upon by scam artists, the Satrianos blamed themselves rather than the predatory practices of the finance companies. ACORN's organizers had to help such victims overcome these feelings. In fact, ACORN's campaign against predatory lending could succeed only by moving victims from the personal to the political. In one-on-one conversations, organizers tried to help victims feel comfortable talking about their problems, conquer their shame, and come to believe they were not to blame and not alone.

Ash explained to Paul that he had paid $4,866 for credit insurance good for five years but financed over the life of the loan; Paul had no idea what the insurance was for—it was for the protection of the finance company—or how much it cost. In fact, he didn't know it had been included in his loan. The Consumer Federation of America called this typical HFC practice the "worst insurance rip off" in the United States. In addition, contrary to what the HFC agent had said, the Satrianos had a $7,500 prepayment penalty, which meant that if the Satrianos wanted to pay off the loan as soon as possible or refinance at better terms, it would cost them $7,500. The Satrianos' contract also included a provision that barred them from taking court action against the company. With the HFC loan, the Satrianos wound up with a three-hundred-dollar *increase* in the very monthly payments they had intended to reduce. Once Ash had explained all this, Paul, normally a mild-mannered man, became furious. The personal became the political.

The Plan and a Leader

On June 15, 2001, at the home of Paul and Mary Lee Satriano, Minnesota ACORN held a press conference to announce its opening battle plan against abusive home-lending practices. Wearing a plaid shirt and jeans, Paul stepped up to the microphone. "More than anything, I want to warn you other consumers about HFC's practices, so I teamed up with ACORN," he said. He ran down a list of HFC's gimmicks, including its credit insurance schemes. He explained that the subprime loans, at first concentrated in low-income and minority neighborhoods, had spread to white working-class neighborhoods. More than nine thousand subprime loans were made in the Twin Cities metro area in 1999, and he believed many of these were predatory loans. The Twin Cities area, he told the press, was one of six in the nation that ACORN decided to concentrate on. The others were Massachusetts, New York, Arizona, California, and Iowa. Just a month earlier, Satriano had felt like a victim. Now he was an activist and an ACORN spokesperson.

Satriano said the campaign goals included educating homeowners and prospective buyers about the dangers and warning signs of abusive loans. As part of its education campaign, ACORN would conduct door-to-door visits and sponsor community seminars about predatory lending, and help those already stuck with predatory loans find relief by working with lenders to refinance at reduced interest rates. "We'll be fighting for new legislation. Let's end the abuse."

After the press conference, Craig Streem, a spokesman for Household Finance, limited his rebuttal to a claim that HFC would change its loan-making criteria, taking it out of the hands of loan officers, and from now on HFC would carefully portray credit insurance as voluntary.[4]

Ash and other ACORN staff—Satriano; Kevin Whalen, ACORN's Midwest regional director; Becky Gomer, Minnesota's head organizer; and Alton Bennett, a board member—were not impressed with HFC's response and began pressuring HFC by filing with the Minnesota Department of Commerce dozens of complaints relating to HFC practices. When the bureaucracy took no action, they planned a town meeting. Bennett invited Minnesota's newly appointed banking commissioner, James Bernstein, to the meeting to hear direct testimony from Household borrowers. Bernstein reluctantly agreed to attend, with the caveat that he would not appear onstage. On Thursday, June 29, 2001, a hundred people filled an airless conference room at Liberty State Bank in St. Paul to hear several ACORN members testify about abusive loan practices.

One after another, they told Bernstein that HFC was charging artificially high interest rates, points and fees, and prepayment penalties, and offering adjustable loans with "teaser rates." They complained about Household's practice of coercing borrowers into using credit insurance—especially expensive single-payment insurance financed over the life of the loan. Many testified that they were not informed of the extra fees for points, credit insurance, and prepayment penalties in their mortgage agreements, or that loan officers lied to them.

Bernstein was so affected by the testimony that he stood by the stage and pledged to investigate the company. He urged people who had similar stories to contact his office so he could determine whether to conduct an investigation of Household. He also advised borrowers to continue making their payments to avoid losing their houses and, if they decided to refinance, not to use the same company. When ACORN helped draft and support a bill that would outlaw loans so unaffordable they had no reasonable chance of being repaid, lobbyists for the banks and financial services made sure the Minnesota State Legislature did not pass the bill.[5] Meanwhile, Paul Satriano, feeling like a celebrity, began preparing the testimony he would present at a U.S. Senate banking committee hearing in Washington on predatory lending.

Nationwide Confrontation

Confront and educate, or just educate? That is a dilemma all consumer rights groups face. Minnesota ACORN was not alone in its effort to educate the public about HFC and predatory lending, but it was the only group in the area prepared to go beyond the tactics used by traditional consumer rights groups. Those groups argued that a campaign that emphasized public education efforts that warned buyers to beware of bad loans might be enough. After one of ACORN's press conferences, Dan Hardy, Mortgage Association of Minnesota's chief of staff, took a similar route, essentially blaming the victim: consumers should look out for "the fine print. Consistently, what we're hearing from consumer advocates is that many of the problems that are caused by predatory lenders could be prevented if consumers were better-educated."

Donner knew that polite consumer education would not affect corporate power and would not build the collective capacity of people in low- and moderate-income communities to fight in a way that would lead to reform. By summer 2001, she was helping local organizers in fifty-three cities, including Minneapolis, organize demonstrations at many offices of HFC, handing out flyers warning borrowers about Household's practices, and holding press conferences in front of homes about to be foreclosed. In Minnesota, ACORN supported a bill that had been introduced in the last two legislative sessions, but it never even reached committee hearings. With state legislation going nowhere, ACORN turned to the cities of Minneapolis and St. Paul and lobbied for municipal versions of its legislative proposals, as well as for resolutions barring each city from investing in institutions that engaged in predatory lending.

In 2001, as Donner was preparing to escalate ACORN's war against HFC, the United States had reached a staggering level of inequality. CEOs of large corporations made 411 times as much as the average factory worker. The United States had become more unequal than at any time since the dawn of the New Deal—indeed, it was the most unequal society in the advanced democratic world.[6]

When HFC announced that it would hold its annual shareholders' meeting in Brandon, a suburb of Tampa, Florida, Donner thought the meeting presented ACORN with an organizing opportunity: a shareholders' resolution against HFC. To explore the idea, she called Scott Klinger, a former corporate manager and financial analyst, who worked with a public interest group called United for a Fair Economy and the Coalition for Responsible Wealth (RW). Founded in 1999, RW's specialty was filing shareholder resolutions seeking to promote a more humane and equitable economy.[7]

Klinger drafted a resolution to present at the next Household shareholders meeting that would offer HFC executives incentives to end predatory lending practices and ensure fair treatment of its customers. Deeply involved in the socially responsible investing movement, Klinger helped ACORN find Julie Goodridge, president and founder of NorthStar Asset Management, Inc., an investment advisory firm specializing in socially responsible investing. She was willing to introduce at the shareholders' meeting a resolution calling for executive compensation to be tied to clear and measurable efforts to fight predatory lending.[8] Another investment firm, Domini Social Investments, allowed ACORN to use its proxy to get an ACORN leader into the meeting to add her voice to the debate.

The morning of May 7, 2001, twenty-five ACORN members from the New Orleans chapter bussed overnight to Brandon, Florida, to appear bright and early outside the Household shareholders meeting and greet shareholders as they arrived. The HFC building, tucked in among nondescript office parks and strip malls, was, as *St. Petersburg Times* columnist Robert Trigaux noted, an "unlikely site for ground zero of a national ACORN protest campaign against Household." ACORN's Lanny Roy of New Orleans, bullhorn in hand, shouted: "Household Finance . . . you're no good . . . don't rip off our neighborhood!" Others shouted, "Predatory lender! Criminal Offender!" One ACORN member dressed in a full-length shark costume gyrated to the shouts. As more press gathered, ACORN leaders held a mock ceremony awarding Household a shiny, money-stuffed plaque that read "Shark of the Year."[9]

Household's executives had arrived even before the protesters and had hidden in the building, protected by rooftop security guards and hard-faced police, as if they were expecting an attack by armed guerrillas. Julie Goodridge walked past the demonstration with a smile, showed Household's security guards two forms of identification, and entered the building. When the meeting got under way and she presented the ACORN shareholder resolution, the vast majority of the 350 shareholders demonstrated their hostility with groans and shouts of disapproval.

Goodridge was not surprised that the resolution lost, since shareholders rarely approve a resolution opposed by management. But ACORN's leaders regarded as a victory its garnering 5 percent of the vote, a level of support that guaranteed it would appear on the proxy statement the next year.

Media coverage of the action outside Tampa surprised Donner. It was extensive and strongly favored ACORN's case. *St. Petersburg Times* columnist Robert Trigaux documented Household's harsh, inequitable loan practices by recounting the story of Margaret Dickens, a Household victim from St. Louis who was convinced to take out a large loan with excessive fees and unnecessarily high interest rates, and who got "stuck in a spiral of increasing debt."[10]

The shareholder event in Tampa kicked off a series of actions across the country in 2001 and 2002, as ACORN's members called on cities to divest their pension funds of HFC stock until it put a stop to its abusive lending. ACORN worked with local allies from organized labor to pass similar resolutions with regard to union pension funds. City resolutions were passed in St. Louis, Los Angeles, and Chelsea, Massachusetts. Council members in Washington, D.C., Boston, and the Twin Cities also pledged to support such resolutions. In New York City, comptroller Alan Hevesi, a trustee of the city's millions of dollars in pension funds, added his voice to the demands that the company change its practices.

And after friends of ACORN lobbied the man in charge of the finances of New York State, comptroller Carl McCall, he called on HFC to reform its business practices. A potentially alarming adversary, McCall was also the sole trustee of the giant New York State retirement fund, which held shares in HFC worth over $100 million. He threatened to sell the shares if the company did not move quickly. (Later that year, McCall ran for governor with ACORN's support.)

To escape ACORN's national protest and the media's eye, HFC planned to hold its summer 2002 annual meeting in a nearly empty business park in the small, isolated community of London, Kentucky, an hour and a half from the nearest airport. Despite the location, Donner and ACORN would make this HFC annual meeting the biggest event in the town's history. ACORN mobilized borrowers from nearby states as well as from Pennsylvania, Michigan, and Illinois. Their protest garnered news coverage in Kentucky and Tennessee, which had not covered the story up to this point. The shareholders increased their support for ACORN's resolution from 5 to 34 percent, an impressive number for a proposal opposed by management. ACORN's campaign began to get favorable attention in major newspapers—the *Chicago Sun Times*, the *Philadelphia Daily News*, and the *Tampa Tribune*. Even the *American Banker* ran sympathetic stories on ACORN's campaign against predatory lending and Household. The bad publicity led to a drop in Household's stock price.

ACORN's victory came when HFC had announced in July 2001 it would quit selling credit insurance built into its real-estate loans.[11] Still, inside the boardroom, Household's officers thought they could take any punch ACORN could throw.

Class Action

ACORN's staff contemplated a lawsuit against HFC, though litigation has never been a central component of an ACORN campaign. Much more important was to make sure that ACORN members participate so the membership feels empowered. The danger of working with lawyers was that after a lawsuit was filed, people fighting for justice would sometimes take on an attitude of "let the lawyers do it" and neglect the hard work of recruiting and mobilizing members, an essential source of poor people's power. Lawyers by personality and training have a tendency to dominate an organization's strategy, to insist on leading negotiations, and to assume the mantle of spokesperson.

In this case, Rathke and Shea thought legal action could complement grassroots activism by increasing pressure on HFC. Once they were sure that their lawyer, Sarah Siskind from the law firm of Miner, Barnhill and Galland, understood ACORN's approach, ACORN filed a class-action lawsuit against HFC in California in February 2002, charging the company with unfair and deceptive trade practices.

In addition to this lawsuit, the demonstrations, and the shareholder pressure, Donner had one more innovative strategy: she wanted to press state attorneys general, state consumer protection agencies, and bank regulators to take action against

HFC. Donner figured that these state agencies had considerable power over finance companies, since they can sue for deceptive and abusive lending practices if banks and finance companies violate consumer protection and other laws. They also have the power to revoke licenses.

ACORN organizers and members convinced state regulators to attend community hearings to listen to borrowers' complaints, as was done in Minnesota. They wrote letters, made phone calls, and reached out to political allies who would encourage an attorney general to investigate ACORN's complaints. They doggedly pursued state attorneys general and bank regulators with documented accounts of HFC's abuse and deception. Many of these state officials, however, reviewed subprime loans based on the paperwork alone; if the documents appeared to be in order, the attorney general's office assumed no problem existed. In some states, ACORN's complaint records were not kept. Some attorney general offices forwarded the complaints to Household without any follow-up.

To encourage these officials to act more aggressively, Donner with the help of field director Helene O'Brien had local organizers mobilize borrowers to go as a group, unannounced, to a regulator's office, hold a press conference outside, and demand to speak to senior officials to present the borrowers' complaints. Organizers followed up by making appointments with attorneys to meet individual borrowers, who could explain their cases in person.

Some state attorneys worked closely with ACORN to review the legal issues. Kathleen Keest, an assistant attorney general of Iowa, thought ACORN's work in bringing victims of predatory loans to the attention of her office was essential to Iowa's investigation, because victims often fail to file complaints with their state attorney general. "They usually do not know the law, and so don't know that a lender may have violated [it]; they may not feel comfortable talking about financial troubles (especially the elderly); they may just feel they have made a bad decision and will have to live with it," Keest later commented.

Donner understood that few attorneys general (AGs) had the staff to take on a lender the size of HFC, so she tried to mobilize members in many states to get a critical mass of AGs committed to the cause. While ACORN's shareholder action and the local demonstrations kept a spotlight on the issues surrounding predatory lending, ACORN staff networked with several AGs. By early 2002, to Donner's astonishment, thirty-five state attorneys general began working together to conduct a national investigation into HFC.

A big break came in April, when bank regulators in the Washington State Department of Financial Institutions (DFI), working with assistant attorney general David Huey, produced a report based on hundreds of borrowers' complaints. It accused Household and its subsidiaries of violating provisions of the state's Consumer Protection Act, the Consumer Loan Act, and the Insurance Code. HFC, the agency said, misrepresented important loan terms and failed to disclose critical information to borrowers. It found the same problems ACORN had discovered—high loan fees, unfair prepayment penalties, insurance products tacked on and financed over the life of a loan, and loans exceeding the value of the mortgaged property. The DFI had the power to revoke Household's license to do business.

On the heels of this report, ACORN filed another class action in May, this time in Illinois, again charging HFC with unfair and deceptive trade practices. Donner hoped the litigation would magnify the threat of the attorneys general investigation. She also had been working with the press, connecting journalists with victims and explaining HFC's practices.[12] On August 17, 2002, Donner's media work paid off. The *New York Times* business section led with a story detailing ACORN's lawsuits accusing HFC of predatory lending and quoted Household's CEO William Aldinger, who dismissed the suits as groundless: "We are a good group of people, a high-quality team with good ethics." The September 2 issue of *Forbes* magazine ran an exposé on HFC's predatory practices, getting much of its information from ACORN and citing ACORN's litigation. The title of the piece was "Home Wrecker" and its subhead read: "William Aldinger says he built one of the few successful lenders to bad credit risks by managing smarter. People suckered into his mortgages cite other tactics: lies and deceit."[13]

In the fall of 2002, with more and more bad publicity, angry shareholders, incessant demonstrations, and pressure from state regulators, HFC's stock price dropped again. Aldinger was under so much pressure to save the company that he began negotiating a buy-out with London-based HSBC bank, a sale that would be good for ACORN's purposes because HFC would become a unit in a commercial bank governed by greater government regulation.

As ongoing publicity increased pressure on HFC to settle the litigation, the big breakthrough came—the beginning of the end. Less than a month after the *Forbes* story, Paul Satriano got a call from an excited Jordan Ash. "I have good news," Ash told Satriano, now a member of the board of directors of Minnesota ACORN. "Household agreed to a settlement with us and the fifty state attorneys general. It'll be announced later."

The class-action suit would help give ACORN a role in shaping the final AG settlement with HFC, which came a year later, in November 2003. HFC agreed to distribute a record-breaking $484 million to abused borrowers. Iowa Attorney General Tom Miller called it the "largest direct restitution amount ever in a state or federal consumer case."[14] ACORN settled its suit, adding $150 million to the pot for additional relief for injured borrowers by allocating funds to a foreclosure prevention fund (FAP) for Household victims. HFC further agreed to change its practices by reducing points and fees from more than 7.5 percent of the loan amount to a maximum of 5 percent; reduce prepayment penalties from five years to three years on all loans; prohibit making loans for substantially more than the value of borrowers' homes; and end the sale of financed credit insurance and many deceptive sales practices. Household also agreed to provide borrowers with clear information about the costs of the loans at every step of the process and sharply curtail the use of "live check" solicitations to sell refinance loans—the practice of mailing out checks that, when cashed, automatically become loans. The legally binding requirement promised that HFC's loans would be a net benefit to borrowers.

ACORN had forced the nation's largest high-cost lender to change its practices and won back half a billion dollars that had been taken from the lower classes—one of the largest consumer settlements ever. It was a damaging rebuke to HFC. The AG settlement provided an average of two thousand dollars to borrowers, most of whom would never otherwise have recovered any money. Yet ACORN didn't get everything it wanted. For example, HFC could charge five points on its loans—an extremely high add-on—and include a prepayment penalty of six months' interest. But ACORN had scored a huge victory nonetheless, adding up to hundreds of millions of dollars in reduced costs to borrowers every year.[15]

Reminiscent of Richard Nixon, who famously said, "I am not a crook," Household chair William F. Aldinger III had insisted HFC was not a predatory lender. After the settlement, Aldinger conceded: "Our compliance procedures and policies were not as good as we thought."

The Household settlement marked the first time all fifty state attorneys general had worked together on the issue of predatory lending. Beyond helping hundreds of victims, ACORN had engaged thousands of people to demand changes in a large corporation's policies, once again demonstrating that ordinary people can make powerful institutions accountable for their bad behavior. Shea, Rathke, Donner, and the others in ACORN thought the reforms forced on HFC would contribute to making certain practices—though still perfectly legal in many states—*less legitimate* for the industry as a whole. They hoped the settlement would become a template for effective action against predatory lenders in the future. Sadly, that would not prove to be the case.

ACORN did learn an interesting lesson: that class-action lawsuits could not only help individual victims, but also make ACORN more credible, if not understandable, to a media that doesn't comprehend organizing. As Donner later wrote, ACORN's "class action law-suit helped make the campaign more concrete and easier to talk about for the press. Most reporters for daily papers have little time to learn about, much less write about, the ongoing series of actions that has brought a campaign to the point at which they encounter it, but a class action law-suit is a 'thing' to which they can repeatedly refer."

Donner was right. Daily reporters don't have the time to understand the complex issues ACORN addresses, partly because they involve the unfamiliar territory of inner-city life, and also because the sophisticated methods ACORN uses to attack a problem would require a reporter to follow a story over time—time few reporters have.

For Paul Satriano, the victory was bittersweet. The changes forced on HFC came too late for him. Three family deaths in one year put him and his wife behind on mortgage and credit payments. Their house had become home to their widowed son along with his three children, all under age twelve. Paul would soon declare personal bankruptcy. The home he had fought to protect was put up for sale. Although the settlement was the largest ever in a lending case, it did not make all HFC's victims whole. Satriano sometimes felt he had won a war but lost the battle.[16]

As for more lasting changes, Congress, the Bush administration, and the federal regulatory agencies continued to turn a blind eye to the subprime predatory lending problem. In the spring of 2007, when many homeowners could no longer pay their mortgages, hundreds of billions in bonds backed by these mortgages became worthless and triggered a chain reaction that affected international credit markets.

ACORN, as well as groups like UNITE HERE, Center for Responsible Lending, and the National Community Reinvestment Coalition (NCRC) pushed on against the tide. ACORN tried with only partial success to pressure Citigroup to restructure loans rather than foreclose on low-income consumers. ACORN persuaded some lenders to switch from adjustable-rate mortgages to thirty-year fixed-rate loans so borrowers could avoid large interest-rate increases. ACORN has also urged lenders to impose a moratorium on foreclosures, which some 2007 Democratic presidential candidates supported.[17]

To prevent the home mortgage crisis from getting worse and to avert future crises, ACORN in the summer of 2008 lobbied Congress and scored a major victory. Despite strong opposition from the White House and its congressional allies, ACORN and other housing groups made sure the 2008 housing bill that helps victims of the subprime crisis included money for a new $600 million affordable-housing trust fund and $4 billion in grants to restore housing in ravaged neighborhoods.[18]

ACORN had always invested in electoral politics, not with money—it was a poor people's association, but with people power, because it gave the group access to power brokers. But despite its successes, ACORN was always looking for a better political strategy.

In New York in the late 1990s, Dan Cantor, a former ACORN organizer, had been meeting with Joel Rogers, a professor of law, political science, and sociology from the University of Wisconsin, and with an old friend, Bob Master, who was now a labor leader. They were researching the idea of starting a new political party to elect officials from the city council level to the U.S. Senate. They hoped to help catapult ACORN, the union movement, and progressive politics to the center of U.S. power.

Chapter 12

ACORN's Family Party

One bright morning while longtime ACORN activist Dan Cantor and his new wife, Laura Markham, were honeymooning in Scotland in 1989, Laura commented on the merits of the European political system—particularly the triumphs minor parties were having. "Why don't you do something useful and start a third party in the United States?" she asked Dan.

"You can't do it," he replied. "We don't have proportional representation."

"Don't wimp out. There has to be some way to do it."

Cantor had long been thinking about how best to build a progressive political force but had never considered a third party. He had been connected to ACORN since he graduated from Wesleyan University in 1977, first as a community organizer in St. Louis and then as a labor organizer for ACORN's United Labor Union. His father, co-owner of a Long Island auto parts store, worshipped Franklin Delano Roosevelt, and Dan ran for high school student council president on a power-to-the-pupils platform. Politics was in Dan Cantor's blood.

In ACORN's early internal debates about its role in politics, Cantor, Rathke, and others sought an alternative to Reagan-style conservatism and neoliberalism to support their community work. They saw three options. The first option was a candidate-centered approach, where each group on the left shopped around for the better or less evil candidate, usually a Democrat, and jumped on his or her bandwagon; they rejected this approach.

A second option was the Saul Alinsky approach: stay out of the selection process and let the candidates chosen by the major parties fight it out and then persuade the winner with protest demonstrations, letter-writing, and lobbying. But as Cantor would often say in discussions about politics: "Neither of the two parties does an adequate job of representing and advancing the interest of the working class, the poor, and their allies. You need to win power in and through the state. And political parties have proven to be the single most potent way to nonviolently advance an agenda in a modern industrial country."

The third option was a third party. In 1981, ACORN discussed supporting the Citizens Party, founded by Barry Commoner, an eminent professor of environmental science famous for his books and his protests against nuclear testing. He tried to enlist within his new party environmentalist, liberal, and Left groups opposed to President Carter's centrist administration. The Citizens Party program emphasized opposition to Wall Street managers and big business. ACORN had rejected participation because the odds against third parties were so staggering: witness the fate of the Progressive and States' Rights parties in 1948, the Peace and Freedom Party in 1968, and the American Independence Party of 1972. ACORN correctly understood that their failures were not the result of bad intentions or lack of skill: America's winner-take-all electoral system, unlike the proportional representation found in some European countries, gives minority parties no voice in government. A vote cast for the third party is a wasted vote. Even worse, a vote for the best candidate could have the perverse effect of helping the worst candidate win, as in the 2000 Gore-Nader-Bush election. Many disgruntled left-wingers—Democrats and independent voters who preferred Nader to Gore—voted for Gore. They understood that a vote for Nader was like a vote for Bush.

Fusion

For years ACORN had been searching for an answer to this political dilemma.[1] The breakthrough idea came from Joel Rogers, a Wisconsin-based sociology, law, and political science professor and a recipient of a MacArthur Fellowship (the Genius Award). He made a very persuasive argument for a strategy that would solve the typical third-party spoiler and wasted vote dilemmas. The key would be electoral fusion.

In electoral fusion, the same candidate can receive the nomination from more than one political party and occupy more than one ballot line. In other words, with fusion—also called "cross-endorsement"—two or more parties can nominate the same candidate on separate ballot lines, and the votes from both ballot lines are added together.

Throughout the early 1990s, Cantor, who had left ACORN but continued to support its work as a foundation executive, Rogers, Zach Polett (ACORN's national political director), and others worked to build the New Party. They had modest success in such cities as Chicago, Little Rock, Minneapolis, and Missoula, Montana. The party's main base of support was in ACORN, along with various labor unions, especially ACORN-allied locals of the Service Employees International Union.

Any hope of shifting the nation toward electoral fusion, making a European multiparty electoral system possible, stalled with the U. S. Supreme Court case *Timmons vs. Twin Cities Area New Party*. In 1997, the Court rejected the New Party's argument that electoral fusion was a right protected by the First Amendment's freedom of association clause. In a controversial 6–3 decision, the Court permitted states to allow or reject fusion, in effect sanctifying the two-party system as fundamental to the U.S. electoral system.[2]

In the wake of the Supreme Court decision against the New Party, fusion enthusiasts settled on New York, one of only four states in which fusion voting is practiced, as the place to experiment. Besides being a liberal state and a place ACORN had talented staff, including Jon Kest, Fran Streich, and Bertha Lewis, New York had minor parties that actually play major roles.

Kest and Cantor plotted with Bob Master, the political director of the Communications Workers of America (CWA), and an old friend of Cantor's from high school in Levittown, Long Island. Twenty-five years after graduation, they were both still active in progressive politics and lived near each other in Park Slope, Brooklyn. They talked with leaders of ACORN, the Communications Workers of America (CWA), United Auto Workers, New York Citizen Action, and many labor unions and other citizens organizations about building a new fusion party. When polls indicated that a new party whose name included the words "working families" would best attract the people they wanted, the Working Families Party (WFP) was born.

As trim and vigorous as when he organized in the 1970s in St. Louis, New Orleans, and Detroit, and now with a salt-and-pepper beard, Cantor assumed that most of the time the WFP would cross-endorse Democrats but sometimes candidates from the Republican Party and the Green Party, a left-leaning populist-environmental party, as well as running its own nominees. A serious, confident, natural-born leader, Cantor became the executive director of the party, a leading political operative with organizing skills. Bob Master, ACORN's executive director, Bertha Lewis, and Jim Duncan of the UAW became the party's cochairs.

The party grew swiftly, with an annual budget of more than $1 million by its third year and chapters in most parts of New York. During the summer of 1998, in its grungy Brooklyn office one floor above ACORN's, the WFP began recruiting and supporting candidates for public office and lobbying at the state and local level. Cantor made sure the party focused on specific, concrete issues, as he had when he organized for ACORN. Its worker-friendly agenda included well-paying jobs, affordable housing, accessible health care, better public schools, and more investment in public services. And as in ACORN, the party organizers agreed to avoid the hot-button social or wedge issues such as gun control that would divide their constituency.

The challenge for Cantor's party was how to get together an anti–gun control working-class guy who likes to hunt and a suburban mom who is scared to death that her son is going to get killed by an AK-47 at his high school. When recruiting or fund-raising for the WFP, Cantor liked to refer to Pat Buchanan's famous line about how the Left won the culture war and the Right won the economic war. When recruiting new members, Cantor argued: "We're more interested in fighting the economic war, though we try to do so in a way that is attentive to identity politics. We want to bridge the gap between social and economic issues by framing things differently. The living wage is a deeply feminist issue, as the overwhelming beneficiaries of such laws are women. Workers compensation affects African American workers disproportionately, because they are overrepresented in dangerous industries. And massive investment in public schools is one way of being strongly pro-immigrant and pro-family." One big barrier stood in the way of the Working Families Party success in New York: the Liberal Party, founded in 1944 as a vehicle for anticommunist leftists opposed to the Democratic Party who wanted to support Franklin Roosevelt. When Cantor started the WFP, fusion allowed New York voters both to support a Democrat and to send an ideological message. Those who liked the Democratic candidate but abhorred the Democratic Party could vote for that candidate on the third-party, Liberal Party line.

Cantor understood the role Liberal and Conservative third parties had played in New York, accumulating power far beyond their numbers by cross-endorsing major-party candidates, often providing their margin of victory. Republicans such as former U.S. senator Alfonse D'Amato and Governor George Pataki had won thanks to the votes they received on the Conservative Party line. The Liberal and Conservative parties always received the fifty thousand votes necessary to win an automatic spot on the ballot. The WFP would have to replace the Liberal Party as New York's progressive alternative to the Democrats.

Liberal Party vs. the WFP

The WFP got lucky. By 1998, the influential Liberal Party was no longer liberal. With no principles to hold it together, it had become a patronage mill for its chief, Raymond Harding. In the 1993 New York City mayoral race, the incumbent, David Dinkins, New York's first black mayor, was far more liberal than his opponent, Rudolph Giuliani, who defeated Dinkins with the help of the Liberal Party line on the ballot. Harding's relatives received appointments in the Giuliani administration. Harding's action created an ideological vacuum on the left that the Working Families hoped to fill.

The 2000 New York U.S. Senate race gave WFP its opportunity. Both the WFP and the Liberal Party put Hillary Clinton on their line. In one of the strongest showings ever for a third party in New York, the WFP garnered 103,000 votes for Clinton, beating out the Liberal Party, and in the process generating considerable publicity. But Cantor wanted to put a nail in the Liberal Party's coffin. His opportunity would come in the 2002 governor's race.

First, though, ACORN and the Working Families Party had to weather a debacle, the 2001 New York City mayoral race. Most pundits thought that whoever won the Democratic primary would become the next mayor. The WFP endorsed the Democratic candidate, Mark Green, a longtime ACORN ally, who hired Jon Kest, New York ACORN's head organizer, to run his field operation. The election would take place October 11. One month after the September 11 attacks, Green, a Caucasian, found himself in a close and bitter primary run-off against Fernando Ferrer, a Hispanic, who was the Bronx borough president. On a balmy October afternoon a few days before the vote, Green's supporters, including Jon Kest, sat around a table at Nick's Lobster Fish Market, a restaurant that overlooks the water near the end of Flatbush Avenue. Looking for a way to galvanize white voters, the group discussed how they could take advantage of white ethnic voter disapproval of Rev. Al Sharpton, a prominent black supporter of Ferrer. On October 10, leaflets featuring a cartoon of Ferrer kissing Sharpton's ass appeared in predominantly white south Brooklyn neighborhoods, the drawing's implication being that a Ferrer victory would give Sharpton power in City Hall. Green won the Democratic nomination and was heavily favored to defeat the Republican candidate, billionaire Michael Bloomberg, in the general election.[3]

On November 3, four days before the general election, the *New York Daily News* ran a story indicating that Green's field director, Kest, knew about the leafleting tactics and placing him and three others from the Green campaign in a meeting at Nick's where the leaflets were discussed. Outraged, Ferrer called Green, who agreed the leaflets were "racist and despicable" but denied any role in the leafleting. "Four members of your staff were there. You can't claim ignorance," Ferrer said. He wanted Green to fire or discipline someone. "How about suspending Kest?" Green refused.

Those who attended the meeting disagreed about what had happened at Nick's. (Some community activists saw it as an ACORN blunder in its drive to win.) In fact, Kest had no knowledge of the leafleting tactics, but the damage was done. The incident tarnished ACORN and the WFP in the eyes of some black and Hispanic activists ready to believe an organization like ACORN with whites in its upper echelon had slipped all too easily into ugly racial politics. But would it hurt Green?

In the final days of the campaign, Sharpton and several well-known Hispanic leaders shunned Green because of the flap over the leafleting tactics. Bloomberg, in his own advertising and campaign literature, played up the divisions between the minority politicians and Green. Bloomberg spent lavishly and narrowly won. The Sharpton incident may have cost Green the election. It certainly damaged ACORN's reputation in some parts of the African American community.

The bad publicity and accusations of betrayal were painful to Cantor and Kest. But they understood, as Rathke did, that although mixing community organizing with partisan electoral politics could help win victories and build the organization, it was fraught with danger.[4] The compromises and deal cutting needed to accomplish goals sometimes trumped principle. Engaging in politics was a complicated, messy, high-risk, occasionally morally ambiguous but high-return strategy for people seeking to advance their cause while maintaining as high a ground as possible. It's one of the reasons most community organizing groups fear it. Cantor and ACORN's leaders were sure they could take these blows as long as they built deep roots throughout the state.

The 2002 governor's race was an opportunity for ACORN and the WFP to erase the 2001 mayoral setback. With the help of former New York City mayor David Dinkins, Cantor and other leaders of the WFP persuaded city comptroller H. Carl McCall, also the popular state controller, to snub the Liberals in his quest for the governor's office. Harding, still the Liberal Party boss, was forced to put McCall's opponent, Andrew Cuomo, the son of the ex-governor, on the Liberal line—a move that became a disaster when Cuomo dropped out of the race a week before the Democratic Party primary and McCall swept to victory. The Liberal Party fell far below the fifty thousand votes necessary to win an automatic spot on the ballot, virtually destroying its political clout. This time the high-risk, high-rewards nature of electoral politics paid off for the WFP. Cantor and ACORN had banged the last nail into the Liberal Party coffin, and the WFP replaced the Liberal Party as New York's most important third party.

Cantor and Lewis were hoping 2003 would be a pivotal year for the emerging Working Families Party. With its credibility growing, Cantor found it easy to convince many New York City Council Democratic Party candidates to run on the Working Family line in addition to the Democratic Party line. Also, ACORN's activists had made amends to Al Sharpton, based on their common political outlook. Letitia James, a former public defender and assistant attorney general, decided to compete solely as a WFP candidate in the upcoming November elections against a Republican and Democrat in the Thirty-fifth Council District. In 2001, James had received 42 percent of the vote on the Working Families Party line but lost to James E. Davis, a Democrat. If she won in 2003, it would be the first time since 1977 that a minor party elected one of its own members to the New York City Council.

After thirty years of organizing, NY ACORN was on the verge of becoming the city and state version of Rathke's national vision: a large, powerful, dues-paying, multi-issue, multiracial, cross-class membership organization, with local chapters engaged in a variety of tactics, including politics.

ACORN and its executive director, Bertha Lewis, soon plunged into one of the most contentious battles in Brooklyn's history. It would involve nearly every politician in New York. Friendly community leaders would be at each other's throats. Celebrities would line up on both sides, including architect Frank Gehry; actors Heath Ledger, Steve Buscemi, and Rosie Perez; writers Jonathan Safran Foer, Jonathan Lethem, and Jhumpa Lahiri; sport stars Jim Bouton and Bernard King; and rapper Jay-Z. It started when Bruce Ratner, a wealthy New York real estate mogul, bought the New Jersey Nets and decided to move the basketball team to Brooklyn. ACORN, looking to ameliorate New York's housing crisis, would be at the center of the controversy with its credibility on the line.

Chapter 13

Atlantic Yards, the Nets, and the Battle of Brooklyn

> We have a great team surrounding [Lebron James]. Hopefully he will come to Brooklyn, but he's my friend first. I wouldn't do that to him if we didn't have a chance of winning.
>
> —Jay-Z, part owner of the Nets and a Brooklyn native

> More than anything, in an era of increasing housing segregation, Atlantic Yards will be one of the only neighborhoods in Brooklyn where families of all backgrounds will be able to really live and grow together.
>
> —Bertha Lewis

New York ACORN's executive director Bertha Lewis remembers when she first heard about developer Bruce Ratner's plan to "revitalize" a decaying Brooklyn neighborhood. It was at a 2003 rally for Letitia "Tish" James, a Working Families Party candidate for a City Council seat to be determined in November. Ratner, chief executive officer and chair of Forest City Ratner Companies (FCRC), intended to move the pro basketball New Jersey Nets to Brooklyn to play in a new twenty-thousand-seat arena, the crown jewel of his planned $2.5 billion development, Atlantic Yards.

Until 1987, Bertha Lewis had no intention of becoming an activist. Struggling to make ends meet, she just wanted an affordable apartment for herself and her son. She had never even heard of ACORN. The oldest of eight children, Lewis was born in a migrant camp in rural St. Johns County, Florida, in the segregated South. The daughter of sixteen-year-old Frances Lewis and a man she never knew, Bertha was identified as "colored" on her birth certificate and was raised in a close-knit, loving family by her mother, grandmother, and aunt Julia. After Bertha was born, Frances worked as a housekeeper in nearby St. Augustine. The family moved north to Lancaster, Pennsylvania, where the three women picked cotton for the Dutch Mennonites and three-year-old Bertha attended a Mennonite preschool. Before she reached kindergarten, she not only had learned to read, write, and do arithmetic, but also had absorbed the Mennonite values of hard work, honesty, nonviolence, and pacifism.

When Bertha was nine, the family moved to a cold-water tenement with a coal-burning stove in a working-class segregated Philadelphia ghetto. The neighborhood was so infested with mice and rats that residents would leave snow chains on their tires to prevent the rats from chewing them up. When public housing projects were built, Frances refused to apply for a unit, telling Bertha that going on welfare, or "relief," was shameful. When the family needed more money, Bertha had to go into the fields and pick strawberries, blueberries, and tomatoes. Her uncle Ed Wallace, a dockworker, became her stepfather and a devoted parent.

Bertha Lewis's hardworking young mother had ambitions for her oldest child. She would tell Bertha, "My job is to work, yours is to go to school." An avid reader, Bertha took her schoolwork seriously, excelled at it, and didn't get into trouble. In Philadelphia, her mother worked as a seamstress and waitress while her aunt and grandmother continued as farmworkers. An African proverb appropriated by Hillary Clinton says it takes a village to raise a child, meaning that children thrive only if they get support from extended families, friends, and community institutions. Bertha had a village, and she would thrive.

Although Lewis grew up during the civil rights movement and absorbed many of its lessons about social change, she didn't became involved in community activism until she was thirty-two and living in New York. In 1984, she rented an apartment in a deteriorated building at 672 East 136th Street, perched on the edge of the South Bronx alongside the Bruckner Expressway. The highway, built by Robert Moses, cut diagonally through the heart of a once vibrant but now decaying neighborhood called Mott Haven. Jonathon Kozol in his book *Amazing Grace* documented the hardscrabble life of the children who lived there. Most of the apartment buildings in the neighborhood were leveled to make room for the expressway, run down, or abandoned by their owners.

Two years after Lewis moved in, her landlord abandoned the building. To keep a roof over her head, Lewis, a single parent with a thirteen-year-old son, formed an association to run the building. The fifty tenants assessed themselves rent of eleven cents per square foot of apartment space to pay for improvements in the common areas. The city Department of Housing Preservation and Development decided to assist them rather than force them out. "We don't want to send anybody to shelters," said Harold M. Shultz, an assistant commissioner, reasoning that such grassroots efforts would help restore the housing stock in poor areas of the city.

On July 27, 1987, the city took over the property for nonpayment of almost $240,000 in property taxes. But under city law, the holder of the mortgage, Tiffany General Contracting Company in the Bronx, had four months to settle the taxes. Five weeks before the deadline, Tiffany owners Roland Conde and J. Oscar Santangelo paid the back taxes and bought back the building. One big problem: Conde and Santangelo had never visited the building. They presumed it was empty.

When Conde discovered the tenants, he ordered them to leave. Lewis and the others refused. The new owners claimed they had a right to renovate the building without the residents in it because they had redeemed the apartment house from the city in November believing it was officially abandoned. Conde claimed that the building was still unsafe. In fact, there were technical violations, but the building was not dangerous. Conde went to court.

The stress on Lewis and the other residents was severe. Emotions were running high. They retained, for free, the famous civil rights lawyer, William Kunstler, who argued at the hearing that the building was essentially safe, that several residents had leases issued by a former owner, and that the residents had paid rent to a city administrator for a year. The occupants' self-help repairs, or sweat equity, entitled them to remain. Judge Howard F. Trussel of Bronx Housing Court disagreed. On April 11, he ruled that the residents were "illegal occupants" and ordered them to surrender the building immediately and pay fifty thousand dollars in use and occupancy fees. Lewis and the other occupants, however, were not going to leave.

Kunstler hurried to his office to prepare legal papers. He would claim that the tenants had been denied due process and cite factual and procedural errors in Judge Trussel's decision. While Kunstler prepared his case, Judge Trussel ordered the city marshals to remove the occupants. Kunstler rushed to the appellate court.

On July 7, when city marshals armed with a housing court order arrived to evict Lewis and the other occupants, they found a group of people who had settled in for a siege. Twenty-two Guardian Angels blocked their way. Barbed wire topped the locked wrought-iron entrance gate. Banners proclaimed, "Our house or our death," and "We built our house and it ain't for being homeless." From their fire escapes to the streets to the courtroom, the residents were prepared to wage war with the owners of the building. The owners called the occupants squatters. The occupants called themselves homesteaders. Only a last-minute court stay of the evictions prevented violence from breaking out.

The residents vowed to keep on fighting. Lewis, who had become a leader of the building's residents, warned Conde, "You're going to have to come in here and violently take us out." The appellate court ordered twenty-three separate trials to determine the residents' status, ending the eviction proceedings. For ten years, Lewis and the other residents of 672 East 136th Street, with almost no support from the city government, remained as homesteaders and converted the building into decent, affordable apartments. Their work even helped stabilize the Mott Haven area.

In 1987, Lewis was following her passion and making ends meet producing off-off-Broadway plays at the Greenwich Village Church. Getz Obstfeld, the executive director of the housing organization Banana Kelly, who had helped Lewis, suggested she apply for a job with ACORN. It wasn't long before she became New York ACORN's executive director.

Atlantic Yards

Bertha Lewis was one of WFP candidate Letitia James's key supporters and a valuable political ally not only because of her personal charm and political savvy, but also because she was a veteran political organizer with an important constituency base. At the September 4, 2003, rally, James railed against Ratner's Atlantic Yards project. A wealthy and powerful figure in New York politics, Ratner had hired celebrity architect Frank Gehry to design the massive project, which included twelve skyscrapers as high as sixty stories jutting up out of the ground at odd angles along Atlantic Avenue, and four more towers bending and circling the sparkling glass-walled arena. Supporting the project were basketball legend Bernard King and the rapper Jay-Z.

Stretching over twenty-two acres at the congested intersection of Atlantic and Flatbush Avenues, Atlantic Yards would affect at least four tree-lined neighborhoods of mom-and-pop shops, walkable streets, and long-term poor and working-poor residents, along with historic two- and three-story brownstones, many occupied by newly arrived professionals. For Letitia James, a politician with street smarts and a shrewd in-fighter in City Hall, opposition to such a massive scheme seemed like a no-brainer. A lifelong South Brooklyn resident, James was educated in city public schools, Lehman College, and the School of International and Public Affairs at Columbia. Several of the affected neighborhoods—Prospects Heights, Fort Greene, and Clinton Hill—were in the council district that James was hoping to represent, whose residents were a mix of young white professionals, African Americans, Caribbeans, Orthodox Jews, Hispanics, and gays.

Poised and attractive, Tish James vowed to the crowd at the rally to fight Ratner's development, citing environmental concerns, traffic gridlock, displacement, wasteful government spending, and the government's abuse of its eminent-domain powers. "It's too large to be in the middle of a low-rise brownstone community," she roared over the rally's PA system. "We need housing on a human scale where children can play in a yard and neighbors can look out for each other."

Newspaper reports claimed that the project would create 1.9 million square feet of office space, 300,000 square feet of retail space, six acres of open space, and 4,500 units of housing—more office space than the Empire State Building, and more total commercial square footage than the old World Trade Center. The total square footage was equivalent in floor area to three Empire State Buildings. Seventy buildings on six blocks around the site would be condemned and razed. Ratner boasted that Atlantic Yards would be the largest project in Brooklyn's history and the third largest in New York City's.

Gehry, one of America's most famous architects, designed Ratner's project as a planned residential community smack in the heart of land eyed by the Brooklyn Dodgers before that team bolted to Los Angeles in 1957. Since the early 1900s, the Dodgers had represented blue-collar America, the children of immigrants. The movies in the 1930s and 1940s were full of Brooklyn characters with their distinct persona and accent. The Dodgers—"Dem Bums"—were a source of pride, an up-from-the-bootstraps team in contrast to the pinstriped Yankees. Brooklyn borough president Marty Markowitz, who had solicited Bruce Ratner to buy the Nets and bring them to Brooklyn, regularly claimed that the Nets, like the Brooklyn Dodgers fifty years earlier, would bring the borough together.

New York Times architecture critic Nicolai Ouroussoff praised the project because it would "radically alter the Brooklyn skyline, reaffirming the borough's emergence as a legitimate cultural rival to Manhattan." He concluded his paean: "What makes the design an original achievement is the cleverness with which he [Gehry] anchors the arena in the surrounding neighborhood. What is unfolding is an urban model of remarkable richness and texture."[1] Another *New York Times* architect critic, Herbert Muschamp, praised Gehry's "Garden of Eden," the "arena surrounded by office towers; apartment buildings and shops; excellent public transportation; and, above all, a terrific skyline, with six acres of new parkland at its feet. Almost everything the well-equipped urban paradise must have, in fact."[2]

But ACORN's Bertha Lewis was skeptical. To her, Atlantic Yards looked like disguised gentrification, another fancy urban revitalization scheme that would evict the poor to benefit the rich. Since the 1940s, New Yorkers, especially minorities and the poor, have watched politically connected developers and public officials tear down neighborhoods to build cultural centers, office complexes, luxury apartments, public housing, and superhighways. To urban planners such as Tom Angotti, professor in the Hunter College Department of Urban Affairs and Planning, it looked too much like the megaprojects that made the name Robert Moses, New York's former planning czar, an obscenity in many neighborhoods.[3] It was exactly the kind of top-down urban planning that Jane Jacobs, author of the 1961 book *The Death and Life of American Cities*, warned against. It lacked human scale. It destroyed life at the street level. It would push out the poor.

Ratner understood that if both Tish James and Bertha Lewis opposed the project, he would have a big fight on his hands. James had defeated her Democratic and Republican opponents in the November 2003 election with an overwhelming 77 percent of the vote—a huge victory for ACORN and the Working Families Party. Thirty-three of the fifty-one members of the City Council who ran on the Working Families party ticket won, listed on the Democratic and the Working Family's lines. The WFP and ACORN's power was on the rise. James's landslide victory and the increasing power of the WFP and ACORN didn't bode well for Ratner's project.

A week after James's November election victory, one of her supporters, Patti Hagan, a smart, frizzy-haired leader of the Prospect Heights Action Coalition and former fact-checker for the *New Yorker* magazine, told Lewis how much she had enjoyed working with ACORN during the election campaign and said she knew ACORN would join the opposition to Ratner's arena plan. After some discussion, Lewis told Hagan that before she could take a position, she had to do some research and meet with ACORN members: "Our members decide, but I'll definitely get back to you."[4]

Selling Out, or Buying In?

Seven months later, on an overcast day in June 2004, Bertha Lewis attended another rally, this one in Brooklyn's Borough Hall, an Ionic-columned Greek-revival structure topped with a golden figure of Justice. On a stage packed with New York's most important political, labor, community and religious leaders, Lewis stretched her arms into a V, forefingers pointing skyward. To the audience of 1,300 people, she bellowed, "What do we want?"

"Jobs! Housing! Hoops!" the crowd chanted.

To the surprise of many, ACORN announced its support for Ratner's Atlantic Yards sports arena and urban development plan.

Outside Borough Hall, protesters—mostly middle-class activists—accused Ratner of "Manhattanizing" Brooklyn and questioned ACORN's motives for backing the project. Many of these protesters had recently moved to Brooklyn from Manhattan for more room and less congestion. They represented thousands of Brooklyn residents worried that the megadevelopment would overwhelm existing neighborhoods. Why wasn't ACORN—the leftist poor people's organization known for public confrontation campaigns against corporate abuse, gentrification, and political corruption—outside on the picket lines protesting against political cronyism and developer greed?

The protesters accused ACORN of selling out by supporting a deal that would funnel huge government concessions to a private development that would increase population, burden traffic, alter the Brooklyn skyline, and bulldoze many residences through eminent-domain condemnations. Their suspicions were heightened when they discovered that Ratner, like several other city business figures, had donated money to ACORN.

What had happened between the time that Lewis first heard of Atlantic Yards in September and this moment in June?

Soon after the November 2003 election, Lewis began meeting with Jon Kest, sixteen neighborhood leaders (including Pat Boone, president of New York State ACORN), and Ismane Speliotis, the director of New York ACORN Housing Corporation. Speliotis was a nine-year ACORN veteran with degrees from Barnard College, Columbia University, and Pratt University. Like the opponents of Atlantic Yards, Lewis and Kest agreed that the project could be a disaster. But they also saw it as an opportunity to make a big dent in New York's affordable-housing crisis, gaining a lot of credit for ACORN, and boosting ACORN's power. First, ACORN needed to do some research and check with the members. As the leaders reviewed news articles that were appearing in the downtown Brooklyn newspapers, Lewis was impressed that the opposition to Atlantic Yards was getting most of the press.

They consulted with city planners, reviewed the city's housing data, set up meetings, and talked to ACORN leaders who lived in Brooklyn. From years of community organizing, they knew the rental vacancy rate in Brooklyn was less than 3 percent. New York City's population was projected to jump 16 percent over the next twenty-five years, reaching 9.5 million by 2030. Brooklyn and the Bronx were projected to surpass their mid-twentieth-century population peaks. The housing crunch was creating an affordability crisis. More than a quarter of a million families were on waiting lists for Section 8 rent assistance vouchers and public housing.

During November and December, the ACORN staff brought the issue to the membership. As always, participation was ACORN's key weapon against the widespread cynicism and despair that exists in the communities where it organizes. To make sure that members were familiar with the issues, Lewis, Kest, and other staff and leaders began knocking on doors in East New York, Bedford-Stuyvesant, and Brownsville to find out what ordinary residents knew about the project. They held one-on-one conversations with members, helped schedule meetings, and assisted the leaders of the ACORN chapter in drafting agendas. At the meetings, leaders set up role-playing scenarios and "what if" discussions: What's our plan? What if Ratner refuses our plan? What if poor folks who are not members of ACORN begin organizing against us? Who supports Atlantic Yards? Who's against it? If we support it, how much will it cost the organization? If we are against it, can we defeat it?

The most important questions were: Is this the type of issue that ACORN ought to work on? How will it help ACORN members and the poor? What can we win for our members? How long will it take to win? Will it build ACORN membership? Will it make us stronger?

Lewis had been doing this kind of organizing for more than ten years. She saw the process as a way to train ACORN's leaders and members to become well-informed, skilled, and self-confident activists. By now many of them had the skills to understand ACORN's strategic approach to campaigns. Although Lewis often played the role of spokesperson, she had also trained a core of twenty leaders, among them Pat Boone, Marie Pierre and Maria Polanco, who were quite capable of speaking for themselves. Typically black and Hispanic, poor and working class, without any college credits, they would nevertheless impress their neighbors as well as journalists with their knowledge and sophistication about complex issues.

Also in the mix was Lewis's relationship with Ratner; they were not strangers. She had organized a demonstration against Ratner four years earlier over hiring practices in stores like Target and Chuck E. Cheese in the Atlantic Center Mall he operated in Brooklyn—near the proposed Atlantic Yards site. The protesters had wanted the stores to hire more kids from the community and to pay living wages. When the police came to throw the rabble-rousers out, ACORN's people kept shouting from the sidewalk. They soon reached an agreement, and since then Lewis had learned how to deal with Ratner. She knew he was tough, reasonable, and willing to negotiate. And Ratner knew ACORN could be a serious barrier if it opposed Atlantic Yards.

Bruce Ratner was a 1967 cum laude graduate of Harvard University and a 1970 Columbia University Law graduate. His father, Albert, founded the real estate company, Forest City, in 1921 in Cleveland, and built it into a hugely successful company. With his father's help, Bruce Ratner established himself as a critical force in Brooklyn's renaissance by developing some of the most bold (although unattractive) commercial projects during the preceding seventeen years. Ratner brought together the city, the state, and the *New York Times* to plan an $850 million, Renzo Piano–designed newspaper headquarters across from the Port Authority bus terminal. Real estate power brokers were constantly amazed at Ratner's successful government-supported schemes. "He's the master of subsidy. No one does it better," says Fred Siegel, a professor of history at Cooper Union in New York who focuses on urban issues. "That's not a flat-out criticism of him. It's just that he never builds without someone else taking the risk."[5]

Ratner was the anti-Trump—publicity shy, nearly invisible. None of his buildings had "Ratner" engraved on them. His appearance belied his tough nature. He thrived in the city's high-priced real estate market. In the deep trenches of city politics, he was as uncrushable as a New York cockroach.

Yet another side to this real estate tycoon was his civic mindedness. Before becoming a developer, Ratner had been director of the Model Cities Program under Mayor John Lindsay and then served in Mayor Ed Koch's administration as New York City's commissioner of consumer affairs from 1978 to 1982. His brother, Michael, headed the Center for Constitutional Rights, the public interest law firm founded by radical lawyer William Kunstler. Bruce's sister, Ellen, created a left-wing radio syndicate and was one of Fox News's token liberals. At the unveiling of the Atlantic Yards plan, Ratner stated: "Great urban planning incorporates many different uses into a cohesive neighborhood—and truly great urban planning invites the public to participate in the space, whether they work there or live there or they're drawn there to visit." Ratner, a self-described "old lefty," often distinguished himself from another major Brooklyn developer, Donald Trump's father, Fred. Ratner would say that the Trumps never thought about the broader interests of the population and were concerned only about the bottom line. Ratner said he would never turn his back on the larger community's interests.

By January 2004, ACORN's housing expert, Ismane Speliotis, had come up with a plan to use the Nets arena project to stretch the city housing subsidy programs so more poor people could afford to move to and remain in Brooklyn neighborhoods. Kest and Lewis wanted to make a deal with Ratner because they believed he had the clout to get his project approved. Ratner had the money to influence politicians, and Governor George Pataki was his college classmate. Lewis, in discussion with staff and leaders, argued, "It's better to win something than go into opposition and just yell and scream and ultimately lose."

Lewis believed ACORN had a responsibility to steer gentrification to benefit poor and working-class residents. She argued that ACORN's members, like most poor people, didn't want to live in low-income ghettoes. Neighborhoods that only house the very poor—what sociologists call "high poverty" areas—have the worst schools and public services, as well as the highest crime rates. The question was whether a neighborhood could be "improved" without its long-term low-income residents being pushed out. The plan ACORN might negotiate with Ratner, if successful, would result in a mix of well-off, middle-income, and poor people living side by side. By creating hundreds, perhaps thousands, of new jobs that would pay low-income residents living wages, Atlantic Yards would ultimately help improve the lives of Brooklyn's poor and working-class residents.

The leaders and the staff agreed that an unprecedented demand for 50 percent affordable, nonmarket housing would have to be ACORN's bottom line. With their demands ready, Lewis called Ratner to set up a meeting. As usual, she was blunt: "ACORN might support your project if you're willing to build a significant number of truly affordable housing. I mean significant, not the 20 percent stuff. We're thinking half. Poor people, working people, we want half—you can't just do luxury."

Making a Deal

To test the waters, Lewis led about three dozen activists in late January 2004 into Ratner's windowless boardroom high over downtown Brooklyn. Sitting across the large oak conference table, one of the Forest City executives asked the group, "Is Bertha going to start something?" As usual, Lewis was charming. Instead of confronting Ratner and his executives, she calmly proposed a partnership that would preserve profits for Ratner and provide major benefits for disadvantaged Brooklynites. Ratner's people also had to contend with Speliotis. Energetic, cheerful, and attractive, with wavy brown hair and big brown eyes, Speliotis would surprise Ratner's negotiators with her brilliance, especially with numbers.

"If we can pull this off," said Lewis, "it would represent a breakthrough, a model for big-city development projects. We'll help sell the Atlantic Yards project to government agencies, community groups, and the media." In exchange, ACORN continued to insist that 50 percent of the proposed 4,500 rental housing units be below market—an unusually large share of subsidized housing for a private development project. Jim Stuckey, the lead manager for Atlantic Yard, said no. He insisted that anything more that 20 percent was not economically viable: "There's no precedent for 50 percent, period."

At the meeting, Ratner looked relaxed, casually dressed with an open collar and round glasses. He radiated a rich man's ease and self-assurance. When he heard Lewis's proposal, he smiled, as he often did, with his entire face, the gesture engaging his high brow, warming his eyes, and signaling that a deal was likely. After this meeting, negotiations continued.

Over the next three months, ACORN would organize more than forty meetings about Atlantic Yards, mainly in neighborhood gatherings attended by twenty-five to thirty members, plus a boroughwide meeting attended by hundreds of residents. The staff also drafted a series of questions to use in a telephone poll to two thousand members to hear their views on what ACORN should do. "You heard about the Nets moving to Brooklyn?" staffers asked. "What would you like to see happen?" Altogether, the process involved more than 3,500 members participating either by phone or at a meeting.

While many of ACORN's members were leery of the Nets arena project and most opposed eminent domain, their overwhelming concern was the lack of affordable housing. As Bertha Lewis put it at a staff meeting, paraphrasing members' feelings, "Stop the rampant gentrification." In the end, on March 15, 2004, New York ACORN's board of trustees gave the green light to negotiate a plan.[6]

In an effort to carve out a place for low-income families in this mammoth development project, ACORN, now along with several allies, began trying to bang out a deal. ACORN wanted a legally enforceable Community Benefits Agreement (CBA) with Ratner and his Forest City partners. Ratner did not need ACORN in order to get his initial governmental approvals for the project. But he believed he needed ACORN's political clout and its endorsement of an affordable-housing program to help promote the project with the public and several City Council members, and to make sure key members of the state assembly would include funding for the project in the state budget.

The 2004 November elections increased ACORN's influence, especially among the political pros. The WFP turned out 168,719 votes for U.S. senator Chuck Schumer's reelection on the WFP line. "This party has the organizing capacity to be a triple threat for national Democrats," said Schumer. "They can bring disaffected 'Reagan Democrats' back into the fold, they attract independents, and they provide a place for crossover Republicans. They work very well with Democrats. That's not to say they do everything we want, but they see a common cause."[7]

Painstakingly, Speliotis and ACORN's lawyers, Ratner's lawyers, and the accountants went back and forth to create a kind of deal that had never been done before. Ratner's people thought 50 percent was outrageous. Speliotis wanted some complexes affordable to families earning as little as $18,400 a year. How many studios? How many one-, two-, and three-bedroom units? The deal was on, then off, then on, and back and forth. At times during the negotiations, Ratner's people argued that ACORN'S demands were too costly and would undermine the project's viability. The ACORN negotiators knew that developers typically argue that "the numbers don't work" to fend off demands for more parking spaces, affordable units, open space, public art, and other benefits. "The story could be that a progressive developer gave so much away to ACORN that it sapped the life out of the project," was another Ratner complaint. Meanwhile, the price of the development plan rose to $3.5 billion.

While the negotiations took place, Lewis and ACORN were not putting all their hopes for more affordable housing in Atlantic Yards. She and Kest had been busy negotiating with other groups to build a citywide coalition to support affordable housing. On February 2, 2005, despite bitter cold, more than five thousand New Yorkers gathered at City Hall chanting, "Build it! Fix it! Save it!" They held up signs and banners announcing the name of their union, church, or community-based organization and cheered speakers voicing their demands. Lewis had organized the largest rally for affordable housing in decades.

"How can people live in the city without affordable housing?" asked United Federation of Teachers president Randi Weingarten, who was also the head of the powerful Municipal Labor Committee. Pointing out how difficult it is for children to learn or teachers to teach if either or both lack adequate housing, Weingarten said, "The mayor talks a lot about making the city a great place to live. But it can't just be a great place to live for millionaires or billionaires."

Lillian Roberts, head of District Council 37, the city's largest public employee union, called affordable housing "one of the most pressing needs in New York City today."[8] Lewis pointed out that, "for the first time, you have the building trades joining with the community because they are the ones who erect the city's housing and they can't even afford to live in it. It's their issue too. It's tremendous."

As the rally ended and the crowd began to disperse, Brooklyn's Rev. Herbert Daughtry, who was in discussions with Lewis about Atlantic Yards, shouted, "We will not quit. We will not give up. Go tell Mayor Bloomberg. Go tell Governor Pataki. Tell every legislator. Every lawmaker. Go tell it everywhere. We will not stop. We will not give up until every New Yorker has a house to live in. When you go to sleep tonight, dream housing. When you get up in the morning, think housing!"

In March 2005, Ratner, his right-hand man Bruce Bender, a fast-talking charmer, and his press aide, Lupè Todd, set up a meeting with Kest and Lewis at a Starbucks across from Councilwoman James's district office to try to finalize negotiations (James was still leading the opposition to Atlantic Yards). Joining them was the prominent *New York Daily News* columnist Errol Louis. When James walked into the coffee shop, she looked surprised to see Kest and Lewis. ACORN had supported James's election in 2003, but here were their leaders meeting with her arch opponent, Ratner. Why were they meeting here? James wondered if a deal was in the works.

Soon after this meeting, and after a year of negotiations, ACORN struck an unprecedented deal with Ratner. Mayor Michael Bloomberg endorsed it. The centerpiece was the 50 percent set-aside for affordable housing in one of the world's most expensive cities. Never in any U.S. city had a private developer built a large apartment project—an integrated, mixed-income, planned residential community—where half the residents paid market rate rents and lived side by side with the other half, whose housing was subsidized. It was rare for low-income community groups to be part of a planning process for a large development. It was exceedingly rare for the developer to agree to sign a legally binding agreement. As Lewis would write in a letter to the magazine *City Limits*: "In an era of increasing housing segregation, Atlantic Yards will be one of the only neighborhoods in Brooklyn where families of all backgrounds will be able to really live and grow together. That's because ACORN insisted, and Forest City Ratner agreed, that the affordable units be spread throughout every rental building at random on every floor. In Atlantic Yards, if the elevator works for the rich folks, it will work for the poor folks. For the first time in a project like this, low-, middle-, and upper-income people will live—literally—together. And unless you put your pay stub on your front door, your neighbor will never know whether your unit is market price or below."[9]

Potential Benefits for ACORN

The agreement with Ratner and his Forest City partners embodied in a Community Benefits Agreement (CBA) would provide poor and working-class people with more affordable housing, more cultural activities, and more jobs. In the convoluted jargon of housing subsidy programs, the agreement guaranteed that units would be affordable to families at five income levels-—very low, low, moderate, low middle, and high middle. Twenty percent (900 units) would be reserved for families making less than $31,400 a year; Of that group, 136 units would be reserved for families making less than $25,120 a year. Thirty percent (1,350 units) would be reserved for families with incomes up to $100,480 for a four-person household. "Tiering is a critical component of the program," said Speliotis, director of New York ACORN's housing corporation. "Without it, developers will rent to those families with the highest incomes, those closer to $100,000, not $30,000." Speliotis insisted that ACORN be given the responsibility of marketing the units. "Nobody is going to care as much as ACORN that the appropriate people are marketed to, reached and housed," she said.

Rents would be subsidized by the New York City Housing Development Corporation, a state public-benefit corporation that planned to use a combination of bonds and reserves from investments to finance the subsidies.

To keep the displacement rate low, the agreement stipulated that displaced property owners would be fairly compensated and that displaced tenants would be given a new, comparable apartment at their existing rent in the new complex. Minority-owned and women-owned construction firms would receive 20 and 10 percent respectively of the construction contracts, and public housing residents and low-income people from the immediate area would have priority for any jobs.

Ratner also promised that space would be set aside for a health clinic and day-care center and that the arena would serve as a community resource, housing high school and collegiate sports, games, tournaments, graduations, and community activities. He would later agree to build an additional six hundred to a thousand affordable condo units either on or off the project site, significantly increasing in the number of for-sale units available to working families in Brooklyn.

ACORN wasn't the only player in the negotiations. Among the seven other signatories of the agreement were the Downtown Brooklyn Neighborhood Alliance, led by the prominent civil rights activist and pastor of House of the Lord Church Rev. Herbert Daughtry, and the New York State Association of Minority Contractors. The eight groups were essentially made up of black members. James Caldwell, the president of Brooklyn's BUILD (Brooklyn United in Leadership Development), said it would be a "conspiracy against blacks" if Forest City did not win the right to build Atlantic Yards.[10]

At a press conference on May 19, 2005, ACORN, represented by Lewis, along with New York City mayor Bloomberg and Ratner, announced the agreement. Lewis was known for expressing her activism with a potent personal and theatrical flair, from her clothes—lapis lazuli earrings and matching gold-trimmed gown—to near-poetic turns of phrase (she once contrasted brownstone people, yuppies, to brown people). She had accused Bloomberg's administration of "educational racism" during a fight over school-staffing issues in 2003, but on this day she grabbed the mayor's head between her hands and publicly sealed the deal with a kiss.

After the press conference, Lewis said she believed that this deal would have a domino effect, because it would be used as a model to show other developers that the interests and needs of the local community can be served. Few people with experience in grassroots work thought that ACORN could have won any more concessions. On the progressive DMI Blog, Brad Lander, the director of the Pratt Institute, a leading authority on community development, and a critic of Atlantic Yards wrote: "[ACORN] did better than I thought they would."

But most of the opponents of the project—the community groups representing existing residents and small businesses—thought that, if anything, ACORN had compromised too much. While many of the critics applauded ACORN's housing plan, they thought the project was fundamentally flawed. Tish James, who continued to lead the opposition, felt she was left out of the negotiations and did not believe this was the best agreement ACORN could have gotten.

A Polarized Battleground

Opponents would gather around the most vocal and effective adversary of the Atlantic Yards, Develop Don't Destroy Brooklyn (DDDB), which was led by Daniel Goldstein, a former graphic designer in his early thirties, the son of an investment fund manager. Goldstein had bought a condo on Pacific Street overlooking the defunct rail yards. When he saw a "This Neighborhood Is Condemned," poster pasted on a lamppost, he became anxious and determined to stop the development.

Goldstein suspected, with some justification, that ACORN's allies were what he called "shell organizations."[11] For example, according to a report in the *New York*

Daily News, BUILD had no membership income for 2004 and only $10,000 in revenues. For 2005, however, the group reported a whopping increase in its budget to $2.5 million and another $2.5 million for 2006. Most of that came from Forest City Ratner. Just two of the eight signatories to the agreement—ACORN and the New York State Association of Minority Contractors—existed as incorporated entities before the negotiations. What Goldstein did not understand was that ACORN's deep roots were sufficient to give the Atlantic Yards project street credibility.

Goldstein called the CBA process a "sweetheart, back-room deal that bypasses the democratic public approval process."[12] To some extent, he was correct on that score as well. Because Forest City Ratner was building on state-owned property, it was exempt from the usual approval process. As a longtime ACORN ally, Ron Shiffman, wrote in opposing the project: "A private developer shouldn't be allowed to drive the disposition of publicly owned or controlled land without a participatory planning process setting the conditions for the disposition of that land."[13]

The big issue for the opposition was eminent domain and displacement.[14] While Ratner had first announced that only 100 people would have their homes taken by eminent domain, DDDB conducted a door-to-door survey that found the number closer to 850. Many homeowners said there was no excuse for government to take their property just so a big time developer who made large campaign contributions could run roughshod over their property rights. A young architect who had lived in the neighborhood for ten years and was a potential victim of eminent domain was quoted in a community meeting saying, "This is an abuse of eminent domain. If they can take my home under these pretenses, they can take anyone's."

Goldstein soon became the only tenant in his building—the only person listed on the outside buzzer. When he left the building, the elevator stayed on the first floor until he returned. "They can't build this project without my little apartment, and we have a very strong legal case," he would insist. "Owning this condo gives me more power than the City Council."[15]

For a while, despite the opposition, it looked like Ratner would get the government approvals and vindicate ACORN's decision to partner with him. But Ratner, FCP, and ACORN had underestimated Goldman's tenacity. After three years of assembling in living rooms and church basements, Goldstein's group began to gain allies such as the Pratt Institute Center for Community and Environmental Development and another longtime ACORN ally, David Dyson, the pastor of Lafayette Avenue Presbyterian Church in Fort Greene, whose church had provided the space for ACORN's first office in 1982. Said Dyson: "We're trying to prevent the misuse of eminent domain, trying to increase the number of affordable housing units, trying to decrease the number of high rise luxury office buildings. Those are the kinds of issues that a community group should have, but the Reverend Daughtry—who's also an old friend—and our friends at ACORN are trying to cut a personal deal so that they can be brokers over whatever little piece or crumb of this pie falls from Ratner's table."[16] Goldstein also used a smart public relations ploy, getting a bandwagon of local celebrities and authors to join the opposition, including Heath Ledger, Jonathan Lethem, and Steve Buscemi.[17]

Just when it looked like Atlantic would move closer to fruition, something unexpected occurred. On July 19, the Empire State Development Corporation (ESDC) gave its nod of approval for what had grown from a $2.5 billion to a $4.2 billion project and released a 1,400-page environmental impact statement. The state's environmental impact study laid out all the potential effects of the proposed Atlantic Yards project for the first time, and to the opponents they weren't pretty. The project would worsen the already tangled web of traffic. It would cast a huge shadow over the surrounding neighborhoods, while street-level signs would create more neon at night in the concentrated commercial corridors on the project's western tip. By August, pacesetting opinion makers in the *Village Voice*, *New York* magazine, and the *New Yorker* characterized the project as a mistake, helping to galvanize the opposition.[18]

With public opinion appearing to go their way, Goldstein and his allies had two big opportunities to defeat Ratner's plan. They would have to mobilize their supporters in the upcoming September 2006 primary elections to send a message to pro-Yards Brooklyn politicians. Then they would have to mobilize their supporters at the October public hearings required by law. The elections did not go their way; the pro–Atlantic Yards candidates in two congressional districts won, while Goldstein's ally and an outspoken opponent of the project, Charles Barron, lost.

Class and Race

Tensions came to the boiling point at the public hearings. Supporters and opponents from unions, local block associations, community boards, and business groups filled the 880-seat auditorium at the New York City College of Technology in downtown Brooklyn. Both sides took turns applauding, booing, and interrupting one another. Opponents mounted a mordacious refrain of catcalls when borough president Marty Markowitz described the project as "a wonderful addition to Brooklyn."

Those supporting Atlantic Yards put the subtext of race front and center. A fifty-one-year-old Brooklyn resident advanced to the front of the hall. "I'm here to speak for the underprivileged, the people that don't get the opportunity to work, the brothers that just came over out of prison," he said. "Those who opposed the plan were not true Brooklynites." As to traffic congestion, he said, "That's nothing." But "stopping this project would force young black men into a life of crime." Staring at the opponents to Atlantic Yards, he said, "You go back up to Pleasantville." Like many black residents attending the hearing, he saw Atlantic Yards as a beacon of hope.

A few black leaders opposed the project, but most blacks in Brooklyn supported Atlantic Yards. Opposition leaders like Goldstein were clueless when it came to effectively reaching out to the older, more established network of black community activists. In May 2006, Goldstein had shot an e-mail message to a *Daily News* columnist, attacking ties between the groups that supported Atlantic Yards and what he termed their "wealthy white masters," referring to Ratner's corporation. The reporter publicized the message, stirring an outcry from Lewis and other black supporters. Goldstein made a half-hearted apology, calling his remarks "unfortunate." But the damage was done.

Nevertheless, opponents like Tish James, who is black, saw a cynical race ruse. She accused Ratner of intentionally stirring up racial divisions, typecasting upscale white residents as the main source of resistance and as numb to the needs of black Brooklynites. James and other critics may have been theoretically correct when they said that a better-planned project could provide more affordable housing, with less harmful impact on the area. But that option was not available.

Although Bertha Lewis emphasized the class issue, she did not shy away from the matter of race. On more than one occasion, she called her opponents "white liberals."[19] Although she would publicly apologize, in her heart it was partly about race.

In the urban trenches, race and class intersect. As Brad Lander, the director of the Pratt University Center for Community Development and an advocate for low-income housing, commented: "This is not about race per se. But when you layer on that the people who live near Atlantic Yards are more likely to be whiter and wealthier, and the people who live farther out are more likely to be people of color without good jobs or housing, the race elements have become stronger."[20]

According to census data, the number of whites living near the project site—in neighborhoods like Fort Greene, Boerum Hill, and Prospect Heights—had grown steadily in recent years. Those new arrivals were affluent and highly educated, especially compared with mostly black residents of the nearby public housing projects who were concerned about jobs. As white yuppies boosted the area's median income, they forced up housing prices. In Fort Greene, for example, which bordered the project site to the north, average apartment prices rose faster from 2004 to 2005 than in any other Brooklyn neighborhood. When Forest City sponsored an information session on July 2006 about the project's subsidized housing, the forum was packed with thousands of the area's black working-class and poor residents.

Controlling Gentrification

Lewis felt ACORN had no choice but to support the project. The housing crisis for the poor and working class was getting worse. Rents were sharply increasing. More professionals settled in the outer boroughs. A February 2006 survey released by New York City housing officials confirmed what ACORN already knew. While household income fell by 6.3 percent from 2001 to 2004, the median monthly rent increased by 5.4 percent from 2002 to 2005. As Brad Lander said, "Rents are up, low-rent units are almost impossible to find, and people are struggling to pay the housing bills."[21]

For years, ACORN had tried to stem the tide of gentrification. But the combined forces of market pressures, real estate industry political influence, and the political elite's undermining of rent control fed gentrification. New York rent control had been so watered down by political compromises that the number of tenants protected by its regulations declined each year. In addition, owners of New York's famed Mitchell-Lama buildings, a program which spurred affordable working-class housing, were withdrawing from state regulations so they could increase rents.

A March 2006 ACORN study only exacerbated ACORN's concern. The study examined eighty-seven new development projects in various stages of progress in downtown Brooklyn, containing 5,934 housing units. ACORN's report found that only 201 units, or just 3 percent of the total, were affordable for moderate-income people, and only 4 percent for low-income families. In almost all those projects, city tax dollars were subsidizing luxury development in the form of 421a and J-51 tax abatements for purchasers of luxury housing. The result: between 1990 and 2000, the African American population of the neighborhood that included Brooklyn's downtown, Fort Greene, Brooklyn Heights, and Boerum Hill decreased by 17.2 percent.[22]

Francis Byrd, a Democratic district leader from the area who opposed Atlantic Yards, understood ACORN's dilemma: "Certainly, there's a sense among many folks who have seen this happen before that putting up a fight with a developer won't get you anywhere. So whatever little you can get is the best you can hope for."[23]

In December 2006, supporters and opponents turned their focus to the coming vote by the Public Authorities Control Board (PACB), which would have the final say. This obscure board required approval from all three members—Senate majority leader Joseph Bruno, assembly speaker Sheldon Silver, and Gov. George Pataki's appointee. Pataki, whose term ended December 31, was an enthusiastic supporter of the project.

Ratner had made an earlier concession to Silver when he cut the amount of Atlantic Yards office space, so as not to compete for tenants that Silver would rather see in his downtown Manhattan district. Now, as most people were preparing for their December 2006 holiday vacations or engaged in last-minute Christmas shopping, opponents pressured Silver to postpone final approval. DDDB delivered thousands of letters from city residents to Pataki, Bruno, and Silver urging them to delay approval until their lawsuit was finalized. On December 19, on the steps of City Hall, several civic organizations, including the Municipal Art Society, the Regional Plan Association, the Citizens Union, and the Natural Resources Defense Council, rallied for a postponement of the final vote based on the project's lack of financial transparency and failure to address traffic and other environmental concerns.

The next day, the PACB voted to approve Atlantic Yards. To sweeten the deal, Forest City offered an eleventh-hour concession. At least two hundred of the market-rate condominiums would be subsidized and made affordable to first-time homeowners, and $3 million would go toward improving parks near the development. For Lewis the approvals were just the beginning of the end. The deal with Ratner helped ACORN organizationally and politically, which would add weight to ACORN's next battle.

Goldstein was not prepared to give up without a fight; he would now rely on his lawsuits. The opposition's criticism had merit. A private developer shouldn't be allowed to drive the disposition of public property. But ACORN was not powerful enough to stop Ratner's project, force a different type of planning process, and then guarantee the different process would bring a better result. In fact, urban development planning was usually less than ideal, and the poor were typically left out.

While Brooklyn had become the place of choice for many upscale households, more than 20 percent of its 2.5 million residents lived below the poverty line. In a place where the working poor and even the middle class were already being driven out by rent gouging and gentrification, arguments from the gentrifying class about its right to preserve its neighborhood were not very compelling to ACORN. As Greg

Blankinship, cochair of ACORN's Prospect Heights/Crown Heights chapter had argued all along: "Downtown Brooklyn is growing, and if it's growing, let's get a piece of the action. Let's get something for the low-income community."[24]

This battle over Brooklyn reflected the tensions between the legitimate concerns of middle-class professionals who wanted their vision of the city to reign, and those of the poor—who needed the new jobs and housing and the integrated neighborhood that a big development project like Ratner's could provide. For her part, Lewis believed her coalition spoke for the majority of the community. In a conservative era, when government had substantially withdrawn from supporting the poor, community groups had to wrench concessions directly from private corporations. "We've been in that community for twenty-two years, while a lot of organizations have come and gone," Lewis explained to her opponents. "Our mission in life and who we are is about protecting that community." She bristled at their self-righteousness. "Most of those people opposed appear to be earlier gentrifyers," she said. "We just think that folks who have been part of the gentrification of the community don't get to define the community."

New York Daily News columnist Errol Louis captured the feeling of many blacks and certainly of ACORN's staff and members: "The most interesting and least-reported story behind the final state approval of the $4 billion Atlantic Yards project this week is the emergence in Brooklyn of a pro-development coalition of private-sector builders and black working-class residents who are leading a tenacious fight to bring jobs and housing to the borough. Standing in the path of progress are middle-class civic groups whose mostly white leaders profess concern for low-income New Yorkers—and even claim to speak for them—but shed the illusion of liberal compassion the minute the poor folk get uppity and start negotiating their own deals for the future of their families and communities."[25]

By the fall of 2008, delays in Atlantic Yards caused by the recent economic downturn, the credit crunch, and legal challenges had emboldened the project's critics. They claimed Ratner had consistently overpromised regarding the project's progress and the number of affordable housing units that would be built. With the basketball arena scheduled to go up before the affordable housing and the ongoing increases in costs, speculation began to grow about the future of the project.

Bertha Lewis was angry and hopeful. "My members would like this to get done as originally conceived. We have to deal with the reality of the lawsuits that have delayed development and the changing economic circumstances. We don't speculate about this. It is work that is actually going on, and anybody who's ever done development would understand." Forest City has demolished buildings and has let out over $42 million worth of construction contracts, with nearly 50 percent going to women and minority firms. "We are confident we have the clout to push the developer to make good on his promises of the affordable housing component," said Lewis.

Unlike many of the Atlantic Yards opponents, ACORN was not an ad hoc, one-issue organization. It did not pin all its hopes for the future on Atlantic Yards. If the project prevails, this victory, although significant, will be a just another step in a long-distance run to a better life for the poor and working class.[26]

In the event that the 50 percent nonmarket housing agreement gets undermined, ACORN will still have gained, because it has garnered lots of publicity, shown elected officials that ACORN can mobilize a constituency, and revealed to the business community that ACORN can be pragmatic in order to win victories that benefit the poor. In addition, ACORN has potentially raised the bar regarding the percentage of affordable housing required in private developments. With the money ACORN raised from Ratner, it employed more organizers to fight for more victories. ACORN hired two organizers to recruit new members from a list of thousands of people seeking affordable housing who attended various events paid for by Ratner. Some of these folks will join ACORN's army of activists and help fight to win the next battle.[27]

The fight over Atlantic Yards was typical of ACORN's mix of political pragmatism and radical ideas. Unlike ideologues on both ends of the political spectrum, ACORN knew that the perfect is often the enemy of the good. It understood the benefits of compromise. "Rather than wait until something happens to us," said Lewis, "we go out and help shape the results." ACORN (the activist, poor people's organization) and Ratner (the rich developer) found a way to work together for the common good.

The battle in Brooklyn tested ACORN's pragmatism and power. Suddenly, however, a titanic juggernaut in the Deep South would force Rathke and ACORN to take on a fight it did not choose. The opposition extended far beyond local politicians and middle-class community activists. It would include the Bush administration, uncaring bureaucrats, and greedy speculators. Hurricane Katrina would unleash devastation more forceful than any ACORN had gone up against before.

Chapter 14

Then, Overnight, It Is Washed Away

As Hurricane Katrina headed toward New Orleans, Dorothy Stukes, a lifelong New Orleans resident, decided to stay. She'd been bunking at a friend's place in the Third Ward not far from Charity Hospital, where her sister Ruth was recovering from two major surgeries. Twelve inches of Ruth's intestine had been removed, and Dorothy did not want to leave her sister behind.

On the afternoon of August 28, 2005, Stukes wavered in her decision to ignore Mayor Ray Nagin's call for residents to evacuate. But she didn't have a car, and the mayor didn't have a plan to evacuate people without cars. The next day, after ferocious wind rattled her house, she figured the storm had blown over. But around two o'clock that day, water began pouring in and kept rising. Stukes worried that if she didn't abandon the house and seek higher ground, she and her friend Adam Johnson would drown. The levees separating Lake Pontchartrain from New Orleans had been breached and the city was flooding.

Finally Stukes and Johnson decided they would try to reach Interstate 10, situated high above the water line. Only five foot four, Stukes began wading through chest-high water. Her dislocated hip and arthritic knees throbbed. After walking an hour and half, she flagged down an SUV labeled "Homeland Security" and pleaded for a ride. The white driver said no. Stukes saw a bottle of water sitting on his dashboard and begged the driver at least for the water so she could take her medicine. The driver refused, but a woman passenger said, "Ma'am, take this water." The car roared off.

Stukes and Johnson finally reached Interstate 10 and quickly joined welfare mothers, nurses, teachers, and service workers trapped in the nearby Superdome. She had fled the danger, but her future prospects were uncertain. She suffers from diabetes, hypertension, and high cholesterol and had few resources to fall back on, as was the case with most New Orleans working poor. She had no savings accounts to pay for a motel room, no car or access to public transportation, and no insurance to cover her personal belongings and the house she shared with her sister in Metairie, a suburb of New Orleans.

At the Superdome, there was no official help and no one seemed to be in charge. Most of the people Stukes met were black and worked in the low-paying service jobs that prop up the New Orleans economy—they picked up the garbage, changed the sheets in hotel beds, and made po'boys. Stukes had worked for fifteen years as a security counselor for the Orleans Parish Schools, where she assisted kids with family problems who were physically threatened by other kids or were victims of school theft. She earned $18,000 a year before taxes. Her friend Adam had worked for twenty-one years in housekeeping for the New Orleans Hilton.

The Superdome had no air-conditioning, electricity, or running water. It stank of human waste, and the troops refused to open the doors to let in fresh air. The heavy hurricane winds had peeled away parts of the roof, leaving two holes to provide the only ventilation. Stukes tried her cell phone for emergency numbers, but it didn't work. In Washington, D.C., the head of the Federal Emergency Management Agency (FEMA), Michael Brown, told the White House he had everything under control. President Bush himself seemed so unconcerned that his staff felt compelled to prepare a DVD of network newscasts to stir him into action.

Stukes heard the mayor on the radio plead with the federal government to "get off your asses and do something, and let's fix the biggest goddamn crisis in the history of this country." But other radio reports gave Stukes the impression that the mayor was confused. Stukes's fear competed with her anger. Our government let us down, she thought. "You have an earthquake in Pakistan and they're over there the next day," she said to an acquaintance. "And we're in the Superdome without air, no way to use the bathroom. They can send help over there, but they can't save their own people? We are taxpayers." She couldn't believe it could take so long to ship in supplies and remove people to safe, secure shelter.[1]

Above all, Stukes was concerned about her family. She couldn't locate her hospitalized sister, her son or her daughter, or her five grandchildren. Nor did she know what happened to the house in Metairie. (She would soon learn that the kitchen ceiling and roof had collapsed, leaving the house uninhabitable.)

On September 1, buses finally arrived to take the survivors to Houston, where they would join 150,000 other evacuees. Stukes became separated from her friend Adam. Before boarding the bus, she was able to charge her cell phone long enough to check her voicemail messages and learn that her daughter and grandchildren were safe. Still, she longed to be with them.

Dorothy's rage at the utter failure of the authorities to protect her and her loved ones competed with her desire just to go home and be with her family. She worried that she would not get her job back because the area where she worked was flooded out. She read that the City of New Orleans was broke. She was broke herself. She didn't know what to expect in Houston. It soon became clear that like so many of the poor from New Orleans, she had lost her job and her health insurance with it. How was she going to take care of herself? she wondered. Stukes would cry, settle down, and then get angry again.

The head of the organization that would soon channel Stokes's fury and give her hope, Wade Rathke, was attending an ACORN planning meeting in Denver with his partner, Beth, as the storm gathered on the weekend of August 26, Like millions of Americans with livelihoods on the Gulf Coast, they flipped the remote between the Weather Channel and CNN. They reluctantly agreed to lay out $350, a significant sum to them, to put Beth on a plane to New Orleans so she could go to their house in the Bywater neighborhood to help their twenty-four-year-old son, Chaco, seal up the house and evacuate before the hurricane hit. After Beth and Chaco packed their personal belongings, they joined the traffic jams trying to get out of New Orleans. They inched forward for the next ten hours, finding a shelter at the Baptist Church in Laurel, Mississippi, a hundred miles away.

Wade called home to encourage his eighty-four-year-old father to clear out. His father was stubborn and rarely took Wade's advice. "We're veterans. We don't cut and run," he said. "That's for tourists and flatlanders." Just before the storm struck, his father reluctantly changed his mind and with his wife and Wade's brother, Dale, headed for a friend's house in Jackson, Mississippi. Wade's twenty-year-old daughter, Dine, now organizing in Florida, had been so busy she had just realized the potential danger. As her e-mails started shooting in, Wade could feel her anxiety a thousand miles away. That night the hurricane slammed into New Orleans.

To the Rathkes and everyone else in New Orleans, after even the worst of hurricanes, you were back home in a couple of days. Not this time. The family scattered everywhere. Dale relocated to Houston, at first staying with friends and then in a hotel room provided by Ameriquest, a national mortgage lender and now one of ACORN's affordable-housing partners. Wade's parents moved to Kansas City to stay with relatives, where Ed was rushed to a local hospital to receive medical attention for his heart. Wade and Beth moved to a friend's house in the Spanish Town section of Baton Rouge, Louisiana; in a week they'd move again.

Not only was Rathke's personal life in turmoil, the enormity of the challenge of Katrina was beginning to sink in. Feeling despondent, he wrote in a memo to himself:

> Local organizing starts on the block and moves from house to house, apartment to apartment as families come together in the neighborhood. People do come and go . . . but the address is there. The family that leaves is replaced by another one, not so unlike the one who left. After years of organizing, we produce lists on voter turnout; lists for those who attend meetings; lists for those who got involved in our issues or attended a fundraiser; lists of people we made phone calls to; and of course, our dues payers and supporters and friends.
>
> And the field of folks are plowed over and over to a richer and richer yield of action and power. A database pushes them all together in categories that allow leaders to survey, committees to call and assemble, and organizers to constantly massage, visit, and move. This rich gumbo produces a mass membership, such as the New Orleans ACORN chapter. Then, overnight, it is washed away.

New Orleans ACORN

For almost thirty years, the members of ACORN and SEIU Local 100, under Rathke's leadership, had been immersed in New Orleans's civic, economic, and political life, fighting for higher wages and against bank rip-offs like predatory lending, blocking the privatization of the municipal water department, and engaging in dozens of other campaigns to make the city livable for its working poor. The list of achievements was long. New Orleans ACORN forced landlords to stop discriminating against the disabled. As part of ACORN's national campaign, the New Orleans chapter taught thousands of working poor how to benefit from the federal Earned Income Tax Credit, which reduces taxes by providing workers with up to $3,846 in extra cash. ACORN partnered with banks to encourage home ownership. A local Whitney Bank vice president explained: "ACORN finds the buyers and trains them. We provide permanent financing for the graduates of its home-buying program at below-market rates." Although these were subprime loans, the default rates were no higher than conventional loans.

In 2000, Beth had become the head organizer for Louisiana and hired a high school teacher, Stephen Bradberry, as the lead New Orleans ACORN organizer. A tall, lean, and handsome African American, Bradberry was looking for a job that would reflect his values and help make New Orleans a better place for the poor to live. His youthful appearance and slight smile often gave people the impression that he was not serious, but he transformed the New Orleans chapter with his energy, vision, and people skills. He built a flying squad of local leaders who negotiated an ACORN partnership with a local university that got New Orleans city officials to ban the dry sanding of dangerous lead-based paint in a low-income residential neighborhood. He organized a citywide education campaign that led to a greater voice for parents in the local schools. Bradberry also set up after-school programs in five public schools. Despite the combined power of the city's business and political establishments, ACORN and Bradberry led a successful ballot initiative to raise the minimum wage in the city by a dollar an hour, a campaign that solidified ACORN's reputation as a David willing to do battle with local Goliaths. In 2005, Bradberry received the prestigious Robert F. Kennedy Human Rights Award for his work with ACORN.

ACORN's reputation as a political force in New Orleans grew when its PAC helped elect several candidates to office, including Marlin Gusman, who was elected sheriff in 2004. In the spring of 2005, New Orleans ACORN was awarded a certificate by the City Council in a special ceremony for its work in the neighborhoods.[2]

The national organization had grown to more than two hundred thousand members and a staff of more than five hundred working in various regional and local offices in more than eighty cities. ACORN's New Orleans chapter had grown to more than nine thousand dues-paying families by early 2005. Sixty-six people—the local staff as well as some of ACORN's national staff—worked in a crowded two-story wood-frame house, a former funeral home that now served as the New Orleans office. It was remarkable that ACORN had accomplished so much in New Orleans given its weak economy. From 1980 through 2003, New Orleans lost more than 50,000 jobs (from 339,953 to 279,056).[3] Bradberry was getting ready to flex ACORN's muscles in the upcoming mayoral election. Then the hurricane hit and ACORN became unmoored, its members lost, the office flooded, its staff displaced.

After the Hurricane

New Orleans became a city in exile. Of the 485,000 residents before Katrina, more than 356,000—mostly low- and moderate-income families—were now part of the great New Orleans diaspora. Much of the American public were glued to their TVs, shocked by the images of starving, exhausted, unkempt people fleeing the Crescent City, having believed that such scenes were confined to far-off places like Kosovo or Sudan. ACORN members along with hundreds of thousands of others who had fled—many like Dorothy Stukes with just the clothes on their backs—were also glued to television news, as well as Google maps, cell phones, and newspapers, trying to discover how much water had flooded their bedrooms and when they could return.

To the tourist, New Orleans consisted of just two neighborhoods, the Garden District and the French Quarter. But what would happen to the modest Creole cottages of Faubourg Marigny, where ACORN's headquarters was located? Or the shotguns and camelbacks scattered throughout neighborhoods such as Bywater where Rathke lived and the Lower Ninth Ward, described by reporter Roberta Gratz as "woven together by a network rich in family history, social connections, and proximity to relatives and friends."[4]

The national office was in chaos. Most of the operations had to relocate to Baton Rouge. ACORN had no plan for coping with such a disaster. When Rathke obtained a map of the flood zones that overlaid ACORN's membership, it showed that the neighborhoods that Katrina made famous, such as Gentilly and Hollygrove and New Orleans East and the Lower Ninth Ward, were all ACORN strongholds. Several ACORN members lived on nearly every block in the Lower Ninth Ward. Rathke, now living with a half-dozen ACORN organizers in a crash pad just outside Baton Rouge, told Beth: "The addresses may be there or they may have washed away. Phones no longer exist, rendering hundreds of call and walk lists immediately moot. Cell phone towers are down and could be for months. Do databases even hold cell numbers? And how many of our families in New Orleans even have cell phones? Few ACORN members have e-mail. Almost any tool we used in the past to connect people with each other is useless. Beth, how do we find nine thousand families?" How was the organization to give voice to members who were now scattered across Louisiana, Texas, Mississippi, and elsewhere? How could ACORN remain a force for the poor when no one could find or communicate with many of its members?

Yet ACORN had an advantage that no other antipoverty organization in New Orleans possessed: a national organization with dues-paying members, elected leaders, a skilled staff, and seven hundred local chapters in more than eighty cities. Even though the New Orleans office was in disarray, ACORN had two national support offices in New York and Washington, D.C., that housed its fundraising and lobbying operations. It also had local chapter offices, activists, and organizers in cities that had suddenly become refuges for the Katrina diaspora. ACORN's people were able to find and house members in Houston, Dallas, San Antonio, Little Rock, Atlanta, Birmingham, and as far away as Seattle, Vancouver, and New York.

ACORN had another asset: it was decentralized, with a highly skilled staff capable of operating on automatic pilot without orders from the national office. Rathke's brother, Dale (a graduate of Princeton, brilliant with electronics and numbers) along with a trusted aide and volunteers from the national staff, relocated to the Houston chapter, set up a communications department, and started running supply lines into ACORN's temporary Baton Rouge headquarters for computers, cell phones, paper, pencils, and Post-its.

Bradberry learned that text messaging works even when cell signals are down telephonically. From ACORN's temporary headquarters in Baton Rouge, he began to text members who had cell phones and quickly received two hundred replies from all around the country. Joe Stafford, twenty-five, a member of ACORN's Uptown New Orleans chapter, and his girlfriend, Carmen, had fled to Houston with their two children, ages ten months and two years, after Stafford lost his father in Katrina's floodwaters. They were staying at a two-bedroom apartment with four other families when he received a message from Bradberry offering relocation aid. Stafford messaged back: "I watched my father die . . . and had to leave his body behind. I don't know where my mother is either. . . . I think she got left in New Orleans. I don't think she left the house, she loved that house, wouldn't leave it. ACORN helped her get that house. That's how we joined ACORN, by getting a house." In a few days he and his family were safely housed with Houston ACORN member Tarsha Jackson. He later said: "I'm so glad we got in touch with ACORN. When I saw that text message on my phone from ACORN, it was a blessing."

A message board on the ACORN website allowed those who had access to computers to reach out to each other and message back and forth. Others were attracted to the site to support ACORN's survival and its work to provide assistance to Katrina victims.

Ten housing counselors from the ACORN Housing Corporation, based in Chicago and elsewhere, flew to Houston to work at the Convention Center and at various hotels that FEMA was using to house evacuees. They assisted evacuees with financial and housing matters, especially those dealing with mortgages, available credit, and their entitlements under the emergency. Working with Winning Connections, Inc. (WCI), a voter contact and telecommunications company, ACORN quickly developed a phone script and a toll-free hotline to help homeowners obtain mortgage relief and prevent foreclosures and evictions. WCI also helped ACORN deliver emergency calls to Houston residents, informing them of the official call for voluntary evacuation ahead of Hurricane Rita.

When buses pulled into the Astrodome in Houston, ACORN members often greeted them, waving ACORN flags and wearing ACORN T-shirts, and quickly identifying members who had been trapped in the New Orleans Superdome.

Leader Recruitment in Houston

Houston was not New Orleans. Where the Big Easy was traditional, slow-paced, and sometimes stereotyped as a Mecca of hedonism, Houston was huge, sprawling, modern, fast-paced, and growing. Houston had developed a vibrant economy around international port trade and related services, while New Orleans had invested in a large port in the Gulf of Mexico and a low-wage economy based on the arts, tourism, and gambling.[5] Bill White, the mayor of Houston, had a reputation for making Houston a safe, entrepreneurial city. New Orleans mayor Nagin did little to alter the city's reputation as the city that doesn't work.

No one was waving flags to greet Dorothy Stukes when she got off the bus at Houston's Reliant Convention Center, next to the Astrodome. One of the first refugees Dorothy encountered told her she had no intention of returning to New Orleans: "They can have New Orleans. It's a toxic-waste dump now." Dorothy, who had found some of her family, desperately wanted to return. Meanwhile, she moved into a four-bedroom apartment on Bennington Road in northeast Houston in a modern building with her daughter, Tamara Small, her son-in-law, Andrew Williams, and their three children.

Soon after Dorothy arrived in Houston, a friend told her about a group called ACORN that was helping people. Stukes immediately met with Ginny Goldman, ACORN Texas's head organizer.[6] Goldman asked, "What happened?" As tears streamed down her face, Dorothy recounted the trauma she had suffered. "It was like being in Iraq without a gun," she said. Goldman, a ten-year ACORN veteran trained by Madeline Talbott, sensed a special quality in Dorothy. She was feisty and friendly, with a story that she told passionately but without self-pity. Goldman thought Stukes might have the vigor and resilience necessary to be a successful activist leader.

"What are you going to do?" asked Goldman.

"I want to do something," Stukes said. "I want to help. I couldn't imagine this could happen in a city in this country, in 2005."

"Well, ACORN is trying to do something for the Katrina survivors. This won't be on the front pages forever. We need to build an organization. You want to help?" asked Goldman, testing Stukes's readiness for leadership. Some people are broken by loss and trauma and some people grow stronger. Stukes was gaining strength. She volunteered to help.

When Goldman met Dorothy Stukes, she saw how disheartened she was. Goldman knew from experience and training that this discouragement came from anger rooted in powerlessness. She had to help Dorothy turn her anger into action that would produce results. Goldman's job was to guide recruits toward the enemy, the people and institutions who had the power to fix the problems that poor people confronted. For Stukes, this was easy; she knew her enemies. They included President Bush and his cronies in Washington and the business world, FEMA and its uncaring staff based in Louisiana, and local officials, including the mayor and his corporate pals. After listening to Stukes's story, Goldman did something that all ACORN organizers are trained to do: she provoked her, and raised her expectations of what she could achieve. Goldman had to steer Stukes's anger toward collective action.

Like other ACORN members, Stukes had no leadership experience, so she immediately signed on to a crash on-the-job training course with Toni McElroy, who had been elected president of Texas ACORN in 2004. A lifelong Houston resident and a history major at the University of Houston, McElroy had retired from her job as a management and customer-service trainer in the Houston Public Works Department in 2002. Her father, George, a Korean War veteran, championed the rights of minorities and the poor as editor of the oldest African American newspaper in Texas. Her mother, Lucinda, taught school. Both parents instilled in Toni a lifelong love of books. Now and then she relied on Aeschylus and Sophocles to help her navigate the complex world of community organizing.

Goldman, McElroy, and Stukes planned a September 9 town hall meeting in Houston. With Goldman and McElroy, Stukes went to the shelters and apartments where the evacuees lived and distributed flyers that said that the purpose of the meeting was "to get information to survivors, hold elected officials accountable and to help rebuild the New Orleans community."[7]

After some coaxing by McElroy, Stukes agreed to cochair the September meeting. At that gathering at Mount Calvary Lutheran Church in a gritty area considered Houston's toughest black ghetto, hundreds of Katrina survivors expressed their rage and grief about immediate needs for housing and jobs and about the possibility of returning to their homes in New Orleans. McElroy, an African America woman with silver streaks running through her black braided hair, set the tone of the meeting. "There is strength in numbers, and you have a strong organization to depend on and that you can participate in so your voice can be heard."

Stukes began to find her voice. She and the other members urged the meeting participants to help build a survivors organization by joining, petitioning, door knocking, and taking part in public actions. "If we talk to the right people, it won't happen again," said Stukes. "We won't let it happen again. We need to speak up for ourselves. If you're poor like we are, they're going to slam a door in your face. If we fight together, they can't ignore us."

At this Katrina meeting, Houston's mayor White, who respected ACORN's work, took some of its ideas to heart. He committed to providing grocery cards to buy food for families sheltering survivors. (ACORN would become one of several groups distributing these cards.) White also agreed to halt evictions of families from local motels. The New Orleans evacuees were buoyed by their success at getting Mayor White to show up and then agree to meet their demands. The victory whetted their appetites and gave them a sense of their potential power. At the urging of Stukes and McElroy, those attending the meeting agreed to form a survivors association. Said one attendee, reflecting the mood of the group: "New Orleans is my home and I want to go back and rebuild my house. I want to be called a survivor."

Organizing a Diaspora

By the end of the first week of September, without a plan, Steve Kest continued to operate on automatic pilot in his New York office, sending out action alerts to ACORN's vast national e-mail list, conducting demonstrations, press events, and call-ins directed at congressional offices demanding the immediate relief and rescue of New Orleans residents. Local staff organized town hall meetings in several cities to identify survivors.

Rathke knew that ACORN had to respond to the immediate human needs for food, clothing, and shelter. He was pleased when he heard that ACORN people from Michigan, who organized a major relief effort, were driving a white Ford step van and making stops at ACORN offices in several cities as it traveled from Detroit to Houston, collecting relief supplies and donations for the ACORN Hurricane Recovery and Rebuilding Fund. After arriving in Houston, they traveled to shelters, churches, motels, and apartments housing hurricane survivors, bringing food, clothes, and medical assistance to evacuees. Meanwhile, thousands of ACORN members in cities across the country continued to open their homes to evacuees.

ACORN also needed a long-term New Orleans recovery plan, but Rathke was scared and confused. "At first I didn't know up from down," he would later confess. "I worried that New Orleans had become a biohazard zone, that houses would have to be demolished, and that it would be irresponsible to help people to return. I was at a loss about what to do, how to organize."

In Houston, Goldman was feeling overwhelmed. To add to her 24/7 job as head Texas organizer, she was helping Katrina survivors as well as organizing them into a fighting force. Soon after she met Stukes, Goldman called Rathke in a state of panic. "What should I do?" she asked. Rathke, whose own life was in chaos, said, "We're not sure. Just sign up members, go organize, do what you do and we'll figure it out as we go along." Confused yet empowered, Goldman would have to rely on her experience and instincts.

Like Rathke, she had to listen to the base, listen to other staff. Rathke assured her that a strategy would develop, slowly and organically. Goldman's Houston office was one of ACORN's largest, most aggressive and successful chapters. But two weeks after Katrina, it became evident that the Houston chapter couldn't continue its normal business as well as absorb the additional burden of helping the evacuees. Goldman had very little time to train and nurture a potential leader like Stukes. The crisis steadily replenished ACORN's membership, and its staff was working overtime to find housing and services for survivors. The press of events was overwhelming ACORN's capacity to influence policy, recruit new members, serve existing ones, support the existing leaders, and train new leaders.

Meanwhile, Rathke talked with as many members, staff, experts, and, in this case, survivors as he could. Among them was a longtime ACORN leader, Paul Fernandez, who was trying to prevent a foreclosure on his flooded home in the Lower Ninth Ward. "I want to return," said Fernandez. "That's what our organization should be doing—fighting to make sure we can return." Rathke and other organizers were hearing the same from other ACORN organizers, as well as from hundreds of evacuees.

Rathke and ACORN's leaders realized that ACORN immediately had to help the tens of thousands of displaced homeowners who, like Fernandez, were in danger of losing their homes due to foreclosure by banks. Most of these New Orleans refugees had lost their jobs and were scattered across Louisiana, Texas, Mississippi, and elsewhere, living in motels, shelters, apartment buildings and with relatives. ACORN organizers rushed to disaster shelters in Houston, Baton Rouge, and other cities to locate these mainly low-income Hispanic and African American homeowners and discover why their homes were being foreclosed when lenders had made highly publicized claims of mortgage relief after the hurricane.

What ACORN organizers discovered was dismaying but not surprising for anyone who has worked in low-income, racially segregated communities. Major lenders had given their middle-class customers ninety days or more to make mortgage payments, but many subprime lenders that had targeted low-income consumers were offering them mortgage relief for only one month.

To expose the industry's double standard, ACORN on September 22 released a report, "How the Sub-Prime Mortgage Industry Is Sandbagging Katrina-Affected Homeowners." After several newspapers and TV stations publicized the report,

ACORN—along with labor unions and consumer groups—demanded meetings with mainstream and subprime lenders and successfully negotiated plans to prevent foreclosures.[8]

While ACORN leaders and organizers began to discuss a strategy to make sure New Orleans residents would have the right and the capacity to return, they discovered that FEMA buses were pulling up at the shelters in Louisiana, outside New Orleans, enticing people to leave for Las Vegas, Utah, and elsewhere with promises of housing, jobs, a better life.

Tanya Harris, a large, energetic, outgoing African American, was living in an overcrowded Baton Rouge shelter when FEMA buses arrived to take people out of the state. She suspected that FEMA had no real plan to help folks once they arrived at their new destinations.[9] Before the storm, Tanya, thirty-three, had been a member as well as an off-and-on ACORN organizer. Her family had been longtime members in the Lower Ninth Ward. Right after the storm while living in the shelter, Tanya spotted Marie Hurt, a nine-year ACORN veteran, by recognizing the red ACORN T-shirt. Smiling broadly, she rushed up and hugged her.

Worried that FEMA was offering to take evacuees to some city where they had never been, where they didn't know anyone and didn't want to go, Tanya decided to organize an ACORN meeting at the shelter. A few people asked what her group was up to and told her they had no interest in starting a new life away from the only home some of them have ever known. Once word got around that ACORN, an organization known to some of the evacuees, was talking about going back to New Orleans, more and more residents got involved.

A few of the people who gathered said they heard that business owners and wealthy residents were being allowed back into the city daily and expressed anger that affluent families had already returned home. Tanya warned the folks not to get on the FEMA buses: "How do you know what's going to happen when we jump on that bus? We need to fight to get people what they need so we don't have to get on those buses, but can stay and rebuild a life here. That means living-wage jobs and trailers in New Orleans or as close to home as possible. FEMA needs to help us to keep in touch with people so we can come back." Tanya Harris liked action and making things happen. She easily remembered facts and could be counted on to make sound commonsense judgments. She rejoined ACORN's organizing staff and quickly became a New Orleans ACORN force in exile.

During September, amid the confusion, ACORN had managed to organize local and national press events and neighborhood petition drives in more than thirty-five cities. Its "Proposal for the Hurricane Recovery and Rebuilding" called for an independent Katrina commission and fair treatment by subprime lenders, who had not offered displaced homeowners the same relief as banks.[10] ACORN members even met with many senior congressional leaders in Washington, D.C., pushing for the right of survivors to have a say in the rebuilding process. They received a respectful and even enthusiastic welcome in many quarters.

To many opinion-makers and TV commentators, the breakdown of President Bush's magic charm as a result of the administration's response to Katrina seemed to open the way for a new national agenda on many issues, especially poverty. Rathke,

ACORN, and the victims of Katrina couldn't wait for the new debate about poverty. But influencing the rebuilding process—largely in the hands of the Bush administration and Republican leadership—would require a much broader organizing effort from ACORN. The waters were receding, but the real battle of New Orleans was still ahead.

Creating the Katrina Survivors Association

New Orleans was not only one of the nation's poorest cities but also among the most segregated. At the time of Katrina, the city was 67 percent African American. Among the nation's hundred largest metro areas, it ranked third in poverty concentration. With a 23 percent poverty rate, it was the twelfth-poorest city in the nation. Its median household income in 2000 was only $27,133. Less than half of households owned their own homes. Of the city's African Americans, 35 percent did not own a car, compared with 15 percent of whites. Housing discrimination and the concentration of government housing subsidies contributed to the city's economic and racial segregation. Three-quarters of the flood-zone residents were black, and nearly 60 percent were living on less than $30,000 a year.[11]

While incompetence and indifference were stalling early government recovery efforts, experts warned that the wrong policies could lead to increased disaster. Business leaders were concluding that New Orleans needed to sacrifice some of the city's low-lying areas—poor, working-class, and predominantly African American—to improve flood protection. In early October, major newspapers quoted HUD secretary Alfonso Jackson as saying that post-Katrina New Orleans would not have as many black people, and that as a result, HUD would not be funding New Orleans public housing at pre-Katrina levels.[12] A consensus was growing within ACORN that it needed to fight for a New Orleans rebuilt for the people who had lived there.

Instead of responding to Katrina with a bold, large-scale public works program to employ evacuees, including the rebuilding of New Orleans, the Bush administration retreated to its "compassionate conservative" philosophy of relying on private charities to fix the problems of the poor. Administration officials urged the U.S. Conference of Catholic Bishops to be prepared to care for a half a million refugees.[13] ACORN and other activist civic groups would have to step into the breach.[14]

ACORN's leadership faced some hard decisions. ACORN's power rested in recruiting individual dues-paying members who would join local chapters and get active in fighting for a better life for themselves. Bradberry, Goldman, and other paid organizers heard the plea of ACORN's members to return home to New Orleans and to have a voice in the future planning of the city. At the same time, members sitting in shelters and trailer parks in various cities yearned to go just about anywhere, and immediately. As one of them said, "We don't care if it is New Orleans or Timbuktu." The organizers asked themselves: How should ACORN balance this long-term goal—to make sure the poor and displaced have a right to return and a real voice in the rebuilding of devastated areas—-with the ongoing short-term need to make sure evacuees spread across the country in camps, hotels, and arenas had food, safety, decent shelter, clothing, and money?[15]

Even before Katrina struck, ACORN's local organizers, including those in Houston and Baton Rouge, had their hands full paying attention to the typical ongoing issues of unaffordable housing, crime, high utility rates, and schools. One thing was clear: continuing to serve members in addition to achieving challenging, long-term goals would require additional funds.

Rathke sat down with his communications director, Kevin Whelan, and they decided to try a new kind of fund-raising, "a shot in the dark" using ACORN's website. Whelan converted the site into a call for contributions to the ACORN Hurricane Rebuilding and Recovery Fund. Shea, the head of ACORN Housing, and Steve Kest, ACORN's executive director, led the effort to reach various allies, who responded by sending thousands of dollars to help relocate and rebuild the national office. MoveOn, the activist political organization with over three million Internet members, put the ACORN Hurricane Fund on its list, and by the next morning $40,000 had poured into ACORN's coffers. Don Stillman, a former UAW staffer and an old friend of Rathke's, called him for the office address because his daughter, Sarah, had won a $5,000 prize at Yale for an essay on ethics and was sending some of the money to the ACORN Hurricane Fund. Capital One, a Fortune 500 credit corporation, led the big donors with $500,000. Ameriquest contributed $100,000, as well as weeks of housing in Houston for dislocated staff. Citigroup and BankAmerica chipped in $100,000 apiece.

These pledges allowed ACORN to quickly rebuild the offices without waiting for insurance reimbursements that would have taken months, to move the staff into temporary housing, and to get the Baton Rouge office to the point where it could handle the operations. Somehow, in the chaos, ACORN paid its thousand staff members.

Wealthy supporters such as the iconoclastic septuagenarian Herb Sandler, who ran Golden West Financial Corporation and the Sandler Family Funds, understood ACORN's urgent need for money. By early October, Sandler, who would soon sell Golden West for $24 billion to Wachovia Bank, would commit over a million dollars to allow ACORN to increase its organizing capacity to reach its members and respond to the crisis. The Catholic Campaign for Human Development and similar church-based programs pitched in to support ACORN offices in the impacted areas. TV celebrity Roseanne Barr would donate the proceeds from her upcoming performances in San Francisco to the ACORN Hurricane Recovery and Rebuilding Fund, part of her long-term commitment to ACORN.

For almost three decades, ACORN had been making headway in the areas of wages, housing, the environment, and other concerns. But now Rathke sensed that ACORN was at a crossroads, and that the road he took could seal ACORN's fate.

In Houston, Stukes was continually plagued with nightmares resulting from her New Orleans ordeal and her frustrating dealings with unresponsive politicians and bureaucrats, especially FEMA staff. Her blood pressure rose when she learned that FEMA was rewarding lucrative no-bid contracts to companies like Halliburton ($125 million) and not to qualified contractors who had worked and lived in New Orleans and wanted to go home and rebuild. FEMA, for example, paid the Shaw Group, a giant engineering firm with ties to the Bush administration, $175 per hundred square feet to install blue tarps on storm-damaged roofs, while the actual installers earned as little as $2 per hundred square feet and the tarps were provided free from FEMA.[16]

On October 7, Stukes led two busloads of members of the Houston ACORN Hurricane Survivor Committee, waving red flags bearing ACORN's logo, to confront FEMA's Houston director, Tom Costello, about his failure to address the survivors' needs. They jammed the foyer of his south Houston field office, demanding that FEMA improve its efforts to help Louisiana hurricane victims. The group persuaded FEMA to make services more accessible, including running a shuttle bus to the FEMA service center, to translate materials into Spanish, and to extend benefits to Hurricane Rita survivors. FEMA also agreed to send senior officials to ACORN's Houston Katrina Survivors Association meetings. After the victory, Stukes waited with anticipation for the October meeting Rathke had planned.

On October 21, Rathke drove to his cramped office on Greenwell Springs in Baton Rouge. The one-story brick building that housed ACORN's local chapter and SEIU Local 100 now had to squeeze in most of the national staff. As soon as Rathke arrived, he convened a meeting with O'Brien, ACORN's national field director; his partner, Beth Butler, Louisiana ACORN's head organizer; Goldman, Texas ACORN's head organizer; Maude Hurd; Steve Bradberry, New Orleans head organizer; Marie Hurt, who ran the Baton Rouge office; and Tanya Harris, Stukes, and other activist survivors. They discussed strategies for implementing a massive effort to reach evacuees and sketched out a plan that only people in ACORN could have imagined.

They all agreed that ACORN needed to focus survivors on their homes in New Orleans rather than organizing them into local chapters where they now lived. The task was complex. Built on ACORN's federated network of offices and the initial efforts in Houston, the plan required finding dispersed evacuees from all over the country and uniting them into a national organization of survivors. The group agreed to hire twenty organizers and canvassers in Louisiana spread between Lake Charles, Baton Rouge, Alexandria, and New Orleans when ACORN could get back into the city, and another twenty organizers and canvassers in Texas and elsewhere, with about half in Houston. The group would fight for the right of survivors to return and continue addressing their day-to-day issues. They would continue to look for members, recruit new families displaced by the hurricane, help all of them with their immediate problems, and mobilize them into a force that could influence New Orleans, Louisiana, and national policy.

Amy Schur, ACORN's smart, detail-oriented national campaign director, was put in charge of coordinating the work of local organizers in various cities in Texas, Mississippi, Arkansas, and elsewhere who had responsibility for helping survivors confront government officials so they could access food, housing, and cash, and find relatives. The canvassers, mostly from the membership and evacuee ranks, hit the hotels, shelters, trailer parks, government agencies, charities, and churches to build a list of evacuees to assemble into the organization.

Later in October, ACORN president Maude Hurd reached out through a conference call to Stukes and dozens of other emerging leaders. They agreed to call themselves the ACORN Katrina Survivors Association (AKSA).[17]

Planning on a Diaspora

Without major government assistance to help poor people return and rebuild, the city's most damaged neighborhoods would lose as much as 80 percent of their black population, according to a detailed analysis by Brown University demographer John Logan. Combining data from the 2000 census with federal damage assessment maps, Logan provided a new level of specificity about Hurricane Katrina's effect on the city's worst-flooded areas, which were heavily populated by low-income African Americans.

Of the 354,000 people who lived in New Orleans neighborhoods where the hurricane damage was moderate to severe, 75 percent were black, 29 percent were poor, more than 10 percent were unemployed, and more than half were renters. Logan concluded what ACORN activists and Rathke had already surmised: much of the city's black population could not return unless their neighborhoods were rebuilt and the government provided relocation costs.[18] It was no wonder that, as soon as the water ebbed, the debate over rebuilding versus razing assumed a racial overtone.

Evictions of tenants were widespread, as landlords sought to clear the path for redevelopment. With the court system in disarray, judges across the region were unsympathetic to the plight of tenants, and in Louisiana they had few rights. With the mayor's support, well-connected developers would be able to buy up the properties from hapless owners and landlords for a pittance. Rathke and the ACORN leaders knew that without some countervailing force, the mayor's planning committee's vision of a whiter and richer city would win by default.

Dozens of groups had become active in the fight to rebuild. They included The Metropolitan Organization (TMO), New Orleans Network, and the Southern Partners Fund. Habitat for Humanity made plans for new housing. Common Ground was gearing up to provide food, clothing, a health clinic, and even emotional support to the victims of Katrina. All these efforts were helpful. As far as creating a political force, however, except for TMO, most of the groups were too small, too poor, or too disconnected from the disaster victims to make a big difference. Most of the local activist groups relied almost completely on volunteers or had, at the most, only one paid staff person.

Smaller groups such as the New Orleans Network and the Southern Partners Fund coordinated with each other, but larger groups like the faith-based TMO and ACORN were not. Sister Christina Stephens, a TMO organizer, told a reporter: "We just haven't seen the presence of [other organizers]. I know they might be doing some things; . . . we're just not rubbing shoulders with that."[19]

Who with political clout could ACORN coalesce with? Other groups didn't have the skills to raise large sums of money and engage in politics. Few had a base of dues-paying members or the interest to mobilize the poor in New Orleans, Baton Rouge, or Washington. Only ACORN seemed to have the capacity to lobby and mobilize simultaneously on the local, state, and national level.[20]

For two months after the hurricane, hardly a day went by when some Washington, D.C., inside-the-Beltway liberal or progressive public interest group or think tank didn't produce a position paper or op-ed piece on what government should do to restore New Orleans. The bloggers, e-mailers and Democratic Party leaders were full of sound and fury but not much action. Local community, civic, and religious groups held press conferences and set up websites. Liberal foundations, the Red Cross, and United Way affiliates were holding meetings and spreading their money around.

Curtis Muhammad headed a New Orleans group called Community Labor United (CLU). He had been a member of SNCC, with roots in the voter registration drives of the civil rights movement. Over the preceding twenty years he had been an activist in New Orleans, and like so many others he was trying to help. Unlike ACORN, however, Mohammad had no staff, a small budget, and little capacity to influence the course of events in New Orleans. When Rathke read an article in the *Nation* magazine about the aftermath of Katrina that ended by encouraging readers to send money to Muhammad's group, Rathke exploded in frustration. He wrote on his blog that Muhammad's group was a

> little bitty thing of maybe a dozen or two activists that has convened meetings off and on for years mostly on Saturdays for a while at Dillard . . . [attended by] well intentioned AFT teachers that are personally involved with Curtis Muhammad, who ran a small local union for UNITE for a couple of years before he retired. . . . But now a wave of water moves through New Orleans and I actually get inquiries about whether or not CLU can help in some way.
>
> Huh? What? They are nice people and we count them as friends and allies, but are we talking about something real there? Of course not! Could they handle money? No reason to believe that. Do they have a base in New Orleans? No, not whatsoever. Heck, I don't know if they could organize a two-car funeral if they were driving both cars. They have only convened forums in the past to talk about stuff. If that was needed, they could do that I suppose, but there are a lot of folks who can do that.

Rathke compared Muhammad and other groups to Ahmed Chalabi, who after years of exile and without a real base in Iraq had received over $35 million in U.S. tax dollars to act as Donald Rumsfeld's front for the people who lived in Iraq and opposed Hussein: "We create representatives for the people for the purposes of the sponsors and the donor community, just like we have seen in Iraq."

The blog caused a fierce storm of criticism from left-wing blogs, important African American activists, and foundation executives. Rathke felt obliged to apologize on his blog and personally to Mohammad. But the incident exposed his resentment of groups who had no base in New Orleans, "who couldn't find the city without a map, were fronting for people they did not know or represent," but were nevertheless getting donations and foundation grants because people couldn't distinguish between groups with and without the capacity to get things done.

ACORN's members and organizers believed that the power brokers and speculators would quickly buy up the land, extort the public treasury, and create a rebuilding plan without input from ordinary residents. If ACORN was to counter these forces, it needed a realistic master plan prepared by professionals. Rathke and Steve Kest reached out to old friends who were experienced professional planners: Ron Shiffman from the Pratt Institute, who had helped Rathke start ACORN's New York chapter; Chester Hartman, founder of the Planners Network, which specialized in supporting community planning; and Dr. Ken Reardon, chair of the Regional and Local Planning Department at Cornell University and the cousin of ACORN's national field director, Helene O'Brien. The final member of the planning team was David Cronrath, dean of the Louisiana State University (LSU) School of Art and Design. Cronrath had experience with community-based design and architecture, sympathized with issues that ACORN was facing in New Orleans, and was looking for a way LSU could become involved in the New Orleans recovery. ACORN needed members of the local political establishment who were not pawns of the business elite. Bradberry roped in Oliver Thomas, president of the City Council, and Cynthia Willard-Lewis and Cynthia Hedge Morrell, both councilwomen in the flooded areas hit hard by the hurricane.

The LSU School of Art and Design, the Pratt Institute, and the Cornell Local and Regional Planning Department agreed to cosponsor the "ACORN Community Forum on the Rebuilding of New Orleans" on the LSU Baton Rouge campus. It would fill the void left by all levels of government who were ignoring the poor and working class in the decisions regarding the future of New Orleans.

On November 7–8, 2005, fifty displaced New Orleans residents, including Dorothy Stukes, met with fifty leading urban planners, architects, and affordable-housing specialists for the forum. Hundreds of Katrina survivors from around the country who couldn't attend took part in the discussions via a webcast and by e-mailing questions to the speakers at the forum. Amazingly, it was the first time any urban-planning experts had asked a group of Katrina survivors what they wanted. It was also the first time Rathke met Stukes. He shook her hand and said, "Darlin', I am so pleased to meet you." Stukes, wearing a red ACORN T-shirt, thought he was "so handsome and charming."

Stukes, Rathke, and the others began the forum with a tour of New Orleans. On the bus, ACORN members introduced themselves to the experts. They all ended their introductions with the words, "I am ready to go home."

Two and half months had passed since the storm. What experts and Katrina survivors saw shocked them. New Orleans was a ghost town. The streets were eerily empty, with mile after mile of partially and totally destroyed homes and stores, fallen trees, abandoned upside-down cars impaled by tree branches, massive heaps of debris and garbage, furniture, carpets, and TVs strewn about the streets, refrigerators lying on top of cars, roofs in the middle of the street, and broken telephone poles. The Lower Ninth Ward and other poor neighborhoods showed almost no sign of any rebuilding effort or any human activity at all.

Inside the homes, they saw sofas, dining-room chairs, and mattresses stained a ubiquitous sludge-brown color. No trucks, front-end tractor-loaders, or workers were removing the dangerous, unhealthy garbage. Peter Werwath of the Enterprise Foundation, which provided billions of dollars in grants and loans to groups that build affordable homes, was stunned by the empty neighborhoods—no residents, no FEMA workers, and no reconstruction teams. He said to his fellow bus passengers, "I am just astounded to see how little has started this long after the fact."

At the time, hundreds of FEMA trailers were sited in dusty parks surrounded with barbed wire on the outskirts of Baton Rouge, far from New Orleans, resembling depression-era migrant camps. One of the professional planners on the tour, Chester Hartman, wondered why FEMA didn't situate trailers in the parking lots of closed shopping centers and big-box stores, putting the displaced residents closer to the city and their old neighborhoods. Trailers with Porta-Johns, bottled water, and generators could have been located on a family's New Orleans lot so that people could return to the neighborhood, begin to protect and salvage their old home, and connect with friends and neighbors. FEMA claimed that it couldn't place trailers near homes because there was no water, sewers, or electricity.

Nor was FEMA doing anything about the mental health needs of victims who had suffered the trauma of losing their homes, social networks, and jobs. Twenty thousand public school students uprooted by the hurricane were still not attending any school. One could see on the faces of the survivors at the LSU forum the pain of losing networks of people who mattered deeply.

Since many of the city's businesses had been destroyed, there were no sales and property taxes. People had lost their cars to the storms, but no public transportation existed to transport them to jobs. FEMA estimated that fifty thousand new housing units needed to be built. But there was no plan. When the buses returned from the tour, ACORN members and the experts it brought to New Orleans plotted together to develop a plan to rebuild the city.

In September, two months earlier, an official, largely white New Orleans elite group had begun this very task— the Bring New Orleans Back Commission (BNOB) appointed by Mayor Nagin to prepare a master plan. The seventeen-member commission included City Council president Oliver Thomas as well as jazz musician Wynton Marsalis (telecommuting from Manhattan), but a small group of white leaders, such as James Reiss, a real estate investor and chair of the Regional Transit Authority, exercised the real clout. They represented the interests of the white-shoe law firms, engineering offices, and local shipping companies.

Reiss, who lived in an exclusive gated community, Audubon Place, was a descendent of an old-line Uptown New Orleans family. Rathke and other ACORN activists had been stunned to read an interview in the *Wall Street Journal* less than two weeks after the storm in which Reiss said New Orleans would have to come back whiter and wealthier. Investors, he said, would not put their money in the city if they could not be assured of reduced crime, a problem they associated with the city's African American residents.[21] "That *Journal* article knocked us on our heels and woke us up to the fact that the new reality was going to be a fight for our lives and our very right to come back," said Rathke.

The most influential power broker was Joseph Canizaro, a wealthy property developer who had contributed over $1 million to Republicans since 1997, was a leading Bush supporter, and had supported Mayor Nagin in the 2002 mayoral election. Canizaro, whom Rathke dubbed "a big-time developer in this middle-sized city," planned to mobilize the support of some of the nation's most powerful developers and prestigious master planners through his connections with the Urban Land Institute (ULI), a think tank for the real estate industry.

In October, just before ACORN gathered at the forum at LSU, Canizaro told the Associated Press: "As a practical matter, these poor folks don't have the resources to go back to our city just like they didn't have the resources to get out of our city. So, we won't get all those folks back. That's just a fact."[22] Nagin and Canizaro claimed that in three years the city would recover only half of its August 2005 population. ACORN's staff and leadership understood this to mean, as Rathke would say, "A Greyhound ticket to another town would best serve the New Orleans underemployed and poorly educated African Americans."

The Urban Land Institute advised the city to focus rebuilding efforts on New Orleans's higher ground and the neighborhoods that were least damaged in Katrina's aftermath. That meant leaving out Gentilly, Hollygrove, New Orleans East, and the Lower Ninth, all ACORN strongholds. The ULI urged the city to return the flood-prone areas, including the Lower Ninth, to wetlands, agreeing with some hurricane experts who said that doing so would reduce the intensity of future hurricanes and keep residents out of harm's way. The government planners recommended that New Orleans shrink its footprint to adjust for a smaller population, using forced buyouts, if necessary, to eject homeowners from the designated neighborhoods.

The participants of the ACORN forum heard David Cronrath, the dean of LSU's College of Art and Design, attack the mayor's urban planners, accusing them of treating New Orleans as if it had been hit with a plague: "It could be rebuilt without regard to citizens who are alive, well, and want to return home. . . . The plague analogy has made it easier to conceptualize the wholesale reformulation of the city—as if all those empty buildings don't have owners with current hopes and future dreams to return." Cronrath called the mayor's commission's plans "drastic and revolutionary physical solutions, . . . a resident's nightmare, not a dream." He labeled them hastily assembled plans that distracted residents from the most pressing issue—"how to efficiently rehabilitate existing houses protected by better levees."

Radhey Sharma and John Pardue, LSU professors from the Department of Civil and Environmental Engineering, addressed the gathering. Sharma, affiliated with the LSU Hurricane Center, told the survivors that their role was important. "We do technical work all the time," Sharma said, "but where are the stakeholders? That's where you come in." Pardue, director of the Louisiana Water Resources Research Institute, said that the research showed that posthurricane environmental concerns, while serious, had been overstated. He added that health concerns should not keep people from coming back to the city; hazards were remediable.

Vincent Wilson, a leader of the ACORN Katrina Survivors Association (AKSA) and a housing contractor turned activist, represented a symbol of hope to the people who were ready to fight for the right to come home. Wilson's brick ranch-style house in the Lower Ninth Ward had been owned by his family since it was built in 1967. He lived there with his wife, Mary Ann, and their son, Zanthony. Inundated with water, it would have to be demolished.

Wilson addressed the experts in a large LSU conference room. He emphasized the urgency of a rebuilding plan that allowed families to return and rebuild their lives and communities. His appearance and voice were completely at odds with the heat of his words. A light-skinned African American, thickly built, wearing black-framed glasses and a nondescript golf shirt, he spoke in even tones. He accused the government of having utterly failed him, having rendered him and his neighbors invisible. He countered the stereotyped news stories by white reporters that the Ninth Ward was home to deadbeats, not taxpayers. "Two-thirds of the Lower Ninth Ward are homeowners," he said.

"We're on a nice quiet, quaint block," Wilson went on. "Everyone on our street for two blocks is a homeowner just like myself. It's the type of neighborhood where people say 'Good morning' or 'Good night.' If you don't greet people on the street, they'll recognize you as a stranger. We are all working-class people and we pay our taxes as any other citizen of this country, and we expect to get something out of the pot."

Inspiration alone was not enough, though, for a people-powered counterforce. It required what organizers call "local handles"—issues that are deeply felt and easy to understand and that can encourage people to demonstrate, lobby, and vote. Dennis Livingston, a union carpenter, community organizer, and graphic designer who had worked with Baltimore ACORN, had a plan with local handles. He said they needed to stop any further deterioration of their flood-ravaged homes. "Government incompetence and inaction," Livingston said, "mean that defective roofs would lead to more water damage from New Orleans rainfalls. Unless the houses are opened up, aired out, and treated immediately, mold from the city's humidity will take over and make the repairs either prohibitive or small-scale biohazards for the returning residents."

A consensus emerged from the conference that if ACORN could marry the families wanting to come home to their properties with some ability to stave off further damage, the old neighborhoods might be saved. It was a long shot—the people were in one place and the properties were in another—but at least it provided the needed local organizing handle. Brick by brick, house by house, ACORN could build momentum that might influence the local, state, and federal governments. But what a task! They would have to proceed despite the federal government's unwillingness to provide financial aid and assure those returning that they would have category five hurricane levee protection.

Rathke, wearing dungarees and a light beige jacket with elbow patches, told the forum participants: "Any policy program or proposal behind government halls and ivy walls could in fact be trumped on the ground, if we could prove the point house by house." Given the obstacles ACORN faced, Rathke's confidence seemed misplaced. Several things had to happen—all at once. ACORN had to put the growth of the AKSA on a fast trajectory so it would become the nation's largest organization of displaced former New Orleans residents; slow down the Bring New Orleans Back steamroller; keep up the pressure on the state and federal government to spend more money on housing, economic development, and the levees; stop the home foreclosures; and influence the February New Orleans mayoral election.

While most people prepared to celebrate Thanksgiving and the winter holidays,

ACORN's staff and leaders prepared to escalate their fight to restore New Orleans for the less powerful. Soon after the Baton Rouge forum, ACORN organized a press conference rejecting the BNOB plan. Rathke called it racist: "They're arguing for abandoning much of the population of much of the city." ACORN members and survivors protested the recommendations of the BNOB Commission's consultants, the Urban Land Institute, which they believed would starve out many of the lower-income neighborhoods' resources for rebuilding and recovery. Many elected officials in New Orleans joined ACORN and others who were denouncing the Urban Land Institute plan. The New Orleans City Council adopted a resolution calling for the rebuilding of all the city's neighborhoods.

ACORN assigned a few more staff to AKSA so that survivors could lobby, demonstrate, write letters, and otherwise fight with politicians, insurance companies, and business power brokers with what Rathke called "their schemes for a smarter, richer city."

ACORN joined the AFL-CIO and consumer groups to pressure mortgage holders not to foreclose on New Orleans homes. Steve Kest, Amy Schur, and field director Helene O'Brien, working with Stukes and other leaders began a plan to bring five hundred survivors to Washington on February 8 and 9 to rally at the Capitol and the White House, meet with lawmakers, and present their case to administration and elected officials. While emergency food and clothing were needed right away, the survivors also needed the kind of advocacy that could organize, lobby, and mobilize people to engage in the kind of political action that could move Washington to act boldly.[23]

Delery Street

Why so many families wanted to return to New Orleans was simple. It was a city of the lonely and disconnected. But it was also a city with numerous extended families with strong social connections. According to the most recent census, of all U.S. cities, New Orleans ranked second to Santa Ana, California, in the percentage of its population born in the state, at 83 percent. Fifty-four percent of the residents of the Lower Ninth Ward had been in their homes for ten years or more, far above the national average. The population in the part of the Lower Ninth where Tanya Harris lived was somewhere between six and eleven thousand, with 60 percent of the residents homeowners. Harris knew that most of the people, especially the elderly, wanted to return. For the lonely and disconnected, it seemed so sadly hopeless. For the displaced with deep roots who had lived in one neighborhood their whole lives, generations after generation—they had a chance to return.

By late November 2005, Bourbon Street and the upscale parts of New Orleans were coming back to life. But the Lower Ninth Ward, the symbolic ground zero in the fight to return, was still in ruins. City officials, citing safety concerns, had barred residents from visiting their homes. Most of those who had lived there, like Tanya Harris's grandmother Josephine Butler, eighty-three, believed that Mayor Nagin and his cronies had kept them out the past three months, in the hope they would sever their ties to the neighborhood, never to return. Following the hurricane, Tanya went to Baton Rouge, while Butler fled with some of her family to South Carolina. But despite the devastation in New Orleans, Butler couldn't bear to be away from the city. After three weeks in South Carolina, she took a bus back to New Orleans and stayed at the Marriott Hotel with her niece, who was a housekeeper there.

On December 1, the city reopened the last closed part of the Lower Ninth for residents to "look and leave." Harris took Butler to her home on Delery Street to see, for the first time since the hurricane, the house built by her late husband fifty-one years earlier. Harris remembered her grandfather sitting with her in silence at the end of Delery Street with the lines from their cane fishing poles in the Mississippi. "We'd watch the giant cruise ships move up and down the river," she recalled. Wearing a white sweater with beaded flowers and gripping her black purse, the thin, sturdy Butler walked nervously to her house, which had floated off its foundation. She bent over to see inside the squashed house. Looking at the shattered windows, the sodden furniture, she started to weep.

Harris and Butler were two of more than a thousand people who came to "the back of town," the name locals gave to the Delery Street neighborhood. Some hugged and kissed. But despite the sunshine, it was a dark and melancholy day. "It's just like going to a funeral," said George Hill, sixty-six, gazing at his house on Delery Street. "We're coming to view the body."

Tanya Harris and other ACORN activists, determined to battle established power, were part of a long tradition of New Orleans activism and populism. For example, back on June 7, 1892, a twenty-nine-year-old shoemaker, Homer Plessy, bought a first-class ticket on the East Louisiana Railroad that ran between New Orleans and Covington and sat in the Whites Only passenger car. When the conductor came to collect his ticket, Plessy told him that he was one-eighth African American, and that he refused to sit in the Blacks Only car. Plessy had been an active member of the Citizens' Committee of African Americans and Creoles, a civil rights group that had planned his direct action to challenge the doctrine of "separate but equal." But an 1896 Supreme Court decision upheld the constitutionality of racial segregation, particularly in railroads, under the doctrine of "separate but equal." Harris was a modern-day Plessy, hoping for quicker results.

In and out of Louisiana shelters and trailer camps, reconnecting with members and building for the struggle ahead, Harris told her audiences: "The city and developers are deliberately attempting to keep you out of New Orleans. It ain't gonna happen. That plan's backfiring."

She believed in the people. "I'm not seeing that laid-back New Orleans character right now," the battling Harris continued. "I'm seeing a fighting spirit. My grandmother would chain herself to that property before she allowed the city to take it. We take our homeowning very seriously."

After that day, the National Guard and New Orleans police kept barricades on every street and barred the public—including ACORN members who lived there—from reentering the Lower Ninth. City officials, with some justification, said they had to begin razing homes that presented an immediate public danger. Speculators were buying land, ensuring that people who lived in the Lower Ninth before the storm could not return.

After city officials announced that they would begin bulldozing 2,500 buildings that inspectors labeled dangerously unstable from flood damage, Harris helped ACORN members chase off a backhoe crew preparing to demolish a home in the Lower Ninth. ACORN also rushed into court. On December 28, on behalf of ACORN member Greta Gladney and others, ACORN won a temporary restraining order against the city of New Orleans to prevent bulldozing and demolition of property until a full hearing could be held on January 6.[24]

Rathke's unswerving optimism began to return when he learned that some four thousand New Orleans ACORN members who paid their dues by bank draft remained steadfast, with very few cancellations. About one-third of the members had been located.

Four months after the storm, as Rathke drove past his office on Elysian Fields toward his parents' house on the high ground near the lake, he passed five miles empty of life, with dead trees, untowed cars parked next to debris, and houses with FEMA crosses. "Every day where there is no activity," he thought, "housing—good, sturdy housing that could and should be rebuilt—continues to deteriorate and is lost."[25]

The mayor's plan gave neighborhoods one year to repopulate or face closing as a residential neighborhood. New Orleans homeowners needed to prove they intended to return and fix up their homes. ACORN planned to establish a beachhead in lower-income areas by cleaning up and gutting the insides of salvageable homes. But it would need someone who could organize crews, train volunteers to do a specialized clean-up job, and make sure the work was done well, quickly, and at the lowest cost possible.

Then Janet Reasoner called Rathke. She had worked for him in New Orleans before she moved back to Wyoming to be closer to her aging mother and father. Immediately after Katrina hit, Janet felt compelled to volunteer, and Rathke hired her to temporarily help staff the Houston office. She talked to her husband, Scott Hagy, an industrial electrician, who had overseen the building of large industrial bottling plants like Pepsi in the United States and abroad. He was a bushy-mustached licensed contractor and had extensive experience in renovating older houses in the New Orleans area. Nagy packed his bag and flew to New Orleans. He agreed to take over the next phase of ACORN's guerilla war. The effort to stop the razing of neighborhoods and to begin their rebuilding would take place in the trenches of an inundated piece of land in the Lower Ninth.

Chapter 15

A Rich Gumbo

> ACORN is organizing to make sure the job of rebuilding New Orleans is done by the people of New Orleans and truly benefits the communities who have been hurt the most.
>
> —Roseanne Barr

Six months after Katrina, the Lower Ninth Ward's landscape consisted of houses flattened into splinters and empty, deteriorating homes. Sludge had mixed with canal water and settled five to eight feet above the ground branding the upright homes with a yellowish-brown water line. A few houses, including Tanya Harris's grandmother's, were swept across the street, uprooted from their foundations. On the front of the houses still standing, a red spray-painted large FEMA *X* was visible. Each *X*'s quadrants showed the date the house was inspected, its condition, how many people lived there before the evacuation, and, gruesomely, the number of dead bodies found. Where children had once played and families had barbecued, now there was scattered debris of toilet seats, religious figurines, and grayish stuffed animals.

Douglas Brinkley, quoted in the *New York Times*, said: "The Lower Ninth Ward is kind of the heart and soul of the African American experience in New Orleans, and what's New Orleans without the African American experience?" Yet it was hard to imagine this area being inhabited again. The city's homeland-security director, Terry Ebbert, told a reporter, "Nothing out there can be saved at all."[1]

The Lower Ninth Ward had been a marshy swamp until the 1800s, when poor blacks and white laborers began moving into the area, located near the French Quarter. Whether it had a future as a thriving neighborhood or turned back into a swamp would be determined by the political battle between the antipoverty activists and the Bush Republicans and their allies.

At midnight on New Year's Eve, as a damp fog spread from the Mississippi River over the Ninth Ward near the drawbridge that lifts St. Claude Avenue over the Inner Harbor Navigational Canal, four families, including Greta Gladney's, gathered in front of their houses on Jourdan Avenue. Joining the families were thirty ACORN organizers and leaders. They had come there to defy the authorities. Gladney, an ACORN member and founder of a local nonprofit community group, was furious that her Ninth Ward home had received a government red sticker deeming it unsafe. She had jumped at the chance to join ACORN's lawsuit to stop the demolitions. Ignoring the red-sticker warning, she signed the waiver giving ACORN permission to clean and gut her home. Gladney joined her neighbors for a New Year's Eve party and protest.

A college graduate with a master's in business administration, Gladney, forty-one, was the mother of three, her first child born when she was fourteen. As the press gathered to hear what the protesters wanted, Gladney said: "People have been asking, 'What's going to happen to our property? When will we get permission to come back?'" Gladney said she was a fourth-generation Lower Ninth Ward resident. "We've made a commitment with each other to rebuild our block." Not all residents would want to return, she acknowledged, but "folks need to make decisions. It doesn't make sense that we've been kept away for four months, and now there's a rush to demolish the houses. The city didn't build neighborhoods in the first place, you know. . . . We will decide."

The ACORN organizers planned the New Year's Eve protest as another step toward galvanizing a movement back to the New Orleans neighborhoods. At stake for the residents was not just the loss of their homes. They also stood to lose a comfortable, neighborly community where for generations they had lived in finely carpentered shotgun cottages, small bungalows, brick homes, and two-story neocolonials. Before the 1980s, fathers with well-paying longshoremen's jobs worked at the Port of New Orleans. By the mid-1980s, that work was gone, as shipping containers replaced most of the longshoremen. Just before the storm the community was working class and poor, with 30 percent of its residents living in poverty largely because many of the waterfront jobs had disappeared. The others were carpenters, sheetrock finishers, and day laborers, as well as professionals. Stores were within walking distance, and mass transit nearby made car ownership unnecessary. Parents and grandparents raised their kids for success. The Lower Ninth Ward was a musical neighborhood where Fats Domino, the Rock and Roll Hall of Famer, had grown up and still lived in a modest yellow-and-black house with his wife, Rosemary, with whom he had eight children.

Beth Butler, the chief organizer for Louisiana ACORN, stood next to Gladney that night. She recalled an episode before the storm when one of ACORN's bulk mailings was returned to the office, marked "undeliverable." Beth wanted the mail delivered and asked the postal clerk to sit down with a Ninth Ward ACORN resident who knew everyone in the neighborhood, and where to deliver the mail. "Her mail goes to her mom around the corner," the ACORN resident explained to the post office official, "and that one is living with her sister. This one moved across town." She located them all.

Loyed Lonzo and his wife, Lois, both in their sixties, had lived near Gladney's house all their lives. Lois recalled the neighborhood as a "family-oriented" place where everybody knew each other. Loyed remembered that "those green trees were always filled with birds and squirrels." Crime occasionally imposed its will on the community, but strong black families minimized the damage. "It wasn't perfect," said

Loyed. "There were violent gangs nearby. We tried to keep it safe. The families were working class, a place where everyone kept an eye on each other's kids, including scolding someone else's children as if they were their own."

Fifty-one-year-old Vanessa Gueringer, a new ACORN leader, smiled and nodded approvingly. "Relatives and friends lived close together, socialized, and took care of each other. I'm saddened every time I come here." Joining Gladney and the others was Tanya Harris, who helped organized the Katrina Survivors Association and this New Year's Eve event. She had grown up in the Lower Ninth. Her parents and grandparents had lived their whole lives there.

After the hurricane, Harris would take visitors through Lower Ninth. "Look how charming that home is. See that, I love that house." Where others saw empty houses off their foundations, she saw a "cute house that could be rebuilt." She would stop her car by a four-foot pile of debris in front of a house. "Don't let that curbside pile disturb you. It's a declaration of courage, pride, and hope. These are signs of rebuilding the Ninth as families clean out their houses. See the white dust? That's drywall. That means that they are almost home."

At the stroke of midnight, while fireworks exploded in neighborhoods in the French Quarter, the four families watched silently as Hagy, the mustached contractor from Wyoming, turned the crank on a generator at the back of a panel truck with a giant ACORN logo on its side: ACORN Mobile Action Center. Suddenly lights winked on in four houses on Jourdan Avenue. Harris and Gueringer hoped these owners of houses on the front lines would cause a stampede to bring back their neighborhood. "The symbolism behind this is that the residents of the Ninth Ward are coming home," said Harris.

These families were the first beneficiaries of ACORN's clean-up, house-gutting program. With a goal of a thousand homes by the end of March, Hagy had quickly put together an ACORN services crew of more than forty, including dispossessed Vietnamese fishermen and their families from Plaquemines Parish, African Americans from the neighborhoods, and Mexicans from Texas who had been lured into town by rumors of higher wages. Donning protective white Tyvek bodysuits, goggles, heavy gloves, and respirators, Hagy and his crews had entered these Ninth Ward homes, starting with Gladney's, tearing down moldy drywall, ripping up flooring, and carting decades' worth of ruined possessions to the curb. They stored salvageable personal belongings, sanitized the structures to prevent future mold growth, and tarped roofs to prevent further water damage and deterioration. As a result, hundreds of ex-residents of the Lower Ninth began lining up at ACORN's door to sign the clean-up waivers.

Working not just in the Lower Ninth Ward, but extending to Gentilly, Hollygrove/Upper Carrollton, and New Orleans East as well, Hagy and other ACORN staff started mobilizing what they hoped would be an army of volunteers to make the point that people can and will live in these neighborhoods. But would enough people return?

Among all the evacuees, 43 percent planned to return to New Orleans, a survey found. But just as many—44 percent—said they would settle somewhere else, while the remainder were unsure. Only one in four said they planned to move back into their old homes, the poll found.[2]

Hoping to slow down the mayor's plans, on January 6 ACORN and its allies packed the City Council meeting. When the council adopted a resolution calling for the rebuilding of all the city's neighborhoods, the crowd erupted in applause. But it was just a resolution. ACORN needed the mayor's active support. Later in the week, while Rathke was lunching with ACORN's executive committee at their usual place, the Praline Connection on Frenchmen Street, several blocks from the ACORN office, Mayor Ray Nagin walked in and came over to the ACORN table to shake hands and pose for pictures. He joked about not wanting to find his picture on the ACORN website, endorsing ACORN's entire program.

Rathke told the mayor, "I just hung up from a call informing me that there was a rumor that the long-awaited new FEMA flood maps were coming out on Monday and that you endorsed them." Rathke was referring to the maps that would eliminate the Lower Ninth as a place for residents to return to. Mayor Nagin replied: "We expected some new maps in a few weeks and more likely months, which would be better—in my view. But this is going to be a long process and nothing is happening Monday. In fact, it might take a year to go through the process." Then the mayor leaned forward and said, "Wade, you are going to like what you see here." Rathke took this to mean that ACORN would get a full year, maybe more, to prove it could save the city's lower-income neighborhoods.

On January 11, at a public meeting the real estate mogul Canizaro presented the Bring New Orleans Back (BNOB) plan. As ACORN had feared, residents would not be able to rebuild in flood-prone areas. Sticking to the Urban Land Institute's framework, the plan included an appointed redevelopment corporation, outside the control of the City Council, which would act as a land bank to buy out heavily damaged homes and neighborhoods with federal funds. Where necessary, eminent domain would turn low-lying areas into greenbelts or wetlands. The plan gave homeowners in each area of the city four months to prove that a "substantial" part of the population in a neighborhood would come back. (It did not define how many was "substantial.") At the end of four months, city planners would hold neighborhood meetings, assess the progress, and then make tough decisions about where to focus rebuilding efforts.[3]

After Canizaro's presentation, the public had its turn to speak. The first Lower Ninth resident said with some anger in her voice, "You want to turn black people's neighborhoods into white people's parks." "They don't want us," said another. At the mention of eminent domain, a few said they would rather die on their land than be bullied into selling or abandoning their property. One resident said the government would only be able to take her property "over my dead body." Another warned, "If you come to take our property, you better come ready!"

For Rathke, Harris, and Stukes, the plan was outrageous. Given a mere four months, even a community-organizing group like ACORN couldn't get homeowners to prove their intent to return, since most did not have a house anymore or a guarantee of an affordable one if they wanted to return.

For Tanya Harris, this was not the first time the white establishment told the black community, "We are doing it for your own good." She acknowledged that the Lower Ninth residents needed to know about all the hazards, but she, like so many others in the black community, was suspicious. She was well aware that in 1927 city officials had flooded two parishes so that the rest of city could be saved; people were promised compensation that never arrived. Hurricane Betsy in 1965 had flooded the Lower Ninth, and city officials had done nothing to revitalize the area. Her grandmother said to Tanya, in the middle of the 2005 flood, "They're doing it to us again." Rathke wrote on his blog: "If Nagin endorses this proposal, it means he either is not running for re-election . . . or that he is conceding defeat early."

The day before the January 14 City Council meeting, ACORN and its allies won a small battle. City officials agreed to a legal settlement binding the city to notify owners if their homes were on the teardown list. Originally, red stickers placed on homes by inspectors were considered fair notification, even for owners who remained evacuated. The city agreed to mail notification to the last available address; publish notices in the paper and on a city website, and take other measures before demolishing a house.

With more pressure, Rathke thought that the dispersed residents might wrangle a year to rebuild. The developers and the power elite, the group Rathke called the "big whoops," could then determine by some set of standards whether an area had demonstrated that it was capable of coming back. If ACORN could create a host of housing settlements, it would be impossible to evict their residents.

By the end of January, Hagy's crews were stripping 3 to 5 homes a day and had completed 575 homes at a cost of just $2,500 each. They were on their way to reaching their goal of cleaning up a thousand homes by March 2006. The clean-up and gut program would pave the way for people to return. ACORN did some of the work for free, but most homeowners became dues-paying members for $120 a year.

Jo Ann Snyder, forty-nine, drove into New Orleans from her temporary home in Lake Charles to watch an ACORN crew gut her house in the Lower Ninth Ward. She stood on her front lawn, watching a volunteer ACORN crew, mostly college students, wearing white protective suits and filter masks. They hauled destroyed furniture, carpets, and clothing to the curb as Snyder yanked every surviving photo from their hands. She could never have afforded to pay for the gutting and cleaning on her own.

Rathke wrote on his blog: "The fight is clear, even if grossly unfair. If we can prove that our neighborhoods can be rebuilt, where they are, and the way people want them, then we win, which means that we get to live in New Orleans, too. Unbelievable! But, whether we like the deal or not, we have no choice but to play, because the stakes are amazing, and fortunately, every house counts. This is a guerilla war in which people are fighting house by house, block by block, to save their neighborhoods." The house-to-house battle had just begun, but Rathke declared: "We are now winning, even against the odds. The more boots we can put on the ground, the better our chances of success."

The Fate of the Baker Bill

Six months after the hurricane, New Orleans had only one-third the number of residents it had pre-Katrina, the vast majority of the city's public schools remained closed, and only half its traffic lights worked. In the Lower Ninth, FEMA aid was nonexistent.

Nagin had lost credibility with nearly everyone for his response to Hurricane Katrina.[4] When he had run in 2001, Nagin was the candidate of business, and he won with 80 percent of the white vote. In 2005, with the white vote unlikely, Nagin would need the black vote to win. At a Martin Luther King Day celebration, he proclaimed that New Orleans would be "chocolate again . . . a majority African American city." Many commentators and residents thought Nagin had just ruined his own chances at reelection.

As important as the upcoming April 22 mayoral primary race was, the Bush administration and Republicans in Congress held most of the funding cards. ACORN had to lobby the federal government to support a plan that would help evacuees return. ACORN wanted the federal government to allocate money to rebuild homes and a flood protection system to keep people safe. ACORN planned to mobilize hundreds of New Orleans survivors to go to Washington for two days of marches aimed at reminding the Bush administration of its promise to help rebuild their city.

On January 24, ACORN and the BNOB group were stricken with what Congressman Richard Baker called a "death blow." Bush rejected Baker's plan to create a federal corporation to purchase and redevelop the thousands of Louisiana homes damaged by Hurricane Katrina. ACORN thought the plan very flawed, but it was the only plan on Congress's agenda. It would have provided $30 billion to homeowners, guaranteeing they would get at least 60 percent of the equity in their homes. ACORN's Washington staff had worked diligently with Baker's staff to improve the bill, which had wide bipartisan support in both chambers of Congress. That money would have helped jump-start the revitalization of New Orleans by encouraging the rebuilding of most of the 200,000 homes. Bush's domestic policy advisors opposed the Baker bill because, as one Bush spokesperson said, it was government meddling in the free market. In reality, there was no market, free or otherwise, in most of New Orleans. Even Baker, who had a 91 percent lifetime approval rating from the American Conservative Union, knew that the only way you get a market when there isn't one is if a government body creates it. White House officials were quoted as saying their opposition to the Baker plan was "ideological."[5]

Ironically, the death of the Baker plan meant that, temporarily at least, ACORN and other groups had more time to fight the BNOB plan that would wipe out the Lower Ninth. That plan to restore New Orleans depended on the Baker money. Without it, the commission was appearing more and more irrelevant.

The dire need for large sums of federal money remained, however. Six months after the storm and flood, New Orleans was, in the words of a *Washington Post* reporter, "Limbo Land. Vast sections of the city were still without utilities. Without electricity, businesses couldn't open; without open businesses, electric bills couldn't be paid. Of the 50 million cubic yards of hurricane and flood debris, only 6 million had been picked up. Dead cars littered the landscape. Few rode the buses and streetcars. Only 17 of 122 public schools have reopened."[6] In the midst of a dire housing shortage, more than 90 percent of the public housing units were still closed.

ACORN continued its war, sometimes targeting the federal government, sometimes the state, sometimes the mayor, sometimes the City Council. Its weapons included lawsuits, the gutting and cleaning program, rallies, and meetings that engaged the poor in planning what the future of their neighborhoods would look like.

Some local and national power brokers started paying attention. The New Orleans City Council president, Oliver Thomas, recognized ACORN as a group "that can begin to train people to take care of this twenty-year rebuilding effort that we have right now." On February 3, Steve Kest negotiated an agreement to partner with the William J. Clinton Foundation to conduct special outreach on the Earned Income Tax Credit (EITC), targeting Katrina survivors in ten cities. The ACORN Katrina Benefits Access Program provided on-the-spot tax preparation and helped direct displaced residents to much-needed federal and state benefits programs for Katrina survivors. "Can you imagine working all week and instead of cashing your paycheck, you rip it up?" said President Clinton at a press conference at which he was joined by ACORN president Maude Hurd. "If you earn under $35,000 a year and you're not claiming your Earned Income Tax Credit, then you're doing just that—throwing away your hard-earned money. The main idea of EITC is still the old idea of the American Dream, that if you work hard and play by the rules, you ought to have a decent life, and a chance for your children to have a better one. I hope this initiative helps more Americans achieve their dreams and reaches those Americans whose lives were shattered by last year's hurricanes."

For most Americans, though, the problems of Katrina were slipping off the radar. To seize the nation's attention, ACORN would try a complicated high-risk maneuver—mobilizing five hundred scattered survivors to Washington, D.C.

Demonstrating in Washington, D.C.

Before dawn on February 7, 2006, Dorothy Stukes gave a hug to her friend Phyllis Smith before they boarded separate buses at Houston's St. Dominic Chancery. Dorothy squeezed into the bus with seventy-five other storm survivors living in Houston. They settled in for a twenty-four-hour ride.

Marie Short Benoit, a schoolteacher, carried a photo album of her Ninth Ward home, which had been reduced to splinters. Unlike many people, she had flood insurance and used it to pay off her mortgage. She was left with about $15,000. Like the rest of the New Orleans public school teachers, Benoit was laid off from her job. Now she had no home, no health insurance, and an uncertain future. She bounced around from house to house, staying with relatives and friends. Benoit got on the bus.

Sharon Jasper said plans for the recovery had ignored public housing. A former resident of the St. Bernard public housing development, Jasper, like Stukes, was relocated to Houston after the storm. New Orleans mayor Nagin had talked about using some of the $6.2 billion in federal grants to Louisiana to rebuild damaged public housing, but Jasper said she was skeptical. "Whenever it was election time, [politicians] came through St. Bernard," Jasper said. "Now it seems they've kicked us to the curb." She got on the bus.

These and hundreds of other members of the ACORN Katrina Survivors Association departed in a caravan of buses from Atlanta, Houston, Jackson, Little Rock, Dallas, San Antonio, New York, Baton Rouge, Lake Charles, and Birmingham. Many were relieved to escape their temporary housing in hotel rooms, trailer parks, newly rented apartments, and spare rooms in cousins' homes.

Meanwhile, ACORN's Amy Schur, who had constantly called Stukes to give her moral support and keep her updated on recent events, prepared Stukes's press release. It began: "We are going to Washington to let the world know how the U.S. government has turned their back on us—the ordinary people of New Orleans who have worked hard all our lives. Katrina survivor: get on board and let's fight for the help we need, and deserve, to return and rebuild our homes and communities." The citizen lobbyist's list of demands included rebuilding the New Orleans levees to withstand a category five hurricane and capping rents for low- and moderate-income families.

After traveling all day and all night to reach the Capitol steps by February 8, Stukes departed the bus feeling tired and groggy. Joining four hundred other survivors bundled up against the winter chill, she marched up Independence Avenue in search of the power brokers. Adapting the lyrics of a Southern civil rights anthem, they sang, "Ain't gonna let no FEMA turn us around, turn us around, turn us around. Ain't gonna let no FEMA turn us around. Gonna keep on a'walking. Gonna keep on a'walking on home."

As they approached Capitol Hill, the displaced survivors, carrying pictures of their flood-damaged houses, homesick and wanting to return to New Orleans, started chanting, "Cut that check—for New Orleans!" and singing, "This little neighborhood of mine, I'm gonna let it shine." As the lunchtime crowd of Capitol Hill staffers gathered to watch the parade of protesters, a young man wearing a trench coat asked another, "Who are these people?" When a woman told him, "We're from New Orleans, sir," the man nodded and began to clap softly.[7]

With reporters all around, flashbulbs snapping, cameras churning, Stukes addressed the group. Though she did not read her speech, she found public speaking easy. She felt that God had put her on earth for this moment. She spoke from her heart and the words flowed out. "Our purpose is to let our voices be heard," she said. "Everybody is forgetting about Katrina. We want enough money so we can go home. We're not asking for a handout. These are our tax dollars we're talking about, that we have paid into the system." Then she rebuked the mayor. "We want all of New Orleans rebuilt, not just parts. And we don't want a Chocolate City. We want a Gumbo City, a city that has a little bit of everything in it," she said. "We've always been a gumbo city. Everybody loved each other. We were neighborly people. That's why I want to go back home. It's where I was raised and where I want my grandchildren to be raised.

"We are here so our voices can be heard, so our lives and our levees can be rebuilt, so we can go home. It's time for you to put down the barricades, let the people go in so we can start checking on our houses so our property won't decay worse than what it is." As for President Bush, she said: "Keep your promise to provide the funds.

We want answers in thirty days or we are going to return." In fact, ACORN had no money to spend on a repeat performance.

In a show of strength, ACORN enlisted key Democratic politicians to participate in a rally to demand additional rebuilding funds; these included Sen. Barack Obama, Senate minority leader Harry Reid (D-Nevada), Sen. Hillary Clinton (D-New York), Sen. Mary Landrieu (D-Louisiana) Sen. Joseph Lieberman (D-Connecticut), Sen. Byron Dorgan (D-North Dakota), and Sen. David Vitter (R-Louisiana), as well as AFL-CIO president John Sweeney. The House Democratic leadership held a hearing at which ACORN leaders spoke before Congress members Nancy Pelosi, Maxine Waters, Barney Frank, Mel Watt, and others. After the hearing the ACORN members fanned out in groups and lobbied scores of members of Congress on their platform for return and rebuilding. The *Washington Post* carried a front-page picture and story of the demonstration, but to the disappointment of the ACORN leaders, it gave no credit to ACORN.

After two days and a long trip, the members were exhausted. For Stukes and most of the other marchers, their plea renewed their spirits. Some thought they were fighting the tide, but they were satisfied that they were doing their best to fight back. On February 10, a photo of Sen. Harry Reid in front of the ACORN banner, whose caption stated that he was speaking at the ACORN Katrina Survivors rally, was the top news story on the automatic news links that popped up on Yahoo.

One week after the D.C. demonstration, which ACORN labeled the Rally for Return and Rebuilding, President Bush requested that Congress appropriate an additional $4.2 billion to repair flood-damaged homes in Louisiana. On the following day, he requested another $19.8 billion to repair flood and hurricane protection systems along the Gulf Coast. In newsletters and e-mails to its members and supporters, ACORN took most of the credit. Whether Bush signed the bill only because of ACORN's demonstration is doubtful, but this highly visible event certainly helped. In another victory, on March 2, FEMA officials, after a negotiating session with ACORN members and organizers, announced a settlement. It would extend its hotel assistance program for survivors for several more months.

Community Groups Collaborate

By mid-March, white FEMA trailers were scattered about the New Orleans landscape, parked in yards or driveways as temporary homes for residents while they restored their houses. Some residents without trailers returned on weekends from their temporary quarters in Baton Rouge, Houston, and Little Rock to gut, disinfect, restore, and rebuild their homes. But a closer look inside the Lower Ninth and nearby wards revealed the distance that ACORN and the others had to go before their message that evacuees had a right to return would resonate. The streetlights didn't work. Debris, including abandoned cars, pockmarked the area. The Lower Ninth still looked as if the storm had just passed. While many houses in ACORN's targeted neighborhoods were gutted, cleaned, and ready for rehab, even more reeked of mold and were rotting from within because ACORN didn't have enough money to keep up with the demand.

Wade and Beth Rathke bought a sleek, shiny 1979 Airstream trailer (popularly known as a zeppelin with wheels), parked it in front of their house, and began their own house restoration. In the ACORN neighborhoods of Gentilly, Bywater, Treme, Uptown, New Orleans East, Hollygrove, on nearly every block, selective house gutting and cleaning continued. ACORN took on more volunteer labor to keep the cost down to an average of $2,500 to a home. Between sixty and a hundred volunteers were helping to clean and gut every week. Signs tacked to wooden power poles read House Gutting and Mold Removal. By the end of the month, ACORN's Home Cleanout Program would reach its goal of saving a thousand homes.

Other local community groups were making a difference, as well. Relying mostly on volunteers, Common Ground, led by the charismatic leader Malik Rahim, operated a clinic that served twenty thousand people and would raise $27 million in donations that it used to distribute food, clothing, blankets, and other necessities to New Orleans's poorest neighborhoods. Common Ground delayed evictions from the hotels where evacuees had originally been housed by FEMA. The IAF network reached out in what Rathke called "a rare collaborative gesture, offering to follow ACORN's lead on issues of housing and mortgage financing."

A national faith-based group, PICO, assembled several meetings of its pastoral base in Washington and helped lobby for more money. The Gamaliel Foundation, which did not organize in New Orleans, supported ACORN's Recovery and Rebuilding Fund. Together with other local groups, ACORN leaders believed they were sending the message that New Orleans residents were coming home to rebuild. Rathke predicted to ACORN's leaders: "When the public sees that block by block people are living back there, they've managed to fix up their houses, they're making progress, there is nobody who stands for election in this city who's going to say, 'Bulldoze that neighborhood.'"

Yet New Orleans still had no comprehensive development plan, no FEMA flood maps that would reassure homeowners about where it was safe to rebuild, no assurances that the levees and canals would be sufficiently fortified, and no federal dollars for gutting and rehabbing homes. FEMA continued to drag its feet. Even after submitting multiple requests, residents in the predominantly lower-income black areas who wanted trailers had to wait far longer than the residents of wealthier neighborhoods. New Orleans public officials also dragged their feet. With some justification, they blamed everything on a shortage of state and federal funding. Even after FEMA delivered the trailers to minority residents, they couldn't live in them because there was no hookup to water and power. Restoring power should not have been a problem in the Ninth Ward, since unlike other neighborhoods where the lines ran underground and power was supplied with extreme care, the power lines in the Ninth crisscrossed the sky, attached to wooden poles.

On April 6, with the city primary election only three weeks away, the City Council passed an ordinance that gave residents until August 31, the one-year anniversary of Katrina, to clean and gut their homes or risk losing them. Harris and Bradberry demanded and secured a meeting with the council set for April 29, just after the primary election.

Preserving the Status Quo

The April 22 mayoral primary was approaching. Twenty-two candidates had lined up to challenge Mayor Ray Nagin, a debonair forty-five-year-old African American who became mayor in 2002 with a black vote of only 20 percent in a majority black city. He moved with grace and talked with charm, and many women called him "Mayor Hottie." A Nagin victory would be a disaster for ACORN and the poor.

Lt. Gov. Mitch Landrieu, brother of Mary Landrieu, the state's U.S. senator, loomed as Nagin's major challenger. He had a reputation as an energetic lieutenant governor, and the Landrieus had built a formidable political dynasty in Orleans Parish since the 1970s, when patriarch Moon Landrieu served as the city's desegregationist mayor. If none of the candidates won a majority of the votes in the nonpartisan primary, the top two finishers would compete in a May 20 runoff election.

Rathke didn't believe Nagin could be reelected, and he wasn't alone. According to most pollsters, Nagin was the underdog.[8] The erosion of Nagin's white support and the Landrieu family's legacy as progressives caused many analysts to predict a victory for Landrieu. Some of ACORN's staff thought Landrieu was the better candidate, but his refusal even in private meetings with ACORN's leaders to campaign on ACORN's platform of the right to return and the right to rebuild the whole city lessened the interest of ACORN's members. With its members divided, ACORN as an organization decided not to endorse. But ACORN needed an election plan to further its strategy of encouraging residents to return.[9]

Concentrating on voter turnout was an obvious choice, but ACORN faced a daunting task. More than half the city's pre-Katrina population, 250,000 New Orleans residents, remained displaced and widely scattered from Baton Rouge to Boston. Katrina had destroyed more than half the city's polling places, and at least seven voting locations were inaccessible to the disabled.[10]

How would state and city officials deal with its displaced voters scattered in other Louisiana cities and states? How would voters prove residency? Would officials remove them from the voting rolls? Even if they remained on the rolls, would local politicians make a serious effort to find them and provide them with absentee ballots or access to voting machines?

Voting in New Orleans

Thousands of New Orleanians risked political disenfranchisement. Back in January 2005, Rathke had foreseen this possibility as both a danger and a strategic opportunity. In a memo to the staff, Rathke summed up ACORN's position on the election:

> The actual outcome of the election may rise and fall on the power of the absentee ballots cast by evacuees in cities around the country. . . . If New Orleans voters can be found and mobilized for this election, particularly in Houston, Dallas, Atlanta, and other large evacuee centers, then the political reality will not be just located on the high ground away from the flooding, but also in the low ground where New Orleans has fled. This would force politicians to have to campaign on their abilities

to bring people home, not their willingness to kowtow to developers, tourism moguls, and uptown wannabes.

ACORN, unlike most antipoverty groups, did not seek charitable tax-exempt status, and therefore it had the option of engaging in elections.[11] No rules or laws prevented its members from using elections to promote their agenda. ACORN had to make sure that the displaced residents voted and that it would be the link between the candidates and the dispersed voters. Relying on ACORN offices around the country, displaced ACORN members and their friends learned how to use the absentee voting procedures. But three weeks before the election, ACORN and the IAF affiliate TMO—another group with a voter registration campaign—found their effort lagging. Nationwide, only ten thousand evacuees had mailed absentee ballot requests.[12]

"Now's your time. Now's your time to make your voice heard," Kimberly Samuels would exhort into a telephone in a cramped, cluttered room in the ACORN Houston office. "You gonna make a difference. We want you to come out and vote. You gotta get off your butt and get out and do something. You just can't complain." Samuels, one of the leaders of the ACORN Katrina Survivors Association (AKSA) and other volunteers, worked the phones to energize the diaspora of hurricane survivors. Some volunteers knocked on doors and distributed absentee ballot applications, voter registration cards, and voter information packets, and organized voter rallies. ACORN created a website with election information.

Samuels knew that many of the displaced residents feared voting by absentee ballot because they didn't trust the process. She was one of them. "I'd rather take a three-hour bus trip to cast my ballot. I just don't trust the absentee process. I didn't want a repeat of what happened to the people in Florida."[13] So just two weeks before the election, Samuels and her compatriots, with a lot of help from Texas head organizer Goldman, planned to take busloads of evacuees living in Texas, Arkansas, Georgia, and Mississippi to early-voting sites in Louisiana.

On April 10, twelve days before the primary, hundreds of displaced Katrina survivors bussed from Houston, San Antonio, Dallas, Atlanta, and Jackson to satellite voting centers in Lake Charles, Shreveport, and New Orleans to cast their ballots on the first day of early voting. Gilda Burbank, flooded out of her Seventh Ward home, captured the spirit of the group. She believed that voting would be an important step in her plan to return to New Orleans permanently. She could have voted by mail from her Houston apartment, but "it makes me feel that at long last something is going to happen. It's the start of getting my life back," she said.

ACORN enlisted slightly more than eight thousand evacuees to vote early. The busing was both practical and symbolic of ACORN's continued message: the residents were coming back. As the election came down to the wire, ACORN generated all the publicity it could to encourage the displaced electorate to vote.

Nagin won 39 percent of the primary vote, beating Landrieu, who had 28 percent. A third leading candidate, Ron Forman, a local businessman, had 17 percent. Because no candidate received more than 50 percent of the vote, Nagin and Landrieu would compete in a runoff on May 20. Blacks cast an estimated 90 percent of their votes for Nagin. He drew only about 10 percent of the white vote.

Election officials were surprised by the overall turnout, and poll workers noted that large numbers of people traveled from temporary homes in neighboring states to cast ballots in person. About 36 percent of registered voters made it to the polls on Election Day, compared with the nearly 46 percent turnout recorded in the 2002 mayoral race.

The newspapers reported with some surprise that twenty thousand people voted early at satellite locations around Louisiana or by absentee ballot—ten times more than was usual in a city election.

Ginny Goldman was quoted in several papers as saying that, if not for the grassroots effort of ACORN, TMO, and others that helped mail in ballots and provide transportation to the polls, "no doubt, the turnout would be embarrassing. The folks in the diaspora tend to be the lower-income families and minority voting bloc. Without mobilizing, they wouldn't have been in this election."[14]

Nagin, the only major black candidate, polled better than expected. Just as his primary was based on race, so would he court the black vote during the general election.[15]

TMO and ACORN duplicated their outreach efforts for the May 20 runoff. ACORN had already reserved buses and organized bus trips to attend mayoral debates in New Orleans and cast early ballots in the runoff election. On May 11, Stukes bused back to New Orleans with sixty other survivors, although she was unsure that either candidate would provide jobs, low- to moderate-income housing, and insurance to help residents rebuild their homes so they could return.

When she arrived in New Orleans, Stukes said, according to an Associated Press report: "Whoever wins, it won't be a good candidate for the black people. Just be a compassionate mayor to work with all of us, to bring everyone back home."[16]

Nagin had tried to tap into the populist tradition of New Orleans but without the substance and aimed solely at blacks. He would say such things as, "I cross the line periodically, but I am you." During the debates, Nagin cursed, dropped final *g*'s, and gibed the more formal Landrieu. Among the ACORN and other evacuees bused in from Texas for a debate, he instantly gained an appreciative and chuckling cheering section. On May 20, in the racially charged general election, Nagin narrowly defeated Landrieu, winning 52 percent (59,460 votes) to Landrieu's 48 percent (54,131 votes). The race split along racial lines, with Nagin winning 80 percent of black votes, an exact reversal of the 2002 results.

Although Rathke understood that Nagin's victory was not good for ACORN, as usual he regarded the glass as half full, a necessary trait for the frustrating work of an antipoverty organizer. It was also a teachable moment, part of the job description for an ACORN organizer. In discussions with his friends and staff he said: "We came out of the election stronger. We protected most of our allies on the City Council and can work with a majority of that body. We emerged in a relationship with the mayor that, though not friendly, has convinced him that he can't move around us and has to deal with us." Rathke continued: "We moved buses of people from Houston, San Antonio, Dallas, Atlanta, Little Rock—thousands of absentee ballots. This was pivotal in the election, particularly in weeding out some of the elite and business interests in the primary election," referring to several City Council members close to ACORN who were elected. "With all our work prior to Katrina to this point, it was impossible for the media to ignore us, from the *New York Times* down to the *Times-Picayune*, and thereby hugely increased the weight and effectiveness of our voice."

One casualty Rathke didn't mention was Dorothy Stukes.

Keeping Volunteer Leaders

Attracting, training, and retaining leaders like Dorothy Stukes is critical to ACORN's success. Dorothy had grown more confident as a public speaker, and the other members of the AKSA respected her volunteer leadership. At meetings she made sure all attendees participated. She gained insight about herself and what it takes to bring about change. At public events, she was usually on message.

Like most survivors of Katrina, however, she suffered from considerable stress. Survivors had experienced a near epidemic of depression and post-traumatic stress disorder.[17] Dorothy channeled her stress and anger by fighting back, action that distracted her from her anxiety. She was often exhilarated, full of hope. Yet she had a hard time making ends meet. Although she was beginning to gain control of her destiny, she remained uncertain of her future. As the matriarch of her family, she felt the heavy weight of caring for her children and grandchildren.

She had become tired and frustrated over the slow pace of the New Orleans recovery. She still didn't have a job. Sometimes she had difficulty concentrating and would cry out from frustration. Every month she worried, Will I have enough money to pay for my medicine? The disruption in her life that Katrina had caused continued to haunt her.

A month before the election, Rathke had called Dorothy and criticized her for speaking publicly about policy positions that differed from those of the AKSA. He tried to be gentle with her, but he was emphatic. Rathke said, "Darling, you are the spokesperson for a democratic organization. You are accountable to the members. You can't just do and say anything you want."

A few days before Election Day, Dorothy called Ginny Goldman to ask if ACORN could provide box lunches for the Katrina survivors on their trip to New Orleans to vote. Stukes explained that some of the survivors were nearly broke. Goldman said that the AKSA was in debt. "I just got off the phone trying to raise for money for AKSA and for travel and lodging expenses so you and other members can go to the ACORN convention in Ohio," Goldman told her. Goldman, a 1997 graduate of SUNY Buffalo, like all the ACORN organizers, made a modest salary, a mere $35,000, and had turned down offers for higher-paying union jobs.

But the refusal made Dorothy mad. She thought of "all the money the Katrina survivors brought in for ACORN, and I haven't seen or touched a dime." She suspected that ACORN staff secretly worked for Landrieu. Maybe ACORN was raising money off the survivors' plight, she thought. She began to lose confidence in ACORN's ability to bring about changes in Washington, D.C. She needed more money.

Although ACORN had made significant strides since the 1970s in its effort to recruit black organizers such as Bertha Lewis, Tanya Harris, and Steve Bradberry and volunteer leaders such as Vanessa Gueringer and Toni McElroy, race remained an issue. Years of segregation and discrimination made many New Orleans African Americans angry and suspicious of white leaders. The hurricane reinforced their belief that they were victims of a conspiracy by white uptown developers. At one demonstration, Stukes said, "They wanted to genocide [black people]." Things were not going as well for her as Stukes had hoped. While she didn't completely attribute her problems to racism within ACORN, she thought race was a factor. After the election, she quit.

Ginny Goldman and Amy Schur, two outstanding organizers who worked closely with Dorothy, were stunned. By all accounts, both worked exceptionally hard during this period, especially supporting Stukes and other leaders. Goldman, who had been organizing in ACORN for nearly nine years, had never experienced the sudden departure of an active and effective leader such as Stukes. She called Rathke for advice, and he helped settle her nerves by putting the Stukes matter in perspective: "Remember, we have 220,000 dues-paying members organized into nearly nine hundred chapters in a hundred cities—and we're growing every month." Rathke reminded her that each city chapter had an activist voluntary governing board of directors of ten to fifteen leaders, and within these cities the nine hundred or so neighborhood chapters had four to five leaders. "That's about five thousand leaders," Rathke said. "And there are hundreds of other leaders. We're bound to have some dissatisfied leaders and members, aren't we?"

Goldman and Shur understood the incredibly difficult pressure Stukes had faced. She had given a great deal of time to help herself and her fellow Katrina survivors. Organizers like Goldman and Shur always feel the tension between acting fast in a crisis and spending time nurturing members and transforming them into leaders. But in the rush of events, when they had a dependable, naturally skilled leader like Stukes, the organizers figured they could neglect Stukes and she would grow as a public figure anyway.

For Rathke the loss was regrettable but understandable. He had been organizing for more than forty years and knew ACORN was not immune to organizational turnover and internal conflicts. Every organization has inner tension. In every membership organization with elected leaders, clashes between staff and leaders occur. Since its early beginnings in Arkansas, ACORN's leaders had come and gone, and some had fought with ACORN's staff over access to membership lists, policy agendas, and dues receipts. Some felt manipulated by ACORN's white, college-educated staff members, whom they saw as dominating decision making. A few leaders felt they were little more than animated props in someone's elaborate political theater. While Stukes was only one player, although a critical one, in a large saga, her departure was emblematic of the difficulties any anti-poverty group will have in sustaining its volunteer leaders like Stukes and raising enough money to train and sustain them.

Stukes left ACORN, but she didn't stop helping people. She became a volunteer with a United Way–funded agency that assisted Katrina victims. She was content in her new position of providing needed services and immediate emergency relief. She felt good when her agency received a grant of $25,000 from the department store Target and used the money to buy school supplies for survivor families.

A Rudderless Ship

Internal tension aside, ACORN was stuck with Nagin as mayor for another four years. Together they faced the massive reconstruction of a city teetering on the brink of bankruptcy, with 60 percent of its businesses closed. In the spring, the Jazz and Heritage Festival drew large crowds, and conventions were booked for summer and fall, but there was still no plan for the exiled New Orleanians to return. Evacuees confronted the deadline to clean and gut their homes or lose them.

During the election season, ACORN had kept alive other campaigns designed to bring evacuees back. Under the slogan "Memorials, not Demolitions," ACORN members kept pushing the City Council to extend the August 2006 deadline. On April 29, Bradberry and ACORN's members convinced City Council members to support ACORN's recommended amendment to exempt elderly residents in the Lower Ninth Ward from the August deadline. ACORN launched its own information campaign on the gutting deadline, placing flyers in businesses along the Gulf Coast, including more than sixty Winn-Dixie grocery stores and Starbucks coffee shops statewide.

The hardships for the survivors persisted. A desperate mother wrote to FinalCall.com News: "My daughter Banetta Adams has been notified by FEMA that she has 60 days to vacate her apartment here in Houston. FEMA says that she will be evicted because she cannot provide proof of her residency in New Orleans. In other words, FEMA is going to put my child and her two children in the street because she cannot prove that the vicious waters of Hurricane Katrina ravished her apartment and destroyed her property. . . . Where is the justice in this?"[18]

As the long hot summer of 2006 approached, opposition to shrinking New Orleans's footprint had forced the mayor to abandon his plans to declare the low-lying neighborhoods a lost cause. The gutting and cleaning of thousands of homes, the marches, the meetings, the voting—all demonstrated a deep determination by many former residents of New Orleans to return. The mayor had claimed his botched BNOB plan was not his plan, but just one of many plans he was considering. ACORN did not claim victory because, even though Nagin supported the right of all neighborhoods to be rebuilt, he didn't have a program or the money for the displaced. More than 200,000 former residents of New Orleans spread across forty-six states still had not returned. Along with ACORN and the business community, the survivors held their collective breath waiting for an official plan that would revitalize their city and allow them to come home.

The City Council and mayor agreed to put the planning process in the hands of a newly created nonprofit group, the New Orleans Community Support Foundation (NOCSF), funded by the Rockefeller Foundation, as well as by grants from the Greater New Orleans Foundation and the Bush-Clinton Katrina Fund.[19] NOCSF would select professional teams to work with seventy neighborhoods and eventually produce a "Unified Plan for New Orleans" to guide the investment of federal dollars in the rebuilding of Orleans Parish and serve as the city's long-term vision. Sixty-five professional planning and architectural firms from across the country applied to become a planning team, including some of the most eminent in the field, such as Andres Duany, a leader of the New Urbanism school of architecture.

How would ACORN ensure that the poor and working-class didn't get shut out of the planning process? Perhaps it could build on the foundation ACORN had started with its university partners—Cornell, the Pratt Institute, Louisiana State, the New Jersey Institute of Technology, the University of Illinois, and the Earth Institute of Columbia. Since the November 2005 conference at LSU, city planners from these universities had been meeting with displaced New Orleanians in the cities where they had been relocated. Ken Reardon, his students from Cornell, and other planners conducted community brainstorming sessions known as charrettes—an effective process that brings people together to design their community. This collaborative effort produced detailed schema for the neighborhoods of the Lower Ninth and New Orleans East, which up to this point had been ignored by the mayor. All this work would not be for naught if they could win the competition.

With yeoman help from Reardon, Shiffman, and Cornell and Pratt's interns, especially Andrew Rumbach, the collaborative submitted an application under the rubric of the ACORN Housing Corporation and their university partners. It was a long shot, because they were competing against sixty-eight nationally recognized architectural or planning firms.

On July 18, the unforeseen happened. The New Orleans Community Support Foundation (NOCSF) announced that an independent panel of nationally recognized experts had chosen ACORN Housing to be one of sixteen "official" New Orleans neighborhood planning teams, qualified to advise neighborhoods. Residents of the neighborhoods would meet, pick the team they wanted, work with the team, and submit the neighborhood designs to the mayor and City Council sometime in the fall. Their design would be integrated into the Unified New Orleans Plan. To Rathke, this victory could not be overstated: "It means the people's voices are being heard."[20]

After a series of meetings, residents from the Lower Ninth Ward and New Orleans East easily chose ACORN to be their team. This was not surprising given ACORN's networks, its planning team's capacity, its history of attending to the low-income needs of the city, and its housing development capacity.

On July 22, a restive crowd at the K&B Plaza Building gathered to meet the planners and learn about the process. The meeting got off to a rocky start when Jack Stewart, a local historian active in the downtown Lafayette Square District, interrupted the officials running the meeting and accused the city government of coming up with plan after plan that didn't result in action. "Is this another exercise in futility or is this going to be something meaningful?" Stewart shouted out from a crowd of about seventy-five people straining to hear the representative from NOCSF who was running the meeting. One speaker pushed back and challenged Stewart and the other neighborhood activists at the meeting to get involved. Stewart and the other attendees were told that the sixteen teams, including ACORN, were qualified to advise neighborhoods, and now it was up to the neighborhoods to decide which teams they wanted. To choose the teams they were encouraged to come to a community forum on August 1 to hear presentations by the various firms. Rathke was confident that ACORN would be chosen to plan the Lower Ninth Ward and even New Orleans East.

On August 1, 2006, the foundation held the first in its series of public meetings. Groups representing more than seventy neighborhoods were invited to meet the planners and then select the one to help determine everything, from where to build houses to the design of public parks to the width of sidewalks. The upscale neighborhoods were the best organized. The meeting was a mess. Only those who got there early, sitting in the four or five chairs nearest a facilitator, had any chance of hearing a single word of what was being said. Then the groups of neighborhood residents, many of them still displaced, heard directly from the planning teams to get a sense of which ones they might want to work with. After the presentations, residents were instructed to vote for the firms they wanted to represent their neighborhoods through on-line voting that ended August 7. According to Steven Bingler, the architect in charge of the planning process, "The planner's responsibility is not to make the decision, but to empower people to make decisions for themselves and their own communities."

While this kind of democratic planning was consistent with ACORN's philosophy, to the average citizen the process felt more like being in *Alice in Wonderland*. After three hours of confusion and frustration, Rathke, who was attending the meeting with several ACORN staff and leaders, left, telling his colleague Mike Shea, "I believe that going to a worm dig might be a better use of my Sunday." Two hours later, everyone left.

No one could explain how any plan would become a reality, since the federal government had not committed the money to build the housing, create the jobs, and restore the levees and coastal wetlands needed to protect against future flooding—all of which were fundamental to making a visionary plan a reality. Moreover, the planners and architects controlling the process, such as Wayne Troyer and Robert Tannen of New Orleans and Andrés Duany of Miami, didn't understand this kind of participatory planning and were known for what Nicolai Ouroussoff, the *New York Times* architectural critic, called "the kind of cookie-cutter visions that have been sapping the vitality of American cities for decades." Ouroussoff was profoundly correct when he criticized the city for forfeiting a chance to consider how infrastructure could be used to bind communities—rich and poor, black and white—into a collective whole.[21]

Ouroussoff was also correct when he blamed city planning's problem on "the anti-big-government campaigns that gained momentum in the Reagan era, leaving ever more infrastructure, from parks to phone systems to schools, in the hands of private corporations. But the aversion to broad planning is also based on a neo-liberal belief that it is impossible to build any large-scale urban project without destroying the fine-grained fabric of city neighborhoods," a critique similar to the one he had registered against the activists in Brooklyn who opposed ACORN's support of Atlantic Yards. Perhaps most importantly, the power relationships between the poor and working class and the white businessmen remained inequitable, unless those groups quickly formed themselves into a power block, which wasn't going to happen.[22]

While the process would prove educational for some neighborhood activists, thousands of residents who needed housing, food, clothing, and jobs had little time to engage in this time-consuming planning process. But this flawed process was better than the earlier one set up by Nagin that marginalized the poor. Despite the chaos and a faulty process, ACORN got one of the highest vote totals and was now in charge of the process in the Lower Ninth and New Orleans East.

Fighting against a Deadline

The survivors from the Lower Ninth and New Orleans East, most of whom had not yet returned, still faced the August 29 deadline or risked seizure under eminent domain. ACORN's Steve Bradberry, Tanya Harris, Vanessa Gueringer, and others had repeatedly asked the City Council to postpone the deadline until at least November 2006. ACORN had 9,000 member families in New Orleans when Katrina hit, yet almost one year later, ACORN had connected with only 2,500. If the deadline wasn't extended, most of the other families might not have homes to return to, no matter what kind of plan ACORN came up with.

At a crowded City Council meeting on August 4, 2006, Loyola University of New Orleans law professor William Quigley, accompanied by two dozen members of ACORN and Common Ground, warned the council members that the August 29 deadline was unconstitutional because the city had failed to properly notify absent owners. The ACORN members held a large banner that declared "NO To Plan To Steal Our Land!" and signs that proclaimed "Hands Off Our Property" and "Save Our Homes." Council president Oliver Thomas pleaded with the crowd: "It's not a land grab by the city. We did something we thought we could use as a guideline."[23] ACORN member Joy Hess, whose Lakeview home was ravaged by Katrina's floodwaters, said ACORN had hundreds on its waiting list to gut and clean. More than five thousand volunteers had helped with the project, including students on spring break, and workers from the AFL-CIO and the Canadian Autoworkers Union.

The council held one more meeting on August 18 to decide the fate of the August 29 deadline. Representatives from ACORN, All Congregations Together, and the People's Hurricane Relief Fund implored the council to extend or repeal the deadline. Matt Hew of Common Ground said several of the nonprofits that had been gutting homes at no charge had four-month waiting lists. "Some aren't even answering the phones," he said. "There are so few volunteers. The deadline wasn't tied to resources." Despite their pleas, the City Council took no action. The council and mayor insisted the gutting law in April was necessary to force people to clean up moldy and muck-filled homes that threatened the health and recovery prospects of their neighborhoods. It was the council's last scheduled meeting before the deadline.

Stephen Bradberry's telephone at New Orleans ACORN continued to ring off the hook. His office had received more than a thousand requests for the free house-gutting service offered by ACORN since he appeared on an NPR broadcast in late August to talk about the program. He added these requests to the hundreds on his waiting list. The same was happening to other nonprofit agencies, although some had to close their waiting lists for lack of volunteers. Displaced New Orleanians were calling after hearing Bradbury's on-air comments that the city had imposed an August 29 deadline for homeowners to get themselves on a gutting and cleaning list to avoid demolition. In addition, should the federal government and the insurance companies ever come up with the money, their houses would be ready for rehabilitation.

Vanessa Gueringer, a lifelong resident of the Lower Ninth Ward and a member of ACORN since 2001, waited anxiously as the anniversary of Hurricane Katrina approached. If ACORN couldn't force the city to back down, the city would seize whatever homes had not yet been cleaned up or reclaimed in order to resell or demolish them—without even notifying the former residents. As the chair of ACORN's Lower Ninth Ward homeowners group, she felt passionately that holding to the August 29 date was outrageous.

At the last moment, ACORN and other groups persuaded the City Council to amend the deadline so that all the Lower Ninth residents were exempted due to hardship. Any homes scheduled for gutting and cleaning by ACORN (and fifteen other groups) would be deemed in compliance and exempt from any seizure order. For homes not yet scheduled for clean up, the city agreed to attempt to contact the owners twice in sixty days before proceeding to take possession of the property. Gueringer told the press: "ACORN didn't get everything it wanted with this compromise, but at least it stopped the bulldozers for now. But what about New Orleans East and other parts of the city? We've literally got neighborhoods with thousands of homes where we've been able to get, maybe, one family back. Lower-income families can't even afford the transportation to come back here. Now at least we've gained a little more protection for struggling families we are working with."

Two New Houses

So many stories proliferated about the disaster that it was difficult to get the national media to pay attention to the ACORN story. Knowing that the press and TV would descend on New Orleans in droves for the first anniversary of Katrina, Bradberry, Harris, Gueringer, and other ACORN members worked feverishly to mount a compelling event on August 26, 2006, three days before the first anniversary of the storm.

ACORN members, supporters, government officials, and a few reporters showed up. Josephine Butler and her granddaughter, Tanya Harris, greeted the spectators on Delery Street in front of the land where Butlers' home had stood, the area of the Lower Ninth that had suffered the most damage when the levees broke. Her mind's eye saw the one-story, compact white, green, and pink front-to-back-hall style, the shotgun houses built on tiny lots and separated by chain-link fences, and the once vibrant street full of life, with several churches and a nearby juke joint for dancing.

Those at the press conference were told that 1,250 homes had been bulldozed. The area looked more like a junkyard for demolished cars than a potential neighborhood. There was no water, electricity, or people. The few houses that stood were shells with missing doors and broken windows. Harris announced a program that startled some of the onlookers: ACORN was beginning a restoration program with LSU to rebuild or renovate three homes in the Lower Ninth every thirty days. ACORN would have to obtain the funding, provide the labor, draft the rebuilding plans, and cut through the red tape. "Our goal is to help people help themselves and inspire others," Harris said. "We want to give them that first flicker of hope. Our strategy is to do things ourselves and force the hands of government."

Butler and her granddaughter each picked up a shovel and drove it into the dirt, breaking ground for what they hoped would be Butler's new home at 2310 Delery Street. "Nearly sixty years ago, my grandfather, one of the area's pioneers, built his first home on this lot," Harris said. Although they were scattered after the storm, Harris believed the former residents would regroup in large enough numbers to make the street come alive again. "Today, we mark a new beginning for the Lower Ninth Ward and New Orleans. Once those houses are up," she continued, "I guarantee you people will be back."

For many observers across the country, the Lower Ninth Ward came to symbolize the failure of the nation to save New Orleans for all its former residents, not just the white and the well-to-do. Yet given all the obstacles, the task seemed far beyond ACORN's capacity. Moreover, many planning experts warned that what ACORN was doing was unsound planning. Instead of neighborhoods, areas like the Lower Ninth would typify the jack-o'-lantern effect, in which renovated homes were interspersed with blighted and abandoned structures. Bill Reilly, executive director of the Louisiana Recovery Authority, publicly warned, "My worst fear is for the homeowner to take his nest egg, invest it back into the home, and two years from now, look to the right and to the left and see vacant lots."

"The jack-o-lantern effect doesn't scare people in the Lower Ninth Ward," Harris retorted in response to a reporter's question. "Let's get that straight. These people understand what it is to be in an undeveloped area. My grandmother was here when there were gravel streets and just a couple of neighbors on every block."

One year after Katrina, most of the work of rebuilding New Orleans still lay ahead. ACORN's demonstrations, lobbying, voter registration, gutting and clean-up program, and the ACORN Katrina Survivor Association had helped gain additional federal and state funding and proved that many New Orleanians wanted to return and rebuild their city. ACORN had led the fight to halt eminent domain in the Ninth Ward and, like many other civic groups, helped former residents secure government aid, and even provided a job-training and placement program. ACORN accomplished what few groups could. It stopped unfair lending practices, halted the city's rush to take property by eminent domain, and won a greater voice for residents in the rebuilding process by putting together a professional support group of architects, planners, engineers, environmentalists, lawyers, and housing developers. The group designed a comprehensive rebuilding program for the city; it became one of the city's official neighborhood-planning teams and then went to work to implement the plans in two of the poorest neighborhoods, the Lower Ninth and New Orleans East. Still, many experts and local leaders, including the American Planning Association executive director Paul Farmer, remained troubled by ACORN's action and the city's inaction on the footprint question. They thought the city needed to shrink its developed areas. Most of the white power structure agreed. The looming question was still, For whom will the city be rebuilt?

Fired

For the poor in New Orleans, the future looked ominous. The Bush administration's Department of Housing and Urban Development took steps to raze the public housing projects. The agency claimed that the complexes, built in the 1940s and 1950s, were dilapidated. But former tenants and housing advocates disagreed. The plans to demolish the projects would outrage many, including Nicolai Ouroussoff of the *New York Times*. This housing in New Orleans, he wrote, "ranks among the best early examples of public housing built in the United States, both in design and in quality of construction." Of the complex called Lafitte, he wrote: "Low-rise apartments and narrow front porches, set around what were once beautifully landscaped gardens, are intended to encourage a spirit of community."[24]

Rathke and ACORN's organizers thought HUD's decision was reprehensible, but ACORN was tied up in too many other matters to take action. In October another blow to the poor fell: ACORN lost the New Orleans recovery consulting job.

The notice came in mid-October, just three days after ACORN's planners held a key community forum. Residents excitedly spelled out their planning goals: give pre-Katrina residents first priority in purchasing redeveloped property in their neighborhoods; restore and establish after-school programs; address Katrina-related mental health needs; create community policing systems and encourage police officers to live in the neighborhoods they patrol; keep public transportation routes flexible.

Now the New Orleans Community Support Foundation (NOCSF) dismissed ACORN. The notice cited ACORN's potential conflict of interest. Despite its excellent plan and process of community involvement, it was replaced, according to officials, because ACORN Housing would also be a property developer.

Bradberry and Vanessa Gueringer were furious about ACORN's dismissal. They suspected that past clashes between ACORN and local community leaders on issues was the true reason. Several local leaders, fearing ACORN was gaining too much power, quietly lobbied against it. The termination letter from Wayne Lee, chair of the NOCSF board, expressed the "utmost respect" for ACORN's work in New Orleans and urged its continuing participation as a "stakeholder" in Lower Ninth Ward planning.[25]

NOCSF decided to ignore the overwhelming support ACORN got in the voting process used by NOCSF to decide which consultants should be hired for planning. Officials replaced ACORN with consulting teams already planning other parts of the city.

Because ACORN had too much on its plate already, the staff decided not to pursue this battle but to concentrate on its development plans for the Lower Ninth and New Orleans East. Approximately a quarter of Rathke's SEIU Local 100 members lived in these two sectors, and almost a third of the ACORN membership lived in the Lower Ninth Ward. Using the designs developed by its planning team, ACORN would concentrate on building and rehabbing homes in those areas so people could move back.

The project to develop the Unified New Orleans Plan, slated to conclude by mid-January 2007, proceeded apace. Without ACORN's active involvement in the planning, however, upper-income white residents dominated the process. For example, on October 29, when people gathered around tables at the Ernest N. Morial Convention Center to further the Unified plan, 75 percent of the 350 participants were white, and 40 percent had an annual household income of more than $75,000. All but a few participants at the meeting wanted the plan to reduce the number of places to rebuild.

Katherine Prevost, one of the few Ninth Ward residents who came to the meeting, left the session angry because the group refused to direct money toward the hardest-hit areas. "We're the ones that got the water, but we're not going to get all the funding? If the people in an area didn't get water, they don't need the funds as much as people in other areas. I just feel like they're living off the ones that got water. If it never flooded, we wouldn't have these funds."

Nagin didn't show up for the meeting, but he publicly continued to urge residents not to plan on rebuilding in low-lying areas or in those where levee protection was weak, code for the Lower Ninth Ward and two sections of eastern New Orleans. Still, his administration had not stopped issuing building permits in any section of the city. To most people the planning process was incomprehensible or just a bad idea.

Meanwhile, thousands of residents angrily waited for the government housing assistance President Bush had promised. A November 18 *New York Times* editorial titled "Katrina's Purgatory" warned about the dangerous choice survivors faced: "The normal hard decisions of real estate are amplified a thousand times by the possibility that a house in an empty neighborhood in a broken city could be worthless." Further, "the average government award in Louisiana is $60,200, and it will cost more than that to replace your house." That dilemma assumed there was government money available. According to the *Times*, at the end of November 2006, the number of residents approved for funds was only 5,000—out of nearly 78,000 applications. Only an infinitesimal 28 Louisiana families had received their share of the federal dollars intended to help them fix up or restore their homes. Why? Mostly because the Bush administration had taken nearly six months just to request the necessary rebuilding funds. Then Republicans sat on their hands until June 2006 before approving the legislation.

On top of the delays, many families that wanted to rebuild could not find contractors. Even if they could, most couldn't afford the high prices for the scarce building materials. If they could afford the high prices to rebuild, they couldn't afford the skyrocketing insurance rates. In addition to those problems, victims like Dorothy Stukes who missed bill payments or couldn't find jobs hurt their credit records. These folks couldn't get loans or had to pay high unaffordable interest rates on any loans they needed.

There was some good news for low-income renters. On Wednesday, November 29, 2006, ACORN won a landmark legal victory on behalf of Katrina survivors. A federal judge ruled that FEMA must immediately resume providing housing benefits to eleven thousand families who had been unfairly denied aid. FEMA had been providing families with critical housing assistance, then illegally cut their housing funding with no clear explanation, and then told the storm victims they could reapply. One ACORN plaintiff, Carmen Handy, described her dilemma in court: "The reasons I have been given for the termination are not what is in the documents and/or the reasons change each time I call. Every time I call back, the person answering the call knows nothing about what the previous person told me." Very few got the money because of what the judge called a "Kafkaesque convoluted application process."[26]

In December 2006, John Edwards formally launched his candidacy for the presidency in the Lower Ninth, dramatizing his antipoverty theme and that of a nation divided by economic inequality. In contrast, President Bush in his January 2007 State of the Union speech would fail to mention the Gulf Coast or anything about a needed recovery effort. Shortly after his speech, the U.S. Senate's Homeland Security and Governmental Affairs Committee held hearings in New Orleans. Nagin accused the FEMA director of reneging on his agreement to pay $334 million for infrastructure repairs. State officials accused city leaders of failing to provide required documentation. Donald Powell, the president's coordinator for the Gulf Coast recovery effort, pledged long-term support. A protester yelled: "Stand up for justice! We want somebody to stand up for justice!" before being dragged out by the police.[27] Justice could be found only on the deserted streets of New Orleans, where courageous volunteers and organizers stood up for those most afflicted by the tragedy.

Delery Street Revisited

Tanya Harris anxiously awaited the ground-breaking ceremony on February 22, 2007, on Delery Street. It should be big news, Harris felt. The media, including the *New York Times* and TV stations, had said they would show up. Plaques were bought for the volunteers and dignitaries like Congresswoman Maxine Waters. Richard Ford, the novelist would make a speech. For Tanya Harris, this day was also personal.

Under a glowing sun, the Rev. Leonard Lucas Jr. opened the festivities with a blessing of the homes. "ACORN took a stand initially to say, 'Stay in your homes.' You can come back to the Lower Ninth Ward." ACORN made the city bring in water, turn on the lights and made the city say yes when the city said no." Marsha R. Cuddeback, an architect from LSU, said: "The project represents an extraordinary tale of grassroots reconstruction, collaborative learning among diverse stakeholders . . . to serve as a catalyst for positive change." As she spoke, the press appeared and TV cameras began setting up. Ken Bacon, Fannie Mae's executive vice president of Housing and Community Development, confirmed that "many evacuees want to return to the neighborhood where they raised their children and an area they are proud to call home." Richard Ford called the project a "valiant and hopeful house raising," a reference to the barn raisings of early America when neighbors pitched in to help one another construct buildings on newly settled land. He turned toward two ACORN members and said: "There's a lot of cheap talk we hear every day about whether this community will come back, can come back, should be allowed to come back. But if it's going to come back, that will depend a lot less on politicians' talk, or land developers' greedy plans, or on 'the economy,' whatever that means, and instead it will depend on people like you two, who let their feet and their hearts and their determination do their talking, and who know that 'community' is not just a word on a sign."

With that, Reverend Lucas handed over the keys to two remarkable women and their families who were committed to rebuilding the Lower Ninth Ward. They had been next-door neighbors for twenty-five years, and now stood on the property where their original houses had survived for decades before being destroyed. The two women hugged, laughed, and cried with happiness. To some it seemed like a miracle.

One of the women was Gwendolyn Guice. "I can't stop bawling," she said, overwhelmed by the support and the outcome. The other was Josephine Butler, Harris's grandmother. "A lot of people are just sitting back, waiting and seeing. This'll help draw people back," Harris said. Vanessa Gueringer, chair of ACORN's Lower Ninth Ward chapter, summed up: "Rebuilding on Delery Street says to the world that the Ninth Ward is coming back."

ACORN and ACORN Housing had finished building the first two new homes in the Lower Ninth Ward since the hurricane. These new houses—a milestone—were a big step toward ACORN's vision of rebuilding a whole new residential development in the Lower Ninth. Delery had become ACORN's line in the sand.

Building the two houses had required the kind of creative partnership a nonprofit group needed to build affordable housing. Financing came from Countrywide Bank, HUD, Fannie Mae, and Morgan Stanley Chase. Louisiana State University's School of Architecture designed the houses using a new hurricane-resistant, energy-efficient concept. LSU students and youngsters from Covenant House volunteered. Men and women from a drug rehabilitation program helped build the houses under a supervised on-the-job training program. (Most of them went on to future jobs in construction.) Volunteers included members from the Canadian Auto Workers Union and the Unitarian Universalist Service Committee, along with the novelist Richard Ford, who lives in New Orleans.

The homes, valued at about $125,000 each, resembled the colorful wood-frame shotgun style, but instead of the traditional cypress wood exterior, they were covered with mold- and termite-resistant siding. They could withstand winds of 160 miles per hour.

The next day the event made the front page of the national news section of the *New York Times* with a big photo of Guice and Baker. The headline announced: "In New Orleans, Progress at Last in the Lower Ninth Ward."[28]

Rathke, Harris, and Shea knew all too well the extraordinary effort it had taken to put this demonstration project together. How often could ACORN replicate this process? ACORN's people could see that the two houses standing alongside each other, gleaming at the eastern edge of Delery Street, sat in terrain shockingly unchanged since the hurricane, when the water rose twelve feet. Surrounding the two new houses were a school building with a collapsed roof, muddy vacant lots, and shattered houses. Street signs were missing. While a few houses in the distance had been brought back to life, gutted homes rehabbed, many businesses and houses stood empty, waiting to be rebuilt. The view from the back porch of the new home built for Josephine Butler included mudholes, a debris pile, fallen trees, and tangles of vines. While the neighborhood was improved, it didn't look very different than in the days following Hurricane Katrina.

Was this a useful model for the future? Skeptics such as Andrés Duany believed that a neighborhood as impoverished as Delery's couldn't be restored without large-scale intervention. Duany, a Miami architect and planner who was playing a leading role in the city's rebuilding efforts, told the *New York Times*: "I think we have a problem of quantity, and anything that can't be delivered in quantity is not a suitable prototype, regardless of the fantastic intentions. The verification is not aesthetics, not the degree of goodwill; it's quantity."[29]

Duany was right about scale, and ACORN's people didn't disagree. But scale required political will backed up by money, which was in short supply. Delery was a long way from being a neighborhood again, but ACORN was bent on building the political will.

The hurdles to ACORN's recovery strategy remained formidable. Few residents had received the financial and physical resources they needed to rebuild their homes. Protection against future storms was not complete. Health, sanitation, water, and other services were insufficient. High unemployment in New Orleans forced displaced residents who lacked savings, insurance, and credit to look for jobs in the areas where they had relocated. Polls had indicated that now less than 50 percent of the evacuees intended to return to New Orleans.[30]

But on Delery Street under Thursday's bright sun, the focus was not on the hurdles. The words of Harris and of Allan Jones, an electrician who worked on the two houses, captured the spirit of the day: "If you try not to focus on how bad everything is, you can focus on what is good," said Jones.

"Could Delery lead the way back?" Harris then asked. "When my grandmother moved to the area nearly sixty years ago, it was a semi-wilderness and a shot in the dark. It was a leap of faith then. It's a leap of faith now."

Faith plus hard work was about to pay off. In December 2006 Nagin had appointed his recovery czar. A former chair of the Department of City and Regional Planning at the University of California, Berkeley, Ed Blakely was a recognized expert in disaster recovery. After watching him operate for two months, Rathke called him "a force of nature." He liked the way Blakely "nailed the uptown and business elites as 'insular' and called them 'buffoons.'"[31] Blakely also demanded that all the money for New Orleans be spent through his office.

A month after the Delery grand opening, Steve Bradberry received a call from Blakely. "I want to meet with you and ACORN's leadership in private, no press."

Blakely came into the meeting and introduced himself. He said that ACORN was the only community-based organization that he intended to meet with personally before he officially announced the new rebuilding plan. He said ACORN had played a critical role in fighting to save the Ninth Ward and especially the Lower Ninth Ward. "I deeply admire ACORN's grit, persistence, and your commitment." He specifically mentioned ACORN's plan for the Ninth Ward and the way it mobilized people, money, and capacity to build the first houses in the Lower Ninth. He poured coffee as he listened to the concerns of Vanessa Gueringer, Gwendolyn Adams, Tanya Harris, and others. Blakely responded by telling them that the Lower Ninth Ward was going to be one of the seventeen recovery neighborhoods. These seventeen limited areas, he said, would become catalysts for further development around them. And to make sure that these areas got rebuilt, he was committing a large amount of infrastructure funds to the Lower Ninth Ward and the area around the New Orleans East Plaza.

"Whether you get the credit or not, you need to know—and you are hearing it from me personally right now—that you have earned the credit by making the fight, and because of that you have saved the Lower Ninth Ward." Rathke would later say, "They might have rescued the Lower Ninth Ward, but for sure they were on cloud nine."[32]

Two days later, ACORN leaders milled around City Hall among a crowd that included public officials, City Council members, and the mayor of New Orleans. Harris was surprised to see that they were the only people there who were not elected officials, public employees, or members of the press. ACORN was the only independent community group invited to the official presentation of the entire recovery development plan.

The front-page picture in the *Times-Picayune* the next day featured Vanessa Gueringer, Gwendolyn Adams, and Tanya Harris pointing at the Lower Ninth on the map at the City Hall unveiling. Another picture caught the mayor bending on his knee in front of Gueringer, fooling around but also symbolizing his respect for ACORN's work. The *New York Times* covered the story with a color picture of Butler's house on Delery Street.

Blakely's original plan did not include a "right to return" for former residents. In an interview with the *New York Times*, Blakely had said that the "lower-income population" now "trapped outside the city" may not be coming back. New Orleans "won't be the same" when the dust settles, suggesting that a new population with more "energy" may replace the old.[33]

Rathke, forever concerned about the line between co-optation and victory, wondered, Have we been co-opted? He wasn't certain, but he knew the price: the future of the Lower Ninth Ward. As he would later say, if "we could bring back 'dat nine' then we could bring everyone home someday."

"Vanessa Gueringer, chairwoman of Lower 9th Ward chapter of the community activist group ACORN, had trouble containing her excitement when she saw the blueprint for her ruined area," reported the *Times-Picayune*. "While vowing to keep the city honest about its proposal, Gueringer said she believes the plan will quell simmering concerns that politicians intend to abandon her neighborhood. 'This is awesome,' she said, adding that she planned to spend all day on the phone sharing the news with her neighbors still displaced in Houston and Atlanta. 'It says to the Lower 9th Ward: You can come home!' "[34]

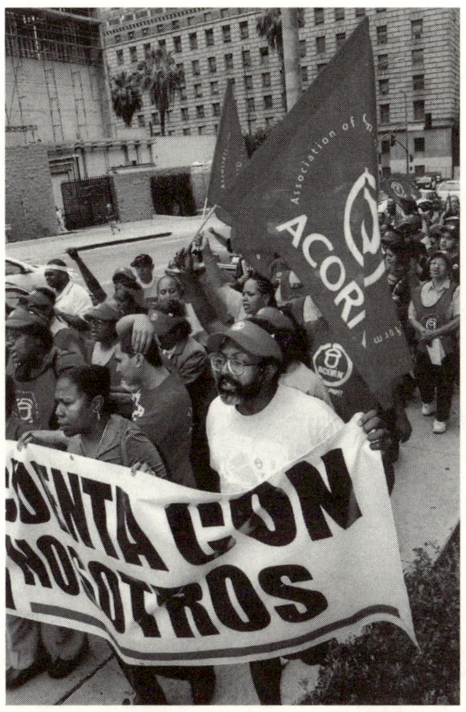

Figure 16. ACORN Housing president Alton Bennett, *far right*, with demonstrators in Los Angeles against a bank engaged in nationwide predatory lending, 2004. (Photo by Valerie Coffin)

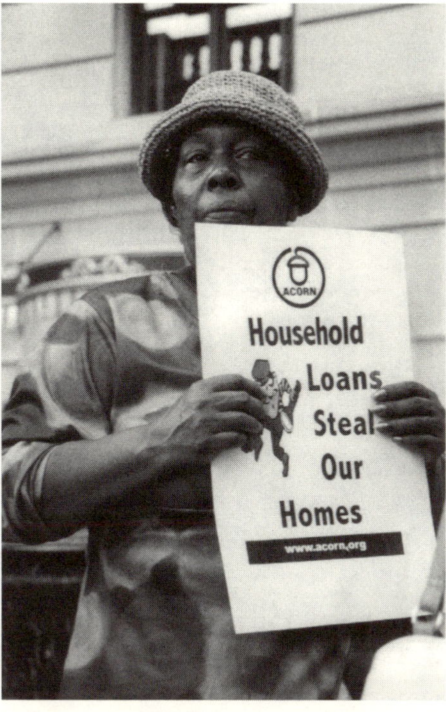

Figure 17. ACORN member protesting HFC lending practices, 2001. (Photo by Valerie Coffin)

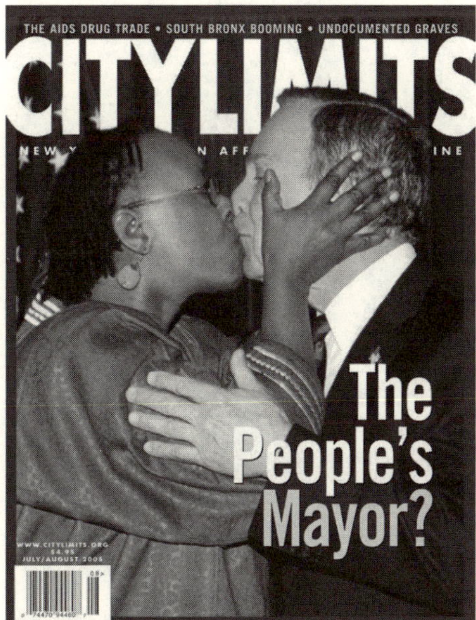

Figure 18. At Brooklyn Borough Hall, May 19, 2005, New York ACORN executive director Bertha Lewis kissing Mayor Bloomberg and developer Bruce Ratner at a media event, a symbolic deal binder between ACORN and Ratner's contentious Atlantic Yards project. (Courtesy of *City Limits.* Photo by Tom Callan.)

NO PARK
NO PARKING
Eminent
Domain
Abuse
FORCES:
US OUT
US APART
US TO PAY
RATNER'S BILL
WWW.NOLANDGRAB.ORG

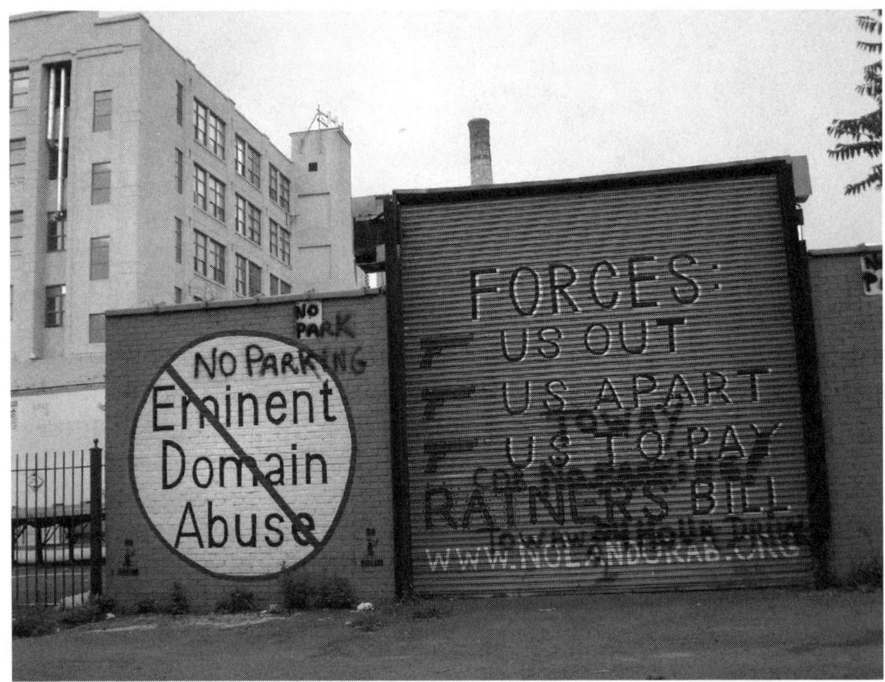

Figure 19. Protest signs opposing the Atlantic Yards development, which would require New York City to take over properties using its powers of eminent domain, 2005. (Photo by Bonnie Friedman)

ACORN says
OHIO
DESERVES
A RAISE
ACORN
MAKE THE
MINIMUM WAGE
LIVING WAGE

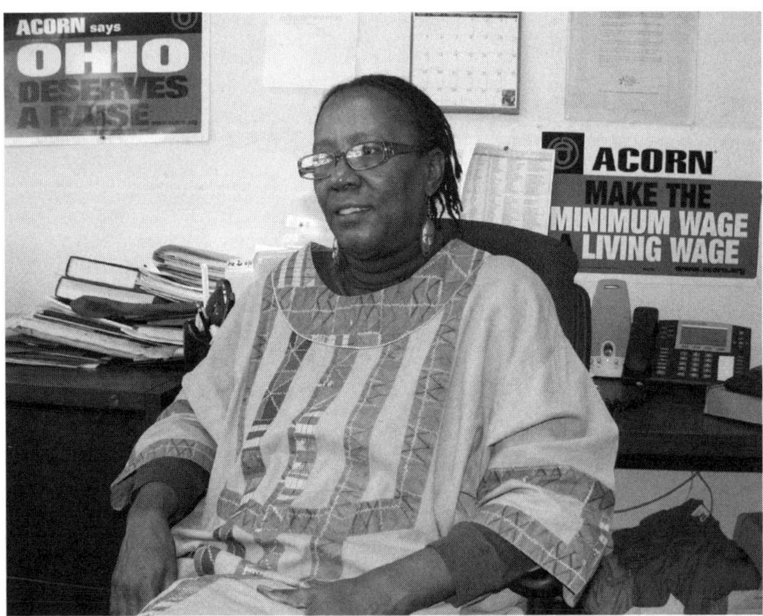

Figure 20. Bertha Lewis in the Brooklyn ACORN office, 2008. (Photo by Bonnie Friedman)

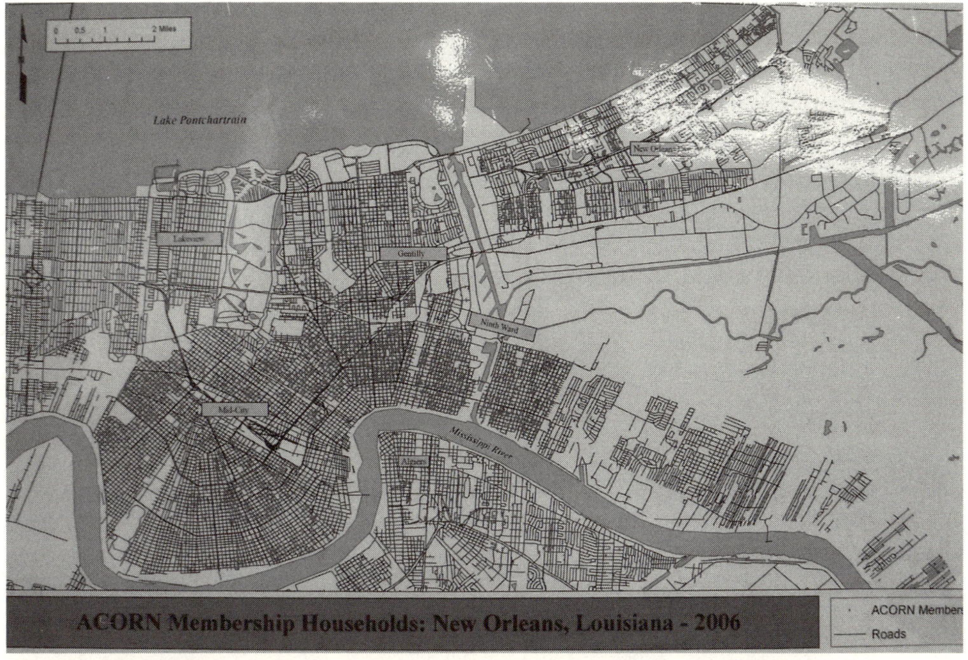

Figure 21. An overlay map of Katrina's flood zones showed that the New Orleans neighborhoods the hurricane made famous—Gentilly, Hollygrove, New Orleans East, and the Lower Ninth Ward—were all ACORN strongholds. Nearly every block in the Lower Ninth Ward was home to several ACORN members. (Photo by Bonnie Friedman, map by ACORN)

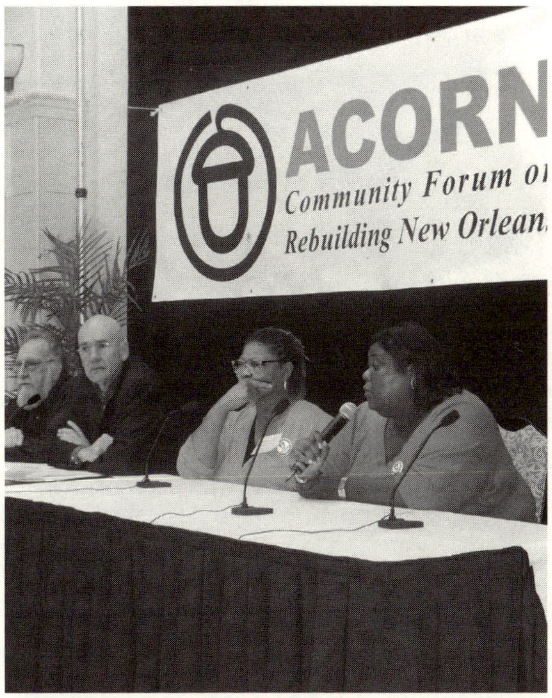

Figure 22. Dorothy Stukes on a panel that includes ACORN organizer Tanya Harris and eminent urban planners Ron Shiffman and David Cronrath, dean of the LSU School of Art and Design, at the Community Forum on Rebuilding New Orleans, November 7 and 8, 2005. The conference marked the first time urban planning experts asked Katrina survivors what they wanted—nearly three months after the hurricane. (Photo by ACORN)

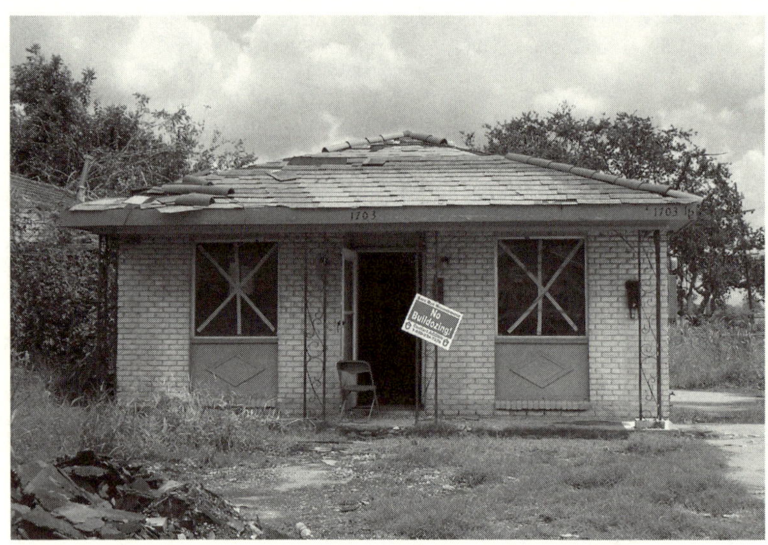

Figure 23. ACORN members on September 27, 2005, a month after Hurricane Katrina hit New Orleans, put up thousands of No Bulldozing signs to discourage New Orleans city and developer interests from writing off their communities. (Photo by Bonnie Friedman)

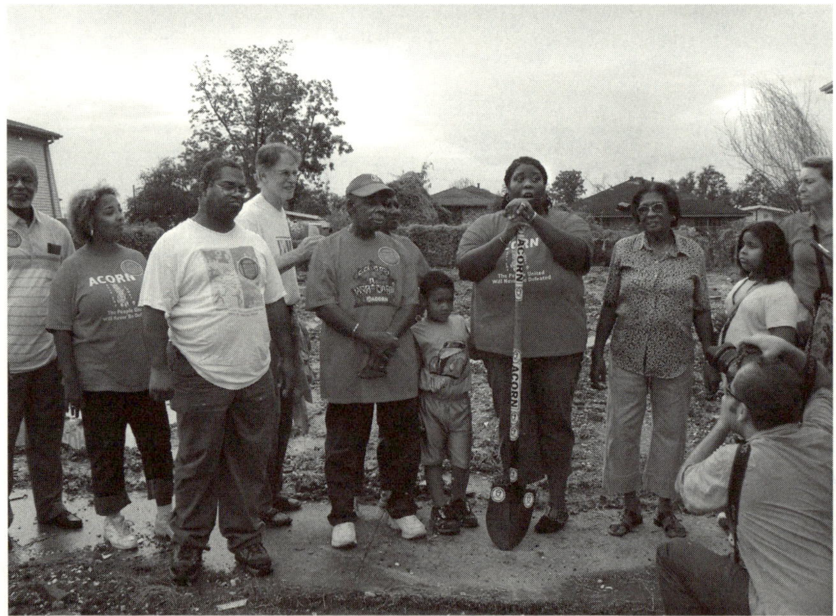

Figure 24. A press conference on symbolic Delery Street, August 26, 2006, three days before the first anniversary of Hurricane Katrina. ACORN organizer Tanya Harris, leaning on a shovel, stands next to her grandmother Josephine Butler in front of the land where Butler's Lower Ninth home once stood. *Left,* ACORN leaders Vanessa Gueringer and Vincent Copper; *right,* Louisiana ACORN head organizer Beth Butler; with Harris's niece and nephew Samuel and Abyssinia Flores. (Photo by Bonnie Friedman)

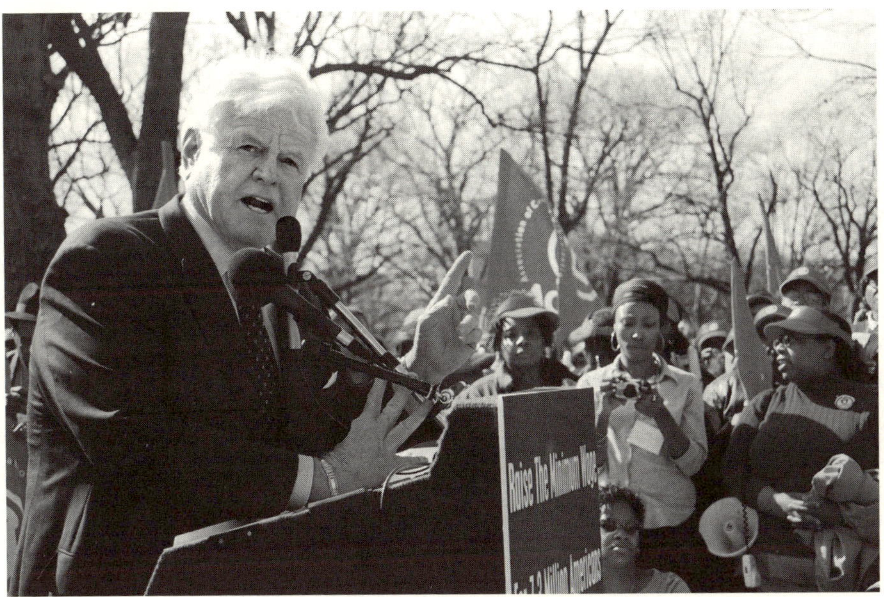

Figure 25. Senator Ted Kennedy addressing an ACORN rally at the 2005 National Legislative Conference Day of Action, Washington, D.C. (Photo by Valerie Coffin)

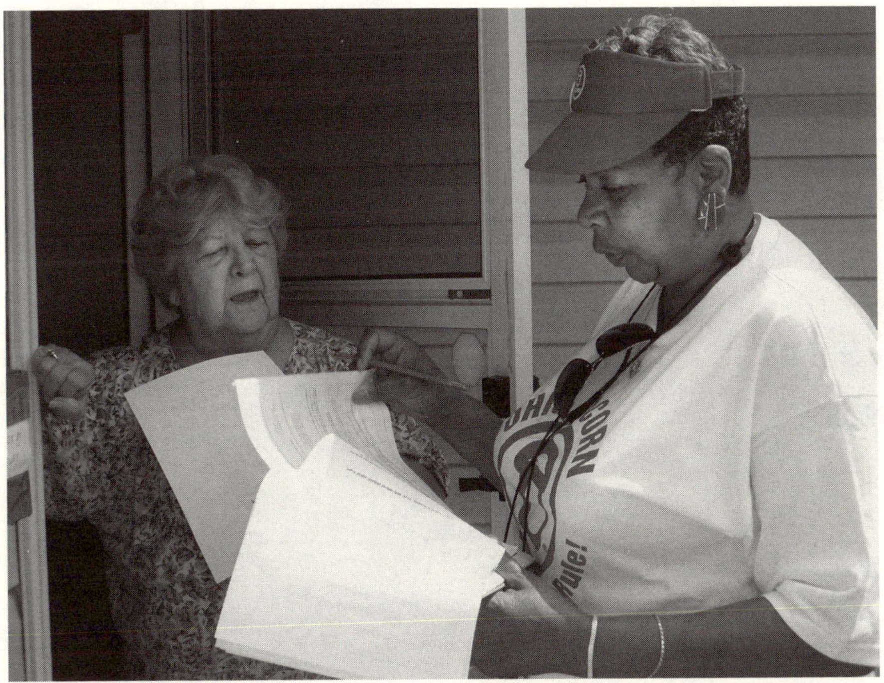

Figure 26. Ohio ACORN member Lashon Campbell Smith going door-to-door registering voters in Columbus, Ohio, 2006. (Photo by Bonnie Friedman)

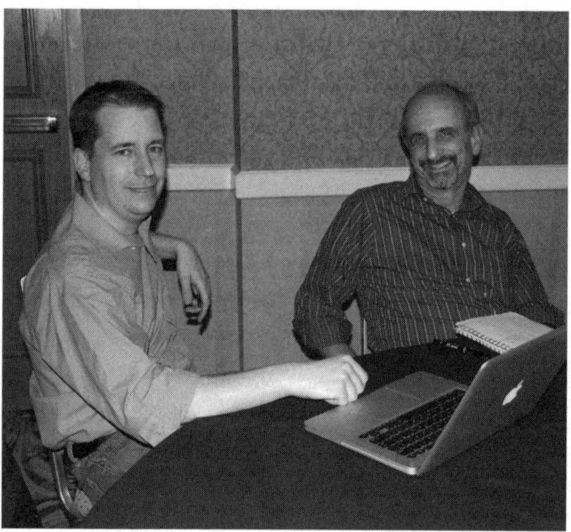

Figure 27. Zach Polett, director of ACORN's political operations, and ACORN deputy political director Kevin Whelan. (Photo by Bonnie Friedman)

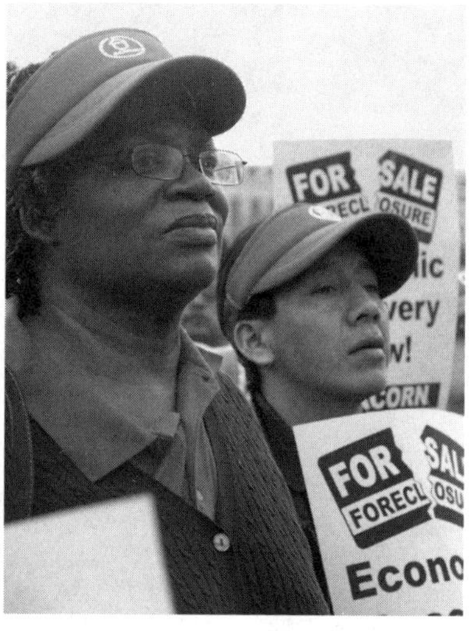

Figure 28. Toni McElroy, ACORN's Texas chapter head and national board member, rallies with five hundred ACORN members on the U.S. Capitol's west lawn, February 9, 2009, to urge Congress to pass President Barack Obama's economic recovery package. (Photo by Valerie Coffin)

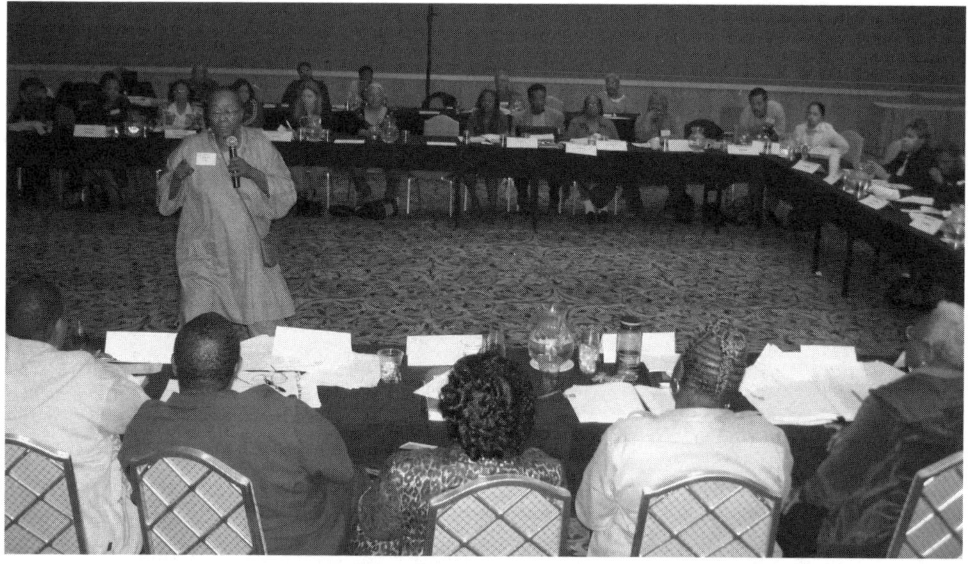

Figure 29. Bertha Lewis addressing the national ACORN board, Las Vegas, April 2009, in the Sahara Hotel's conference hall, eight months after the departure of Wade Rathke. Facing Lewis from left to right are board members Maude Hurd, Rev. Gloria Swieringa, and Carol Hemmingway. (Photo by Bonnie Friedman)

ACORN
Because of Illinois Sen. Barack Obama's record of working for that
, ACORN Votes, a federal Political Action Committee of ACORN leaders, endorsed his candidacy for President.
Porque la labor del Sen. por Illinois, Barack Obama muestra un trabajo por cambios positivos que ayuden a las familias trabajadoras, ACORN Votes, un Comité de Acción Política integrado por líderes de ACORN, refrendó su candidatura para la Presidencia.
2009 JANUARY Enero
SUNDAY
MONDAY
TUESDAY
WEDNESDAY
THURSDAY
FRIDAY
SATURDAY
New Year's Day
Martin Luther King Day

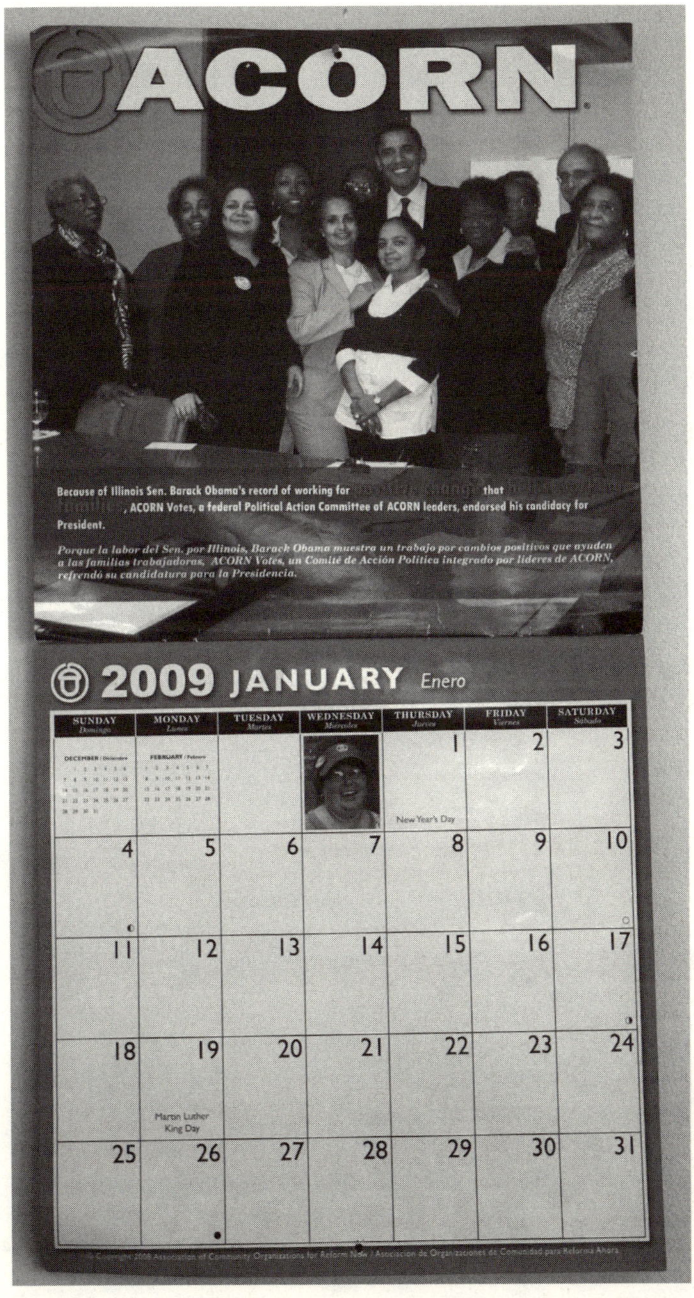

Figure 30. ACORN Votes, ACORN's federal political action committee, endorses Illinois senator Barack Obama for president, February 23, 2008. ACORN members, from left: Marie Pierre (Brooklyn), Vanessa Gueringer (New Orleans), Alicia Russell (Phoenix), Tamecka Pierce (Orlando), Maria Polanco (Brooklyn), Sandra Ramgeet (Boston), Barack Obama, national president Maude Hurd, Toni McElroy (Houston), Zach Polett (Little Rock), Beatrice Jackson (Chicago). "What it came down to," Hurd said, "was that Senator Obama is the candidate who best understands and can effect change on the issues ACORN cares about like stopping foreclosures, enacting fair and comprehensive immigration reform, and building stronger and safer communities across America." (Calendar photo courtesy of ACORN)

ACORN
Value Work!
Raise the

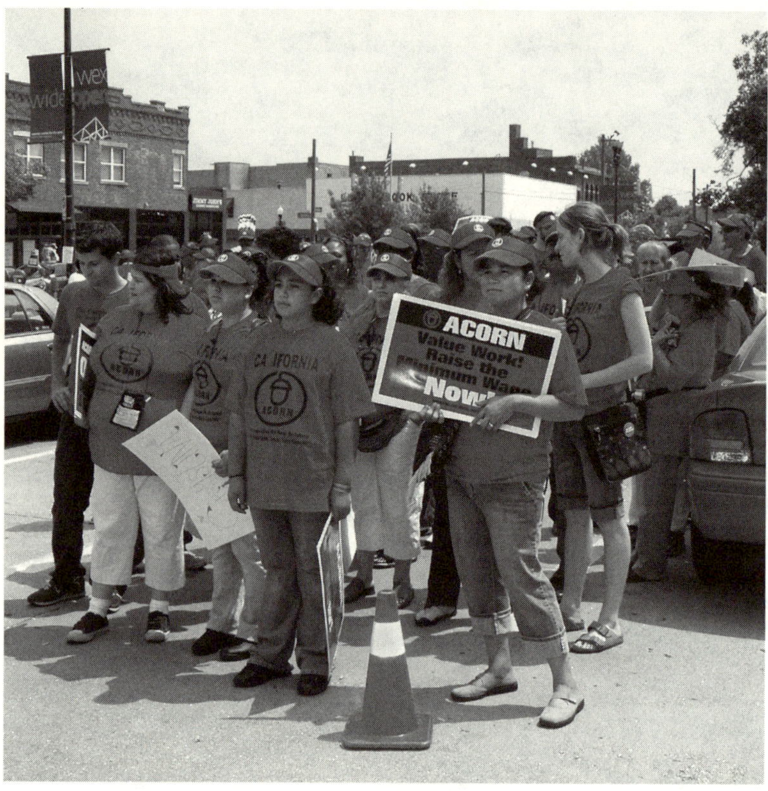

Figure 31. California ACORN members prepare to go into a neighborhood to register voters, 2006. (Photo by Bonnie Friedman)

Today We March,
Tomorrow We Vote!
ACORN

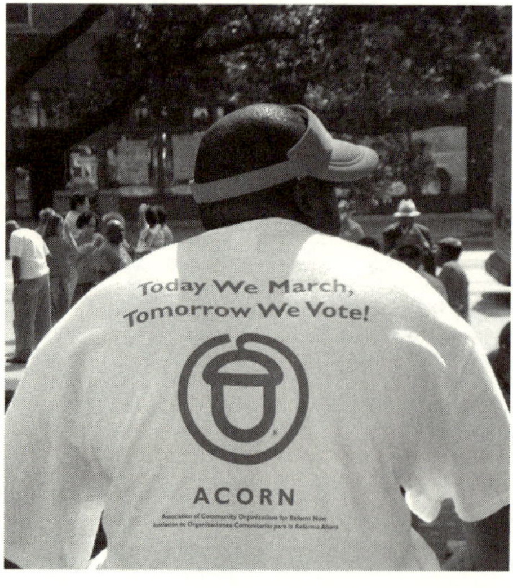

Figure 32. ACORN's success in registering millions of low-income and minority votes made it a target of the Republican Party. During the 2008 election and Barack Obama's first year in office, conservative and mainstream media repeated the false accusations of voter fraud by mostly Republican officials who were trying to destroy ACORN and hurt the president. (Photo by Bonnie Friedman)

Chapter 16

The Right to Vote

> The right of voting . . . is the primary right by which all other rights are protected. To take this right away, is to reduce a man to slavery.
>
> —Thomas Paine, Dissertations on First Principles of Government, 1795

> We have done our level best. We have scratched our heads to find out how we could eliminate every last one of them. We stuffed ballot boxes. We shot them. We are not ashamed of it.
>
> —Sen. Benjamin Ryan Tillman of South Carolina, 1900

After the close and controversial 2000 presidential election, Karl Rove surveyed the political landscape and saw an evenly divided electorate. To ensure that Republicans gained a 1 to 3 percent edge, he needed a plan to energize the GOP's base and slow the rate of Democratic-leaning voter registration. Viewing voter-registration data, he understood the math. Al Gore had defeated George W. Bush with 543,895 more votes and lost the election only because Florida's bungled balloting system threw the election into the Republican-dominated Supreme Court. If people with family incomes under $25,000 had cast ballots at the same rate as those above $75,000, more than 6.8 million additional voters would have gone to the polls in 2000. If only a slight majority of them had voted for Gore, Gore would have won an outright victory. Millions of low-income voters added to the registration rolls could easily decide not only the presidential race, but the outcomes of many races for Congress and for state legislatures as well. For Republicans, stifling voter access became an urgent priority.[1]

While Rove and the Republicans wanted to suppress the voting of minorities and the poor, ACORN's political director, Zach Polett, believed an ACORN national voter-registration drive targeting them could influence the 2004 elections in the opposite direction, giving ACORN's constituency more weight in the coming presidential elections. Working with Steve Kest, Helene O'Brien, and other national staff, he planned a national nonpartisan voter outreach program. On first impression, Polett, in glasses and a rumpled suit and with a slight stutter, could be mistaken for a quiet bookkeeper. His unassuming manner disguises a passionate, brilliant political strategist. He graduated cum laude from Harvard and spent two years at Stanford University School of Medicine before starting full-time organizing with ACORN in 1975 in Arkansas.

Polett understood that voter registration in the United States is complicated and a massive voter-registration campaign risky. Although voting is a right, the United States imposes layers of rules and bureaucracy on the administration of elections. Instead of facilitating registration, which is required by the National Voting Registration Act of 1993 (the Motor Voter law), the government relies on political parties, nonpartisan private good-government groups such as the venerable League of Women Voters, and activist groups like ACORN. Instead of having one uniform set of rules, each state has the authority to set its own.

This delegation of authority to the states to determine voter qualifications and oversee election administration has led to a confusing array of rules that change depending on where one lives. Finding out where to register is not easy. For instance, anyone who tried to register in Florida through the League of Women Voters would be out of luck. Florida's criminal penalties and crippling fines for the innocent mistakes of volunteers shut down the League's registration drives in 2005 for the first time since 1920. A citizen who manages to get a registration form must make sure that the form is on the right kind of *paper*. The registrant's name and date of birth must match Social Security records. If there are typos, the registration will be invalid. Since deadlines differ from state to state, after completing all the paperwork, the citizen must make sure the application is submitted to the county registrar on time, and that the confirmation notice is sent to the *correct address*.[2]

The National Commission on Election Reform Task Force on the federal election system noted: "The registration laws in force throughout the United States are among the world's most demanding . . . [and are] one reason why voter turnout in the United States is near the bottom of the developed world."[3]

Despite these complications, Polett thought ACORN could succeed because of its newly developed close relationship with Project Vote, a nonprofit organization founded in 1982 to engage low-income and minority communities in the election process. Project Vote remains the leading technical support outfit for registration drives aimed at reaching poor and minority voters. (Not surprisingly, continuing his commitment to community organizing, after graduating from Harvard Law School, Barack Obama returned to Chicago to lead a local Project Vote effort.)

Backing for ACORN and Project Vote's campaign initially came from a small amount of foundation money. Funding grew after Polett, who served as Project Vote's part-time executive director, got invited to join a coalition of progressive activists who operated outside the Democratic Party. They recognized the need to register millions of new voters in 2004. Fueled by funds from billionaires such as George Soros and from unions, as well as from liberal-leaning foundations, their voter-registration campaign was able to raise millions of dollars to reach out to historically underrepresented voters.

It was more than the money that gave Polett confidence in his campaign. While ACORN had registered voters since its inception, over time these drives had grown more sophisticated and effective. Based largely on common sense and experience in state and municipal elections, ACORN had rejected voter registration and get-out-the-vote efforts that relied only on leafleting, direct mail, commercial phone banks, and robo-calls to increase voter turnout in African American, Hispanic, and low-income precincts because they proved minimally effective. ACORN's experience showed it could boost voter turnout through repeated face-to-face conversations with potential voters, combined with promoting policies such as campaign finance reform, raising the minimum wage, and opposing hospital closings. (Republicans had used a similar strategy with great success in the 2002 elections.) This combination acted like a magnet to draw poor and working-class people to the polls.[4]

In 2001 and 2003, in cities as divergent as Detroit, Phoenix, Kansas City, and Bridgeport, Connecticut, ACORN's PAC had successfully influenced election outcomes and gained closer relationships with public officials. These campaigns were especially impressive given ACORN's austere budgets for political activity.

In 2003 and 2004, building on its network of neighborhood chapters, ACORN mounted a massive voter mobilization campaign in twenty-six states, including Florida and New Mexico, which would turn out to be presidential battleground states. ACORN's Polett took the head position, while ACORN organizers such as Matt Henderson in New Mexico and Brian Kettenring in Florida would lead statewide campaigns. As a result, ACORN was on a collision course with the Republican Party.

Florida

In Florida, ACORN worked with Project Vote in what they hoped would be a massive voter-registration drive.[5] What made this drive unique was ACORN's simultaneous coalition effort to increase the minimum wage using a state ballot initiative. Kettenring and Florida ACORN volunteer chair Tamecka Pierce, a certified nursing assistant, were aware of the history of voter suppression and the likelihood that ACORN's work would meet resistance by the group's opponents. Pierce and Kettenring thought they were prepared.

Unlike other registration campaigns such as Rock the Vote, which relied on celebrities and advertising to appeal to nonvoters, ACORN would rely on personal contact, a petition drive to put the minimum-wage issue on the ballot, and the recruiting of hundreds of temporary workers to complement its full-time organizing staff and volunteers. In November 2003, Mac Stuart walked into ACORN's Fort Lauderdale office to apply for a temporary job to collect signatures for its petition drive. A bright, handsome, and muscular thirty-eight-year-old Cuban American, Stuart told Frank Houston, ACORN's Florida supervisor for the petition and voter-registration drive, that he was a former police officer and quite excited about ACORN's mission.

After a brief interview, Houston hired him at forty-five dollars a day and ten dollars extra as a team leader. Houston sent Stuart, like other new staff, to Missouri and later to Orlando for training by the experts from Project Vote, where he was carefully instructed regarding Florida laws and ACORN's procedures. Stuart worked hard, wanting to move up to the position of community organizer. He gathered more petitions and registered more people than anyone else on the Florida staff. After two months, Stuart asked for a promotion and was upgraded to a $21,000-a-year job overseeing the Miami voter-registration drive, which included supervising an assistant director and a hundred canvassers. He also had to make sure each member of his team brought in a reasonable number of valid applications.

After a while, however, Polett felt he had to tighten supervision over the organizers to avoid mistakes. Stuart was told that his employment with ACORN was over, and he had to switch from being supervised by ACORN to Project Vote. He was not happy with the change. Every week he had to e-mail to Project Vote a list of the people he had registered, their phone numbers and e-mails, his total tally, and other information. He also had to copy all the voter-registration cards.

Suddenly Stuart started resisting direction. A rumor spread among some ACORN staff that he was meeting with the Chamber of Commerce, one of the groups opposing ACORN's minimum-wage campaign. He refused to follow procedures and constantly argued with his Project Vote supervisor, Frank Houston. He declined to copy voting cards, claiming it was illegal, even after he was assured it was legal. He refused to drop the cards at the Board of Elections in Miami. Later Stuart would say he wasn't respected for his work. He tried to convince other staff not to cooperate with Houston. The atmosphere got so divisive in the office that Houston suspended Stuart, and Kettenring assigned a senior ACORN staff member to investigate the matter.

When Houston had hired Stuart, he should have checked his past more closely. Stuart was not a police officer but had held many jobs, including swimming pool cleaner and sales associate at Home Depot. He had a record of driving with a suspended license, carrying a concealed firearm, and a few drug charges, and he spent time in prison for armed robbery. On August 4, 2004, Houston and Kettenring received the senior staff member's memo titled "Reasons for Termination of Mac Stuart," which laid out four major reasons to fire him, including his willful failure to follow ACORN policies concerning the recruitment and training of employees and his attempt to cash the paycheck of an employee. Kettenring believed that Stuart was "crooked" and "volatile" and supported his immediate termination. Houston notified Stuart he was fired.

Furious, Stuart rushed unannounced into Kettenring's office, yelling that the charges against him were false and that ACORN was guilty of discrimination. He threatened a class-action suit against ACORN. As soon as Stuart left, Kettenring called ACORN's legal counsel.

Brian Mellor, ACORN's attorney, tried to get the Miami-Dade supervisor of elections to investigate Stuart's activities. When Mellor learned later that August that Stuart had tried to cash a check written to Floridians for All, the PAC supporting ACORN's minimum-wage ballot initiative, he thought it was lucky ACORN had fired Stuart. Mellor filed a complaint about Stuart with the Board of Elections and with the rest of the ACORN staff celebrated Stuart's departure.

But Stuart was not finished with ACORN. A friend suggested he get an attorney and steered him to Rothstein, Rosenfeld, and Adler, a prominent Republican law firm. The next thing ACORN knew, Stuart had presented the Board of Elections with approximately a thousand Republican applications that had been collected by ACORN and not turned in to the Board. Stunned by Stuart's claims, attorney Mellor knew how dangerous these allegations were to ACORN's cause. If they became public, ACORN could lose its funding, as well as the minimum-wage campaign. He immediately called his contact at the Board and demanded to know what had happened to his request to investigate Stuart. The contact told Mellor his complaint had been forwarded to the county prosecutor and nothing had come of it. Mellor insisted the Board look into Stuart's Republican applications to determine if they had been collected by him as part of his illegal scheme. To Mellor's surprise, he was told that the thousand applications that had just been turned in could not be investigated because the board had already mixed them in with other applications.

In the meantime, the county prosecutor was aggressively investigating ACORN based on accusations by Stuart that ACORN committed voter-registration fraud. Attending meetings with the prosecutor and producing thousands of documents in response to a subpoena took ACORN staff away from its minimum-wage campaign. Despite this diversion of time, the campaign appeared to be succeeding. The *New York Times* on September 26 reported that in the heavily Democratic zip code areas, new registrations increased to 125,000 from 77,000, a jump of more than 60 percent, while in Republican areas, registration increased only about 12 percent.[6]

Stuart had met with Rothstein, Rosenfeld, and Adler and claimed that ACORN discriminated against blacks and Hispanics, didn't respect his work, and used him as a scapegoat for ACORN's illegal activity. Seeing an opportunity to further their political purposes, the lawyers told him that because he was fired in retaliation for refusing to participate in ACORN's illegal activities, he had a whistle-blower suit.

One month before voters went to the polls, criticism of ACORN's voter-registration work was mounting. Stuart held a news conference, contacted television and print news reporters, and started attracting media attention. He shot off an e-mail to Aliana Periz at WSVN, a television news station in Miami, stating that ACORN committed "voter fraud" and other "illegal" activities and exploited minorities.

At an October 1 news conference, Stuart said, according to *Florida Today*: "There was a lot of fraud committed" by ACORN, and ACORN had knowingly submitted thousands of invalid registration cards and failed to turn in cards from registered Republicans. The *Palm Beach Post* reported on October 8 that ACORN was under state and federal investigation in Miami-Dade County for unlawfully registering former felons to vote.

Rush Limbaugh announced on the air: "We got a story out of Tampa today in the *St. Petersburg Times* about how a group that was formed in the 1970s—you may have heard of them, ACORN—is out trying to register voters two and three times, and they've been caught in the act."

On October 19, Stuart and his Republican attorneys held a press conference announcing that they had filed a whistle-blower lawsuit alleging that ACORN was withholding Republican registration cards, registering ineligible felons, selling voter lists for profit, and "knowingly [submitting] thousands of invalid registration cards." Stuart provided his attorneys with 179 voter applications, many of them for Republican registrants, that he claimed had been collected and withheld by ACORN. The story was widely covered by the South Florida media.

"These are first-time voters from the underclass, and [ACORN] screwed them," said William Scherer Jr., a Republican operative and lawyer who filed the case with attorney Stuart Rosenfeldt. He said the victims of ACORN's misdeeds were a mixed group politically, and all but one of them was black. ACORN, represented by Faith Gay from the Wall Street law firm of White and Case, denied the allegations and countersued the former employee for defamation and libel.

On October 21, the Florida Department of Law Enforcement took the unusual step of publicizing the fact it was investigating ACORN. The FDLE, in a press release, said it had set up task forces to investigate groups "such as ACORN" and prosecute those persons and groups found to have committed voter fraud. FDLE officials said many of the complaints it received involved "organized efforts to commit voter fraud," including voter registrations, party affiliation forms, and absentee ballots, along with accusations that ACORN volunteers and employees "have been connected with the widespread voter irregularities."[7] "So far the only group we've identified with certainty in North and South Florida as having connections to some of the voter fraud issues is ACORN," said FDLE spokesman Tom Berlinger in Tallahassee. In Florida, most voter fraud violations are punishable by up to five years in prison and a fine of five thousand dollars. Gay, ACORN's volunteer lawyer, said she found it strange that FDLE had announced the investigation when it had failed to return ACORN's phone calls offering to cooperate.

The Republican machine was successfully provoking newspapers across Florida to report that ACORN faced criminal investigations in a half-dozen other states over voter-registration and petition signatures gathered by its employees. "I'm disappointed that an organization like ACORN would do this, but I'm not surprised," said Mark Wilson, the conservative head of the Florida Chamber of Commerce, a group closely aligned with the Republican Party and opposed to the minimum-wage amendment.

Stuart's allegations were immediately picked up by conservative news organizations, including the *Washington Times*, a newspaper owned by the right-wing Rev. Sun Myung Moon's Unification Church and conservative Internet blogs. On October 19, the day the lawsuit was filed, Terrence Scanlon wrote in the *Washington Times*: "Increasingly, reports of fake and forged voter-registration cards are surfacing across the nation, and they are prompting official investigations into voter drives. One group in particular has come under scrutiny. ACORN—it stands for Association of Community Organizations for Reform Now—has received wide attention for claiming to have registered more than one million new voters nationwide. But in state after state, allegations are surfacing that ACORN activists are padding the registration books."[8]

On October 27, Stuart appeared on Fox News. Its anchor, Brit Hume, announced a Fox special report, saying: "There are more troubles in Florida today for that left-wing group ACORN. Another former employee has accused ACORN of mishandling voter-registration forms, with the result that Floridians who thought they would be able to vote this year will not be on the rolls." Stuart had become a cause célèbre for conservative journalists and pundits.[9]

ACORN tried to defend itself against Republican accusations of voter fraud. For example, on October 19, Steve Kest, ACORN's executive director, said on National Public Radio: "We've had probably over four thousand people working, doing voter registration for us and, you know, there's a few bad apples. But on the whole, this has been a hugely successful drive in bringing new voters into the process."

Could ACORN keep the Republican accusations from undermining its minimum-wage campaign? On October 29, just four days before the election, a second Florida suit filed by Rothstein, Rosenfeldt, and Adler alleged that ACORN had failed to submit twelve voter-registration applications in time for the general election, depriving their clients of their constitutional right to vote and committing fraud against them. After a press conference called by the law firm, Fort Lauderdale's *Sun Sentinel* ran a sympathetic story about Jude Daniel, a nineteen-year-old Miami resident who thought he was registered to vote, noting that if Daniel tried to vote, "poll workers won't be able to find him on the rolls, even though he filled out a voter-registration form in August." Then, quoting Daniel: "It was important to me. It would have been my first time." Instead, Daniel's voter-registration form was one of 179 found in a box in the ACORN office, according to lawyers representing him. "They'd been sitting in the corner," said Stuart, who turned the box over to his lawyers. "That Miami [ACORN] office is in shambles," said Stuart. The media repeatedly reported Stuart's assertions as evidence that ACORN routinely engaged in fraud. The conservative media added the charge: to "promote its radical political agenda." On October 31, the *National Review Online* cited the Stuart's case as an example of ACORN's shady behavior.

Despite the attacks against ACORN that diverted valuable staff time from its work, ACORN had collected close to a million signatures to place a minimum-wage increase measure on the November 2 ballot in Florida. Nationally, more than ten thousand workers and volunteers, mostly from the targeted community, registered over 1.1 million new voters in low-income African American and Latino neighborhoods. To get the vote out on Election Day, ACORN's staff and volunteers not only contacted newly registered voters but also talked to more than a million infrequent voters encouraging them to vote—a total of 2.2 million voters. On November 3, 2004, ACORN leaders like Tamecka Pierce and Louise Peterson learned that ACORN won a stunning victory when the minimum-wage measure passed by 72 to 28 percent, raising the minimum wage from $5.15 to $6.15, indexed annually to inflation. (The *St. Petersburg Times* cited Louise Peterson and ACORN as among the ten individuals who changed the Florida economy in 2004.)[10]

After the election, the facts about the Stuart matter slowly emerged. In the suit that claimed Republicans were denied their right to vote, nine of the eleven plaintiffs asked to be dismissed from the case. As ACORN's lawyers deposed the remaining two plaintiffs, it became clear that their Republican lawyers had not asked them if they were even qualified to vote or whether they were, in fact, Republicans. One of the two was not qualified to vote, neither remembered completing the voter application used as the basis for the complaint, and both said they were not Republicans and never would have checked off that they were. In addition, Stuart was inconsistent in his deposition testimony regarding how he had obtained the applications in the first place.

Discovery in the other case, *Mac Stuart v. ACORN*, revealed that the applications Stuart had provided his counsel were never collected by or turned over to anyone working for ACORN. ACORN organizers speculated that Stuart had stashed them away to be used in the lawsuit. Stuart failed to produce any evidence to support his allegations. A few months later the Florida Department of Law Enforcement's investigation found no evidence of illegal or fraudulent activity by ACORN. A public records request by Project Vote asking all Florida counties for any documents related to voter fraud elicited just three alleged cases of illegal activity, only one of which involved an ACORN worker.

On December 8, 2005, it was all over. Federal judge James Lawrence King of the Southern District of Florida dismissed *Mac Stuart v. ACORN*, exonerating ACORN of any wrongdoing, and granted judgment to ACORN on its defamation counterclaims. In pleadings filed in the Southern District of Florida, Stuart admitted that his allegations of voter-registration fraud against ACORN were defamatory. Stuart's case collapsed.[11]

ACORN also prevailed in the second Rothstein, Rosenfeldt, and Adler suit. Judge Jose Martinez of the Southern District of Florida dismissed it with prejudice because there was no evidence to make a case against ACORN. The Federal Bureau of Investigation had examined fifty-nine instances of alleged fraud, some connected to ACORN in Florida's Duvall County, and found that all were due to clerical errors by the supervisor of elections.

ACORN and its attorneys tried to put the issue to rest. "ACORN has shown that the claims made against it were false and frivolous, and the dismissal of these claims should vindicate ACORN of any alleged wrongdoing," said one of ACORN's attorneys, Brian Koch. "We are very happy it was found that we are innocent," said ACORN's Tamecka Pierce. "We have zero tolerance for fraud." The exoneration received much less media attention, however, than the groundless claims of ACORN's organized voter fraud.

Florida's Republican-dominated legislature passed a law in 2005 that carried stiff penalties for organizations failing to turn in voter-registration applications more than ten days after they were collected. The law's reporting requirements were so draconian that the League of Women Voters ended seventy-seven years of voter-registration activity in the state because it feared it could not comply and would be bankrupted if there were problems with just a few registration forms collected by its volunteers. A federal judge later blocked the implementation of the law, finding it unconstitutional.

The Florida fraud charges collapsed, but the incidents remained as propaganda fodder for opponents of ACORN, including Republican bloggers and conservative outfits like the Institute on Religion and Democracy and the Employment Policies Institute, as well as the *Wall Street Journal*'s editorial page. They would continue to spread false rumors that the organization had engaged in voter fraud in Florida.

Responding to the GOP-provoked voter fraud accusations, states launched criminal investigations in Wisconsin, Colorado, Ohio, and New Mexico, with ACORN a prime suspect. Mainstream journalists, including National Public Radio, covered the fights over voter registration and participation as a kind of he-said, she-said story, suspending judgment on the relative accuracy of Democrats accusing Republicans of voter repression and Republicans accusing Democrats of voter fraud.

Manipulation in New Mexico

The controversy over voting rights might have continued to generate more heat than light but for the Republicans' vendetta against Matt Henderson, thirty-four, a fourteen-year ACORN veteran and New Mexico head organizer.[12] After graduating from Cornell, Henderson had worked in restaurants and for caterers as a cook. Happily married with no children, he worked ten to twelve hours a day, often riding his bike to work.

His neighborhood, Los Duranes, was in an old part of Albuquerque in the middle of the city, where poor families lived in small old adobe homes and trailers. He believed his group's effort to register poor minority voters was a time-honored way of bringing disenfranchised people into the American democratic process.

Henderson had led ACORN's 2003–2004 voter-registration campaign in New Mexico, which put him squarely in the crosshairs of a tense local fight between the Republican Party and ACORN over voting rights that within two years would lead to a national scandal. Henderson knew local Republicans played rough, but the last thing he expected was a demonstration in front of his office and the threat of a criminal indictment. And he had no idea that his work had caught the attention of Karl Rove and the White House.

In the swing state of New Mexico, Al Gore won by just 366 votes in 2000. Since then, Republicans and Democrats had waged a bitter battle over voter registration. For example, Republicans fought to require voters to show photo identification either at registration or before voting. Democrats and ACORN opposed these efforts because evidence suggested it hindered citizens from participating in elections. In 2003, at the same time Kettenring's effort got under way in Florida, New Mexico ACORN began its voter-registration drives. New Mexico Republicans were sure the result would be fraudulent voting by illegal aliens and others.

By the fall of 2004, the presidential contest between George W. Bush and Sen. John F. Kerry had tightened, and by all accounts, ACORN was signing up many new voters across New Mexico. By August 2004, ACORN and its allies had registered 65,000 people in Bernalillo County, including Albuquerque, a 10 percent increase over 2000.

In early August, a group of Republicans led by county sheriff Darren White marched into the Bernalillo County clerk's office. White asked if there were any "problem" registrations. County clerk Mary Herrera said yes: some three thousand incomplete or error-ridden forms were missing Social Security numbers, post office box addresses, or signatures.

That was enough for White, one of the state's highest-profile Republicans and chair of the county Bush-Cheney campaign. "When they brought me on, it was plain and simple: They said, 'We need to win Bernalillo County,'" White told the *Albuquerque Journal.* On August 5, he dashed off a letter to New Mexico's U.S. attorney, David C. Iglesias, asking him to investigate voter-registration cards that might be fraudulent. A series of "suspect" forms had been submitted in recent weeks, he said in his letter.[13] (The powerful New Mexico Republican senator Pete Domenici had recommended Iglesias, an ambitious conservative former state prosecutor, for the U.S. attorney post in 2000.)

In the late summer of 2002, Iglesias had received an e-mail from the Department of Justice suggesting that U.S. attorneys should immediately begin working with local and state election officials to offer whatever assistance they could in investigating and prosecuting voter fraud cases. In 2004, he received another e-mail urging him to prosecute voter fraud. (In 2008, a report from the inspector general's office found that Karl Rove was in close communication with those who were pushing the Justice Department's harassment of ACORN in several key election states.)

Although most glitches were typical errors by registrants or the people registering them, Republican officials held a press conference, claiming that grassroots groups were producing fraudulent registrations. One of the groups they named was ACORN.

A few days later, Glen Stout, an Albuquerque police officer, claimed he was surprised when he received a voter-registration card in the mail for his thirteen-year-old son, Kevin. The politically conservative Stout reached out to Republican leaders, including Rep. Joe Thompson, an Albuquerque Republican and lawyer. Thompson was about to file a lawsuit against the New Mexico secretary of state charging voter-registration irregularities. Stout agreed to join as a plaintiff.

Stout's son denied filling out an application for the card, and it looked as if his signature and birth date had been forged. ACORN had submitted the application in his name, and local authorities quickly traced the problem to Christine Gonzales, a young ACORN canvasser. Thompson filed a suit in state district court on August 20, seeking a judgment that New Mexico's voter-identification statute, which applied only to first-time voters who registered by mail, should be broadened to include those signed up by groups like ACORN. The law required first-time voters who registered by mail to present identification such as a utility bill or government-issued photo ID.

On August 24, Stout and Thompson stood outside ACORN's Albuquerque offices and, in front of the local press, blamed the group for faulty voter-registration cards. "We have proof," Thompson declared, and produced young Stout's voter-registration form turned in by Gonzales.[14]

Most of those engaged in ACORN's voter-registration process, like community leader William Kyser, understood the process. But snags existed. Though Gonzales's name appeared on the registration card, Henderson knew she hadn't assisted the boy in filling out his registration form, because prior to the incident, he had fired Gonzales for altering other canvassers' forms to get credit for their work.

On September 2, a hearing was to take place before state district judge Robert L. Thompson (not related to the Republican attorney). If the judge ruled in the Republicans' favor, the result would be changes in election rules two months before the election, confusion among voters, and the likely disenfranchisement of hundreds of the people ACORN had registered. Henderson testified that ACORN had no way to contact registrants to let them know they might have to show identification at the polls. People could be turned away and become discouraged from voting if they had to show identification, Henderson said. He cited examples of voters whose identification didn't match their address on the voter roll because they had moved, or because they weren't carrying acceptable ID.

"What's going on now is no different from what was going on in the civil-rights movement of the '60s," Henderson said to the press. "This is about a set of people trying to stop another set of people from voting."

The Republicans' case rested on a few examples of what they alleged to be clearly fraudulent applications. But their case began to unravel when several women whose registration cards were attached to the lawsuit testified that they had registered twice by mistake and that no fraud was involved. The very exhibits used to justify the Republicans' allegations of rampant voter fraud actually showed the opposite: many cards deemed "questionable" by elections officials represented a legitimate attempt by a person to register to vote.[15] On September 7, Judge Thompson rejected the Republican-led efforts to require county clerks to demand identification from voters who didn't register in person with the county. In a press release, Yolanda Peña, a member of ACORN, attacked the Republican Party for inventing false stories about voter-registration fraud. Referring to Glen Stout's son, she pointed out that the thirteen-year-old boy's father was a registered Republican and released copies of the boy's card. The card looked like it had been filled out by a boy, not by an ACORN worker, and could have been a prank. Peña said: "Instead of taking responsibility for this boy's prank, the Republicans used it to try to ram a lawsuit through the courts that would have made it harder for minority voters to vote."[16]

The Republican Party's strategy in New Mexico, like similar campaigns across the country, was to force the predominantly Hispanic and black voters registered by ACORN to show photo IDs in order to vote. "We fought this kind of intimidation in the South in the '60s, and we are fighting it today in New Mexico." said ACORN member David Powdrell. "We are delighted that . . . the Republican National Committee lost in court," added Peña. "Their dirty tricks are racist and un-American."

Far from being cowed by their loss, the dismissal stoked a voter-fraud frenzy among state GOP leaders, who immediately demanded a criminal investigation into voter fraud, with Henderson as their target. Four years earlier, on October 10, 2000, Henderson had been quoted in the press stating that "ACORN made photocopies of all the registration cards it delivered to the county." At the time, it was perfectly legal to do so. By 2004, the law had changed, making that practice illegal, and ACORN no longer made copies.

During the trial, Henderson was asked if he had continued that practice and on his lawyer's advice, he refused to answer. Although the Republicans lost the voter ID lawsuit, on October 1, 2004, the New Mexico Republican Party called on Iglesias to investigate Henderson for perjury and "suspect" practices.

At a televised press conference the same day, Iglesias promised a thorough inquiry. "It appears that mischief is afoot," the U.S. attorney said, "and questions are lurking in the shadows." At the press conference, he announced the establishment of a voter-fraud task force to investigate complaints about election fairness. "There's a lot of information that's of a questionable nature," Iglesias said. "We're getting lots of referrals from people across the spectrum that this election may be dirty. . . . The task force is ready to investigate all legitimate referrals." He acknowledged that his team was already investigating one allegation but declined to give details. ACORN's staff assumed he was referring to Henderson. He also mentioned that the much-publicized case of a thirteen-year-old boy who was registered by ACORN merited investigation, alluding to Kevin Stout.

One important Republican was not satisfied with Iglesias's task force: Mickey D. Barnett, a lawyer who represented the 2004 Bush-Cheney campaign in New Mexico. He had a long history of conservative activism, including opposing unionization, and while serving in the New Mexico senate, he had led the repeal of laws that capped interest rates on payday loans. (These loan companies now charge the working poor up to 500 percent interest on short-term loans.) Barnett shot off an e-mail message to Iglesias urging him to bring federal charges against the canvasser who forged signatures. The *Albuquerque Journal* reported that he berated Iglesias for "appointing a task force to investigate voter fraud instead of bringing charges against suspects."

In addition to the allegations against Gonzales and Henderson, Iglesias's task force took a close look at more than three hundred other matters. Henderson anxiously awaited the result of the investigation. Although shaken and worried, he told the press, "We will never be intimidated by baseless legal attacks."

In January 2005, the voter-fraud task force concluded its work. Iglesias announced there was not enough evidence to bring a fraud case against ACORN. Regarding Gonzales, Iglesias said, "it appeared she was just doing it for the money." No action was taken against Henderson. Iglesias was sure that his bosses shared his view that U.S. attorneys should stay above partisan politics. He was very wrong. Iglesias's decision so frustrated high-ranking Republican officials that they began an extraordinary campaign to remove him that reached all the way to the White House. He became the target of intense criticism by New Mexico GOP lawmakers and political operatives. Prominent New Mexico Republicans, including Senator Domenici, repeatedly complained to chief White House political strategist Karl Rove about Iglesias's failure to bring voter-fraud indictments.

When Allen Weh, the New Mexico Republican Party chair, saw Rove at a White House function in late 2006 and asked him about Iglesias, Rove replied that Iglesias was "gone." On December 7, Iglesias was fired. The White House had ordered Iglesias to illegally prosecute baseless cases against innocent citizens, just to gin up voter fraud publicity. His refusal cost him his job.[17] The spokesperson for the U.S. attorney's office said that Iglesias "has had discussions with officials in Washington, D.C. Based on those discussions, he has decided to move on."

Days before the 2006 election, a U.S. attorney in Kansas City, Brad Schlozman, with enthusiastic support from Karl Rove, brought a voter-fraud indictment against four people registering voters for ACORN, spurring a congressional investigation led by Iowa's Republican senator Charles Grassley. In June 2008, the Justice Department launched a grand jury investigation into whether Schlozman misled Congress about playing politics with civil rights issues.

The facts about voter fraud and voter suppression would have remained under the public radar but for the Attorneygate scandal. The deceit over voter accusations became public in part because of the firing of Iglesias. He was one of eight U.S. attorneys dismissed by Bush's attorney general, Alberto Gonzales. The *New York Times* and the McClatchy News Service began to investigate the Republican allegations of voter fraud and found that they were baseless. On April 12, 2007, the *Times* reported that only 120 people had been charged with the crime in the past five years, leading to 86 convictions. Most of the acts of wrongdoing committed by voters resulted from filling out more than one registration form and by immigrants and felons who voted "seemingly unaware that they were barred from voting," according to an analysis of the federal prosecution records for the 2002–2005 period by Barnard College professor Lorraine Minnite. Her analysis breaks down those prosecutions by type of fraud and type of perpetrator: 44 of 70 convictions are government officials, party, campaign or election workers (compared to 26 voters); and 37 of those 44 convictions are for vote buying. A *Times* editorial noted: "In partisan Republican circles, the pursuit of voter fraud is code for suppressing the votes of minorities and poor people."[18]

After he was fired, Iglesias called voter fraud a "boogeyman" that parents use "to scare their children. It's very frightening, and it doesn't exist. U.S. Attorneys have better things to do with their time than chasing voter-fraud phantoms." Conservatives continued to taint ACORN with charges of systemic corruption ("questionable activities," "investigated for election fraud"), despite the fact that it had never been convicted of a crime or engaged in voter fraud.[19]

Voter intimidation and suppression have a long ugly history in the United States. In every national election since Reconstruction, voters—particularly blacks and other minorities—have been outlawed or intimidated, threatened with violence or turned away from the polls based on their race. In 1900, U.S. senator "Pitchfork" Ben Tillman (D., South Carolina) led one of the bloodiest campaigns against black voting rights. The literacy tests, poll taxes, and bloody days of physical violence following Reconstruction have disappeared, only to be replaced by more modern, less gory schemes. Courageous men and women risked their lives for the right to vote and won the 1965 Voting Rights Act—a defining moment for democracy and equal justice in America.

Since the 1960s, schemes to erode and undermine those victories and suppress voting by minorities became standard equipment in the Republican toolbox.[20] Most recently, voter identification laws and purging voters from the rolls have become legal ways to eliminate likely Democratic voters in swing states.[21]

ACORN's vision of a strong democracy and the importance of engaging the less affluent in the civic process has always included low-income and minority citizen voter registration. Its membership card urges members to do three things: pay their dues, work for the interests of low- and moderate-income people, and vote in all elections. ACORN has assumed correctly that excluding the most vulnerable and least powerful from voting meant excluding them from participating in major public policy decisions and influencing their outcomes.[22]

At the start of 2008, Wade Rathke was sitting atop an organization that had become a formidable force for economic justice and political reform. ACORN's combined "family of organizations," as Rathke called them, had an annual budget of $100 million, over a thousand employees and 400,000 members. The family included two nonprofit tax-exempt corporations that conduct research, policy analysis, and leadership training, two union locals, two southern-based radio stations (KNON and KABF), several publications (including the magazine *Social Policy*), an accounting, financial, and payroll services firm (Citizen Consulting, Inc.), a nonprofit corporation that builds affordable housing and provides homeownership counseling (ACORN Housing), a law office, and a variety of other vehicles that supported its organizing and issue campaigns, such as the Financial Justice Center, the Living Wage Resource Center, and Project Vote.

Bill Clinton, whose foundation provided ACORN with one of its largest donations, just a few months ago was the keynote speaker at New York ACORN's twenty-fifth anniversary banquet at the Citigroup Center. As Clinton approached the podium he passed Rathke's table and told him that he had praised ACORN in his new book, *Giving*, adding, "I gave ACORN a big wet kiss."[23]

Despite the Bush administration's indifference to the fate of post-Katrina New Orleans, ACORN was slowly making progress in its campaign to mobilize survivors who were working to improve the Lower Ninth. ACORN's Vanessa Gueringer was advising film star Brad Pitt, who was developing 150 environmentally fit houses in the ward. ACORN's magnet and charter schools in Chicago and New York were educating inner-city kids. ACORN International, which Rathke had started five years earlier, had offices in Argentina, Canada, Peru, and Mexico, and he hoped to establish membership chapters in the Dominican Republic, Ecuador, Kenya, and Nigeria.

ACORN continued to counsel homeowners and pursue predatory lenders. Soon after wrestling a half-billion dollar settlement from Household Finance in 2003, ACORN coordinated more than four hundred protests and rallies in front of H&R Block offices around the country. ACORN claimed that Block's tax preparers misleadingly siphoned off millions of dollars in tax breaks known as Earned Income Tax Credits, an income supplement for the working poor. After consistent pressure, executives from H&R Block and ACORN agreed to a joint venture to promote the Earned Income Tax Credit. By 2008, ACORN was operating the third-largest nonprofit tax preparation service in the country, with Tax Benefit Centers offering free tax preparation in sixty-two offices and with partners in an additional twenty-four locations, which seemed to refute community organizing theorists who claimed groups should never combine services and organizing.[24]

Despite all the obstacles, by the start of 2008 ACORN and its partner Project Vote were getting ready to embark on a $15.9 million campaign to sign up 1.2 million new voters, this country's largest-ever nonpartisan voter-registration drive. They were prepared to take the risk of the appearance of voter participation errors, because for every one fraudulent ballot there are millions of ballots in federal elections not cast or counted because of complex voter-registration laws, long lines, administrative snafus, illegal voter list purges, and human error. Recognizing that election outcomes change dramatically depending on how many minority voters cast ballots and that increases in minority voting lead to public spending patterns that more closely reflect the preferences of minorities and lower class voters, ACORN's goal was a racially and economically diverse electorate—and the first racially mixed candidate would be running for president.[25]

Chapter 17

Growing Pains

It was March 2008 in New Orleans. The azaleas were in bloom and tourists packed the French Quarter, feasting on Cajun delicacies and taking in the jazz and Zydeco. Just a few blocks away in ACORN's headquarters, Wade Rathke, fifty-eight, met with Helene O'Brien, his chief lieutenant and ACORN's national field director—unaware of the looming crisis. Rathke was sitting atop an organization that had become a formidable force for economic justice and political reform. His friends and enemies had been impressed by ACORN's ten-year expansion from 25 to 103 cities in thirty-eight states and by O'Brien's ability to identify opportunities, recruit organizers, and motivate them.

In the hotly contested primary for the Democratic nomination for president, both Hillary Clinton and Barack Obama agreed to run on New York's Working Families Party ballot line as well as on the Democratic line. Obama, the front-runner for the nomination, had worked with ACORN's Chicago office when he ran a voter-registration drive after law school, represented ACORN in a lawsuit to enforce voter-registration laws, and on a few occasions led ACORN workshops to help train its volunteer leaders. When he sought the group's endorsement during the primary election, he told them: "I've been fighting alongside ACORN on issues you care about my entire career. Even before I was an elected official, when I ran Project Vote's voter-registration drive in Illinois, ACORN was smack dab in the middle of it, and we appreciate your work."[1] During Obama's hard-fought primary election, his campaign had paid $832,000 to ACORN-affiliated Campaign Services, Inc., for get-out-the-vote efforts in Pennsylvania, Ohio, Indiana, and Texas.

ACORN's rapid growth and political influence, however, camouflaged serious unresolved dilemmas that lay just below the surface. Most successful large organizations, even nonprofit and activist ones, depend on dynamic, innovative, risk-taking leaders who mirror the savvy successful entrepreneur who starts a small business and grows it into a large profitable company. Rathke was ACORN's venture capitalist. Unlike most idealistic activists, who sometimes think that good intentions are enough but neglect management issues, Rathke understood that managing a large organization is a complicated business. He considered some of the details a necessary nuisance but wanted control over ACORN's operations. Since his talent and attention focused on building relationships, tactics, and campaign strategies, he delegated administration to others, especially his younger brother, Dale.

Over the years, ACORN had tried to keep up with its growth, budget, and tax status, its multiple offices and headquarters, and its role as an employer, but these efforts were hit-and-miss as the back-office staff scrambled to keep up with all the financial and administrative details. ACORN's attempts to teach head organizers how to manage complex financial transactions and oversee their local staff did not match its excellent organizing training.[2] Responding to the challenges of managing its complex operations, which included radio stations, local chapters, profit and nonprofit entities, state and federal political committees, ballot initiative working groups, real estate holdings, and so on, Dale Rathke, a Princeton graduate, had created a Rube Goldberg machine to manage ACORN's two hundred affiliated corporations. Only Dale, Wade, and, to some extent, ACORN's attorney, Steve Bachman, really understood how the interconnected complex web of entities worked. ACORN's fiscal and audit controls were periodically improved, but Citizen Consulting, Inc. (CCI), the ACORN-affiliated accounting firm, was always understaffed, without sufficient professional oversight, a state-of-the-art cash management system, or sufficient internal controls. This sluggish bureaucracy, among other problems, occasionally failed to get payroll checks out on time, angering ACORN's employees.

ACORN's national board of trustees made up of talented leaders like Maxine Nelson from Arkansas, Alicia Russell from Arizona, Carol Hemmingway from Pennsylvania, and John Jones from Washington, elected by their state chapter members, had ultimate decision-making power. But they often lacked sufficiently detailed and timely financial and other reports to juggle priorities and oversee the corporation's finances. Some leaders needed training in financial matters. In truth, most of the board members were more concerned about ACORN's victories in their neighborhoods than about serving as an audit committee overseeing finances. Only a few members, such as Hemmingway, a board officer, wanted more facts and figures.

Staffing was a continuing dilemma. Recruiting organizers for a constantly growing organization wasn't easy. Yes, there were lots of idealistic young people, mostly college graduates, eager to become organizers, but not all had the experience, management skills, and hard-nosed street smarts to be successful. The low pay, long hours, and often-chaotic lifestyle led to a steady turnover among young organizers. Many of the organizers attracted to jobs with ACORN were white, while the vast majority of ACORN's members and leaders were people of color. Rathke always hoped to recruit some of ACORN's best leaders, who were mostly African Americans, to become staff persons, but the low pay and long hours made it difficult to attract people, especially those with families. Since the 1980s, ACORN had made considerable strides in hiring more minority organizers, and since 2000, ACORN Housing Corporation had been very successful in hiring minority staff. But the organizing staff remained predominantly white. Among the new generation of extraordinary organizers, including Kettenring, Nathan Henderson, Matt Henderson, Kevin Whelan, Craig Robbins, Ginny Goldman, Amy Schur, Katy Gall, Mitch Klein, Stu Katzenberg, Jeff Ordower, Steve Bradberry, Tanya Harris, and Bertha Lewis, only the last three were black.[3]

Although ACORN's organizer-training program had improved and salaries had increased, the group's rapid expansion meant that many of its lead organizers lacked sufficient experience and only volunteers staffed some offices. Organizers worked hard—often too hard—with the result that many quickly burned out after a year or two, especially if they had spouses and children. Rathke and other top staff hadn't adequately addressed turnover. Lewis kept lobbying for funds to recruit, train, retain, and promote more minorities to top staff positions, and was getting impatient with ACORN's progress. With old-timers such as Talbott, the Kest brothers, Polett, and Rathke in their mid-to-late fifties, ACORN needed but had no succession plan.

Like all chief executives, Rathke had the power to carry out decisions made by the board and staff. He was ultimately accountable for the success or failure of ACORN's activities. For years he had led by inspiration, creativity, and persistence. He understood the motives of his staff better than they understood his. The long-term organizers did not submit to his decisions as much as they joined him pursuing a mutual goal of fighting poverty and building a more progressive society. While the by-laws gave Rathke the power to appoint all head organizers of the state and local chapters, the state or local membership board had to ratify his decision. He rarely interfered with a local board's decisions or the organizer's operations. ACORN grew partly because these organizers operated autonomously in a decentralized framework. Their dedication was sustained by a common vision and personal loyalty to each other.

To better lead the staff and manage ACORN's growth, Rathke, in the late 1990s, created a management council made up of those responsible for ACORN's larger operations—executive director Steve Kest; head organizers Butler, Talbott, and Jon Kest; Polett, the political director; Shea, the head of ACORN Housing; Kelleher, chief organizer of Local 880; Liz Wolfe, research director; and O'Brien. Lewis, who labeled the council "the bishops," pressured Rathke to add her, Schur, and a few other senior staff. ACORN's success depended heavily on this creative, talented, flexible, and risk-taking group.

The council met regularly, exchanged ideas, coordinated activities, and advised Rathke, who deliberately structured the group as an advisory board and not a decision-making body, thereby reducing its potential influence. Rathke also kept control by carefully selecting who could attend the national ACORN board meetings.

At the start of the twenty-first century, tension within the board and staff was mounting over Rathke's authority and leadership style. Management council members often felt frustrated by Rathke's command but usually accepted his decisions, happy to do their local work while hoping one day for more influence. Like most of the national ACORN board members, the staff accepted Rathke's decisions. As Garry Wills observed in *Certain Trumpets*, true leaders affect others not vaguely but deeply, taking their followers on a mutually agreed quest. For ACORN's organizers and leaders, that pursuit was a large powerful membership organization capable of improving the lives of the working poor and near poor. But as Wills also said about leaders and followers, "Leadership is always a struggle, often a feud."[4]

For Talbott and other organizers, the feud over ACORN's direction began in 2000 and accelerated after Rathke presented his 2007 plan for the future. Pushed by longtime financial supporters Herb and Marion Sandler, Rathke accepted a grant to address ACORN's internal organizational weaknesses and to develop a long-term strategic plan. The Sandlers, respected for their talent at corporate governance, are founders of Golden West Financial, one of the largest savings and loans in the nation, and among the country's most generous progressive philanthropists.[5] When, where, and how to expand any organization is not an exact science. In calibrating the balance between growth and maintenance, Rathke had historically erred on the side of growth, and it had served him well. Rathke was hoping to use the plan for another surge in ACORN's growth.

Despite the difficulty ACORN had in attracting organizing talent, Rathke surprised and disturbed many of the senior staff when, in 2007, he unveiled his bold expansion proposal. It called for increasing field offices from 100 to 170 cities and increasing membership from 260,000 in 2007 to an astonishing and probably unrealistic 2,500,000 members by 2010. To pay for the expansion, ACORN would raise money through door-to-door canvassing, direct mail, Internet fund-raising, other contractual programs, and a wealthy-donor program. He would increase membership partly by adding members who would pay less than the full dues of $120 a year. In a few years, according to Rathke's plan, ACORN would resemble an AARP for the poor.

Rathke wanted also to tighten the lines of authority. ACORN's structure had six regions—Northeast, Southeast, Midwest, West, California, and Florida. An experienced organizer assigned to each region supervised the state and local head organizers and reported to O'Brien. O'Brien and ACORN's "lifers"—Talbott, Kelleher, Butler, and Jon and Steve Kest—reported directly to Rathke. Under Rathke's new plan, the lifers, instead of reporting directly to him, would report to O'Brien. In short, the new plan increased the power of his loyal field director, O'Brien, and diminished the power of head organizers Talbott and Jon Kest, as well as Steve Kest.

To make matters worse for the veterans, Rathke appointed O'Brien as his successor. Loyal, smart, aggressive, and disciplined, O'Brien had a talent for recruiting organizers and was committed to Rathke's expansion plan. For Talbott, reporting to the less experienced O'Brien would be intolerable, and the thought of O'Brien succeeding Rathke as chief organizer was completely unacceptable. Talbott and many of ACORN's most effective organizers thought O'Brien lacked the strategic skills, charm, and charisma Rathke brought to the job.

Moreover, Talbott believed trying to recruit millions of new individual members was absurd—a strategic mistake that would undermine her own plans. She and the New York organizers had built powerful chapters, not just by recruiting individual members but also by leading powerful coalitions like the Housing Now Coalition in New York and the Living Wage Coalition in Chicago. Talbott thought forging alliances with other groups around economic justice campaigns should be an essential part of ACORN's future.

Talbott and Jon Kest, among ACORN's best organizers, had enormous support among ACORN's local organizers, who looked to them as models and mentors. Although Rathke insisted that his reorganization was critical to ACORN's future success, Talbott and others thought that it was a power grab and that Rathke was being driven by ambition and dreams of an unrealistic legacy.

While Rathke was developing this plan, Amy Schur, Jon Kest, and sixteen other organizers, all with at least five years' experience, held a secret meeting in San Francisco to discuss ways to improve ACORN's operations and to give senior staff a greater voice in staff decision making. Rathke, O'Brien, and their close allies were not invited. Bertha Lewis didn't attend because of several commitments in New York. When one of the organizers at the San Francisco gathering told Rathke about the meeting, Rathke felt betrayed. Schur, Kest, and the others could no longer be trusted. He continued to execute his new organizational plan.

Talbott had hoped that one day ACORN's staff leadership structure would include a council of collegial senior staff who would exchange and vet creative ideas, hone them into concrete proposals, and together present them to the national board. Having lost all hope of this vision, Talbott would soon lead her large Illinois chapter out of ACORN.

Despite the tensions, Rathke was confident he could meet the challenges ahead, overcome the differences he had with dissident staff, and continue to garner the kind of positive stories that had run in the *New York Times* in 2006 touting ACORN's national and local success stories; a June story was headlined, "City by City, an Antipoverty Group Plants Seeds of Change."[6] A *Times* front-page story told of ACORN's Chicago victory in which Talbott's local chapter got the City Council to pass an ordinance requiring big-box stores like Wal-Mart and Home Depot to pay a minimum wage of ten dollars an hour by 2010, along with at least three dollars an hour's worth of benefits.[7]

But a *New York Times* article about ACORN two years later, on July 9, 2008, was one Rathke had hoped never to see. The *Times* published a scoop that had been brewing for a few months based on information leaked by a few disgruntled ACORN employees.[8] Rathke knew about the article but was unable to stop it. He would also miscalculate its consequences. Overnight the right-wing blogosphere was abuzz over the article, which reported that Dale Rathke had embezzled almost $1 million from the organization's coffers in 2000, eight years earlier. Wade had fired Dale from his job as comptroller through at ACORN-affiliated Citizens Consulting, Inc., but kept him on as a special assistant. The various thefts were consolidated and listed as a loan on the books of CCI, a legal way to handle an embezzlement when there is a strong expectation the funds will be returned. Dale signed a promissory note, which included pledges from his parents and Wade for repayment, at 7 percent simple annual interest, and a provision signing over his anticipated inheritance to ensure full repayment.

Although this debt would be repaid, it turned out that Wade Rathke not only hid the embezzlement from ACORN's funders but also did not report all the details to the ACORN national board as he had promised members of the management council he would. He was close to his family, loved his brother dearly, and so did everything he could to protect him. He rationalized to himself and some of the other members of the management council that keeping the embezzlement secret was necessary because the Republicans had just taken control of all three branches of the federal government and he was afraid that the incoming George W. Bush administration would instigate a costly, public, and time-consuming investigation. His fear was heightened by what Rathke thought was an unconstitutional power grab by the Supreme Court in 2000 when it selected Bush as president. Republican harassment had been a recurrent pattern and ongoing fear for ACORN's leadership. While Rathke's case for protecting the organization from those who would destroy it might have explained maintaining public secrecy about the embezzlement issue, his failure to keep his board and foundation donors fully apprised thwarted basic notions of accountability and transparency and threatened to ruin the organization he had founded.

Like a Bomb

When his staff had found out about the embezzlement during the May 2008 staff meeting, many were furious that Rathke had kept his brother on the payroll for eight years after he knew about the theft. When the national board was told, a majority of its members were incensed at Rathke. They believed that once his brother's embezzlement was discovered, Wade should have fully explained the matter to ACORN's board members, who had ultimate responsibility for governing ACORN. Rathke's misjudgment was not just that he covered up his brother's wrongdoing. Many of ACORN's staff, as well as a dozen national board members, bridled at what they saw as Rathke's effort to consolidate his power within the organization and his brother's continued involvement with ACORN's finances.

On May 26, 2008, after the scandal surfaced inside the organization but before the *Times* article came out, the board forced Rathke to resign and fired his brother. Although the Rathke family had entered into an enforceable agreement at the time to pay the money back, ACORN's board believed that Rathke hadn't acted honestly, swiftly, or firmly enough. In the world of scandals, ACORN's missteps don't even register on the radar compared with the swindles perpetrated by top executives at Enron, Countrywide, AIG, and other major corporations who ripped off the government, stockholders, and consumers of billions of dollars, or with politicians who exchange corporate campaign contributions for votes. Georgetown professor Pablo Eisenberg, an expert in nonprofit governance and a critic of some of Rathke's methods, wrote: "In the grand scheme of foundation and nonprofit scandals over the past decade, the embezzlement of almost $ 1 million . . . seems like small potatoes."[9] For ACORN, Rathke's transgressions would turn out to be a tragedy with devastating consequences.

"It was like a bomb. Things just went bonkers," Lewis said to the media. "Nothing like that had ever happened before."[10] Morale among the staff sunk to an all-time low. Some of the veterans, like Helene O'Brien, would soon resign. Many foundation funders were appropriately outraged that they had not been consulted or notified and threatened to cut off funds. As ACORN increasingly relied on income from foundations to supplement dues, local bake sales and other membership-based efforts, it would inevitably come under increased scrutiny. Controversial groups like ACORN, which rely on public trust and external financial support, and which become powerful and effective, have to be above reproach. Progressive foundations sympathize with nonprofit groups grappling with management weaknesses, but they have little tolerance for groups they do not see as having moral force.

Board Action

In an act that reaffirmed the democratic nature of ACORN, the board decisively replaced Rathke with Bertha Lewis because of her proven leadership qualities and her reputation for fighting for more transparency and accountability within ACORN. ACORN's swift action was insufficient for some funders. Blindsided by the disclosure of the embezzlement, a few foundations suspended or ended their grants. One funder, the Campaign for Human Development, run by the U.S. Conference of Catholic Bishops, cut off all funding on June 2. In previous years the Campaign had praised ACORN's work and had given $1.1 million a year to ACORN and its affiliates. Now in a cowardly act, it capitulated to the growing pressure by conservative Catholics who had been lobbying for years to stop funding ACORN, partly because it was seen as favoring abortion rights for poor women.

The Presidential Election and the Attacks

In the midst of the 2008 presidential campaign, the embezzlement provided ACORN's opponents with ammunition. Indeed, because it had been so successful for almost four decades, ACORN had accumulated many enemies—especially business groups, conservative politicians, and the ideological Right, such as the editors of the *Wall Street Journal*, who would have loved to see the organization destroyed. In early July 2008, a *Wall Street Journal* editorial repeated the voter-fraud canard, while warning that a Democrat-sponsored bill to rescue families facing foreclosure, which included funds for homeownership counseling, could provide money to ACORN, "the left-wing activist outfit that was infamous for its bare-knuckle politics." On July 12, three days after the *Times* story exposed the embezzlement, *Journal* columnist John Fund, a persistent ACORN critic, portrayed ACORN as one of Obama's "liberal shock troops," labeling the group "the granddaddy of activist groups" and repeating the misleading accusation that ACORN has a "history of vote-fraud scandals." ACORN had never been involved in voter fraud.[11]

Right after the *Times* story surfaced, the Consumer Rights League—a front group sponsored by the predatory payday-lending industry—issued a statement, reported by Fox News, attacking ACORN for "rampant voter registration fraud."[12] That same week, another front group for employers who fought ACORN on living-wage issues, the Employment Policies Institute (EPI) issued a statement: "This is just one more page in ACORN's corrupt history, which already includes election fraud investigations in at least a dozen states."[13] EPI, funded by the restaurant, hotel, alcoholic beverage, and tobacco industries, and the Consumer Rights League are actually groups created by Washington, D.C.–based Berman and Company, which specializes in "Astroturf lobbying"—phony grassroots organizations for corporate clients. According to the reporting of SourceWatch.org: "EPI's mission is to keep the minimum wage low so Berman's clients can continue to pay their workers as little as possible."[14] Thus, part of EPI's job is to churn out an ongoing information campaign against ACORN for EPI's clients in the restaurant and bar industry, like Outback Steakhouse, Tyson Foods, and Hooters.[15]

Voter Registration or Voter Fraud?

ACORN's voter engagement mission, a part of its core operations, presented ACORN's Zach Polett and Project Vote staff with a dilemma. From their experiences in 2004 and 2006, Polett knew they would face another round of attacks from Republicans and conservative commentators over allegations of voter fraud. Though ACORN substantially improved its training and supervision, they also knew any effort to collect large amounts of information from the public ran the risk of mistakes: missing information, duplicates, or errors by voters or election officials. This challenge to avoid errors is made more difficult in the United States with its crazy quilt of voter registration laws and regulations, which differ state by state and even city by city. There is no cookie-cutter way to register voters, yet mistakes that cause the mere appearance of deceit by ACORN would turn out to be as disastrous as an outbreak of a disease that leads to multiple deaths in a hospital.

Before they opened the doors on the voter-registration drive in late 2007, ACORN and Project Vote staff, led by attorney Brian Mellor, who had worked in Florida in 2004, designed an elaborate quality-control system to police its own workers and brought office managers together for weeks of training.[16] Given the Herculean task of amassing thousands of staff to do the complicated work of registering poor and minority voters, problems would inevitably occur. ACORN recruited more than thirteen thousand workers in twenty-one states to register people in poor and working-class neighborhoods. While the training and oversight was much better than in 2004, it was not airtight. Despite stringent warnings, several canvassers duplicated or faked some of their voter-registration forms rather than do the hard work of approaching strangers and asking them to complete the forms.

ACORN's top managers insisted to its field staff that any questionable signatures had to be reported to local authorities. When ACORN managers suspected that some temporary staff hired for the voter-registration drives were handing in petitions with phony names, the staffers were fired or given warnings and the signatures were reported to government officials, as required by law. ACORN did a fairly good job of managing many of the risks inherent in a massive voter-registration campaign. They thought of everything necessary to avoid voter-registration fraud. With most of its staff devoted to organizing and providing services and with the likelihood of a right-wing assault to discredit its work, ACORN faced another challenge: did it have the public relations capacity to manage the perils of an appearance of voter fraud and other misdeeds?

The National Media's Framing of ACORN

In late September 2008—close to the end of ACORN's drive to register over one million voters, politicians and government attorneys, mostly Republicans, leaked information about problematic signatures to the news media, blaming ACORN for "fraud" rather than praising the organization for uncovering the problem. Despite the fact that neither ACORN nor its employees had been found guilty of, or even charged with, casting fraudulent votes, McCain on national television warned that the November 4 election would be marred by ACORN's election activities. ACORN, he said, is "perpetrating one of the greatest frauds in voter history."[17]

At rallies and press events, John McCain and Sarah Palin, pushed by the conservative base, repeated this charge and demanded that Obama disclose his ties with ACORN, which they described as a "radical" organization. Indeed, throughout the fall presidential campaign, McCain and Palin frequently accused ACORN of "voter fraud" and worked at defaming Obama by linking him to ACORN.[18] A Sarah Palin fund-raising letter stated: "We've always known the Obama-Biden Democrats will do anything to win this November, but we didn't know how far their allies would go. The Obama-supported, far-left group, ACORN, has been accused of voter-registration fraud in a number of battleground states." This narrative fit nicely with the campaign's attempts to tie Obama to a notorious Vietnam-era antiwar activist, Bill Ayers, whom the campaign accused of being a terrorist. The McCain campaign ran a one-and-a-half-minute video that claimed Barack Obama once worked for ACORN, repeated the accusation that ACORN was responsible for widespread voter-registration fraud, and accused ACORN of "bullying banks, intimidation tactics, and disruption of business." The ad claimed that ACORN "forced banks to issue risky home loans—the same types of loans that caused the financial crisis we're in today." (McCain's anti-ACORN attack video was almost a word-for-word duplication of comments made by *National Review* columnist Stanley Kurtz.) One right-wing blogger labeled Obama "the senator from ACORN."

All these attacks, with their overtones of a witch-hunt, hurt others besides Obama. The day after the McCain-Obama debate, several ACORN community organizers received death threats, and the antipoverty group's Boston and Seattle offices were vandalized.[19]

The McCain campaign and the national Republican Party's all-out assault included daily press calls, National Press Club events, and support from Fox News and CNN's Lou Dobbs. Despite ACORN's extraordinary organizing work in cities across the country, in 2007 and 2008, 55 percent of the media stories about the organization dealt with voter fraud, according to a study by Peter Dreier and Christoper Martin of media coverage of ACORN.[20] During October 2008, 76 percent of the ACORN stories focused on allegations of voter fraud, and the reports were mostly inaccurate. The study found that both conservative and mainstream media reported allegations by Republican Party operatives and politicians without seeking to verify these claims or to provide ACORN with equal opportunities to challenge the accusations.

The narrative framing of the ACORN stories demonstrates that—despite long-standing charges from conservatives that the news media are determinedly liberal and ignore conservative ideas—the news media agenda is easily permeated by persistent conservative media campaigns, even when there is little or no truth to a story. Dreir and Martin conducted a content analysis of all 647 stories about ACORN that appeared in fifteen major news media organizations from 2007 to 2008. The news media analyzed included *USA Today*, *New York Times*, *Washington Post*, *Wall Street Journal*, ABC, CBS, NBC, Fox News Channel, CNN, MSNBC, National Public Radio (NPR), and NewsHour with Jim Lehrer (PBS). Using the controversy over ACORN as a case study, the report illustrates the way the media help set the agenda for public debate, and frame the way that debate is shaped. It describes how what the authors call opinion entrepreneurs (primarily corporate and conservative groups and individuals) set the story in motion as early as 2006, how the "conservative echo chamber" orchestrated its anti-ACORN campaign in 2008, how the McCain-Palin campaign picked it up, and how the mainstream media reported these allegations without investigating their truth or falsity. As a result, the relatively little-known community organization became the subject of a major news story in the 2008 U.S. presidential campaign, to the point where according to the study, 82 percent of the respondents in an October 2008 national survey reported they had heard about ACORN.

Stories accused ACORN of causing the mortgage scandal and the government of funneling public funds to ACORN. The study also found that the media, including the mainstream news media, failed to fact-check persistent allegations of voter fraud involving ACORN despite the existence of easily available countervailing evidence. The media failed to distinguish claims of voter-registration problems from accusations of actual voting irregularities. ACORN never engaged in "fraud," which involves intention: a willful act to register ineligible people and then to see to it that they vote. Further, 95.8 percent of the stories alleging ACORN's involvement in voter fraud failed to report the surrounding circumstances, including efforts by Republican Party officials to use charges of voter fraud to stifle voting by low-income and minority Americans. As the media watchdog Media Matters pointed out, the reports on false voter registration often left out two relevant points. The statutes in the states where ACORN registered prospective voters required ACORN to submit all registration forms they received, even when ACORN believed they were faulty. In nine of the eleven states where ACORN's registration efforts were questioned, the law or voter-registration practice required ACORN to submit every voter-registration form, regardless of doubts about its authenticity. For any questionable form, ACORN's quality-control staff had attached a "problematic card report coversheet."[21] As reported by McClatchy News Service and CNN, the law gave ACORN no choice but to flag the form and turn it in or face a thousand-dollar fine. ACORN neither had a policy nor an intention to engage in voter-registration or any kind of fraud. For all the publicity about some ACORN canvasser registering somebody in Florida who called himself "Mickey Mouse," Mickey Mouse didn't vote and couldn't vote. According to experts like Barnard College professor Lorraine Minnite, voter registration and voter fraud are very rare.[22]

Even Drew Griffin, CNN's investigative reporter, who repeatedly took the information flagged by ACORN's own quality-control system and tried to create the impression of an imminent crisis in the elections, eventually got it right: "Our research is showing—this [voter-registration fraud] more looks like a fraud perpetrated on ACORN," not by ACORN.[23]

ACORN's quality-control procedures—phone-verifying every card, flagging problematic cards, and identifying offending workers for local officials—became thousands of Kick Me signs that were used against ACORN in the media and in the legal process. Not one U.S. attorney found any evidence of an illegal vote cast and counted because of registration by ACORN and those working for it. The politically motivated attack on ACORN was part of a long history of intimidation to prevent minority voter enfranchisement. Republican attempts to prevent people of color from voting in the 2008 election were rampant, extending to least nine states. But Republican misdeeds fell below the radar and the truth didn't matter because ACORN's public relations capacity was not up to the assault. "We thought that by being totally transparent—documenting everything we were doing and being the first ones to flag any problems—we would be able to get people to understand what our work was really about," said Kevin Whelan, ACORN's deputy political director. "In retrospect, this was probably naive."

While the United States needs to increase voter-registration rates among African Americans, Latinos, and the poor to honor its democratic promise, ACORN's experience shows that relying on activist groups leads to political vitriol and legal trouble for those involved. In the context of a dysfunctional system and a hyperpoliticized voter-registration environment, it is senseless to depend on groups like ACORN, who end up suffering the repercussions of helping to register voters.

In a democratic society, voter registration should be the government's business. If the government supervised a plan to make large-scale voter registration a reality and removed all the obstacles for low-income voters and voters of color, the controversies over voter registration would diminish. The United States could copy countries as diverse as Brazil and Australia by promoting democracy with mandatory voter registration. With Republicans opposed to increasing voter turnout by people of color election reform is unlikely, partisan controversies will break out before elections, and groups like ACORN will have to raise and spend millions of dollars to make sure the poor and minorities are registered.

Linking ACORN to the Financial Crisis

In addition to charges of voter fraud, ACORN's enemies repeated the accusation that the group had forced banks to issue risky home loans and caused the financial crisis of 2008 because of its long-term support for the Community Reinvestment Act (CRA).[24] This accusation was completely false, a diversionary tactic to take the heat off the unregulated financial services industry and its allies, like John McCain, a long-term foe of government regulation of the financial services industry. The CRA, which outlaws mortgage discrimination and encourages banks to make below-market mortgages, applies only to depository institutions such as commercial and savings banks. Thanks to the government's deregulation mania, many other lenders, including private mortgage companies like CitiMortgage, Household Finance, and Countrywide Financial entered the subprime market. These outfits, which operated without government oversight, accounted for most of the loans that caused the widespread home foreclosures. And like Household's, many of their loans were predatory. Testifying before the House Financial Services Committee in February, University of Michigan law professor Michael Barr reported that banks regulated by the CRA issued only about 20 percent of subprime mortgages. The other 80 percent of predatory and high-interest subprime loans were offered by financial institutions not covered by the CRA and not subject to routine examination or supervision. "The worst and most widespread abuses occurred in the institutions with the least federal oversight," Barr told Congress.

In contrast, the CRA actually penalizes banks for reckless, irresponsible, or otherwise predatory lending. According to Ellen Seidman, director of the Treasury Department's Office of Thrift Supervision from 1997 to 2001, federal regulators warned CRA-covered banks that "badly underwritten subprime products that ignored consumer protections were not acceptable." Lenders not subject to CRA did not receive similar warnings.

Unlike the institutions that offer unregulated predatory subprime loans, banks that make CRA loans are required by federal regulation to verify borrowers' incomes to make sure they can afford the mortgages. In 2006, the Federal Reserve reported that just 11.5 percent of mortgages made by CRA-regulated institutions were high-cost loans, compared with 33.5 percent for lenders not covered by the CRA. Janet Yellen, president and CEO of the Federal Reserve Bank of San Francisco, criticized those who blamed CRA lending for the subprime crisis: "Most of the loans made by depository institutions examined under the CRA have not been higher-priced loans, and studies have shown that the CRA has increased the volume of responsible lending to low- and moderate-income households."

ACORN joined other consumer advocates and lawyers to promote the notion of "assignee liability," arguing that companies that buy and profit from loans bear responsibility for acts committed when those loans were originally made. Without it, the mortgage originators, who typically hold loans briefly before they sell them, can make fraudulent or risky loans without suffering any consequences.

ACORN had tried to stem the subprime crisis as early as 1999 when it pursued Household Finance Corporation, spurred state attorneys general to investigate it in 2002, and forced Household to compensate victims of its predatory subprime practices. ACORN and its counterparts were able only to stick their fingers in the crumbling dike of U.S. finance. Their warnings were prescient, but their opponents too strong.

At a time of growing indigence and inequality, conservatives and Republicans like John McCain worried more about ACORN's mistakes (and its successes) than about the real menace of poverty amid plenty. Indeed, conservatives who criticized ACORN appeared to think that poverty was hardly a problem for the United States in 2008. In fact, more than 36 million Americans lived below the official poverty line—about $20,000 for a family of four. One out of five U.S. children lived in poverty, the highest rate by far among the world's highly industrialized nations. In some big cities, more than one-third of all children lived in poverty. The average income for households at the bottom fifth of the income spectrum is only a little more than $13,000.[25]

Fixing ACORN

The attacks by McCain and the Right, Obama's indifference to the attacks, the withdrawal of financial support by some major foundations, and the need to reform ACORN's management in the wake of Wade Rathke's ouster put Bertha Lewis in the cross-currents of controversy. Not only did she have to battle the attacks on her organization from the outside, but also Lewis had to manage the leadership transition and stabilize ACORN internally.

Immediately after she took over, twenty-three friendly foundations urged ACORN to make needed changes, such as addressing plans for financial accountability, securing a new auditor, and removing Wade Rathke from all duties within the organization. To get control of all aspects of ACORN's operations and turn around its reputation with ACORN's funders, Lewis hired highly qualified outside consultants—attorneys and CPAs who specialized in nonprofit law and accounting. The Sandlers provided ACORN with a full-time expert management consultant, Mark Gritten, a former corporate executive. Lewis instructed them to dig into ACORN's operation and make recommendations to restore ACORN's credibility, increase its effectiveness, and satisfy the demands of ACORN's funders. The old staff fully supported Lewis, including Zach Polett, the political director and a close Rathke ally who agreed to help with fund-raising and political strategy. Lewis held dozens of meetings with staff, board members, foundation executives, corporate sponsors, and representatives of other progressive networks to develop a plan for the future.

On another front, a dispute broke out between Rathke and Lewis over office space at the headquarters in New Orleans and over Rathke's control of property and of the dozens of ACORN's affiliated corporations he had set up. They included ACORN radio stations, ACORN International, *Social Policy* magazine, and the Wal-Mart Alliance for Reform Now—a coalition whose aim is to force Wal-Mart to be accountable to community standards and values.

In addition, Lewis needed to confront a divided national board. The majority of the board leadership, including longtime board president Maude Hurd, supported Lewis's decision to sever ties with Rathke and move on. Another faction of the board, led by ACORN's New Orleans chapter, valued Rathke's work and thought he should remain with ACORN. A third faction, who for years had tried to wrest control of ACORN away from Rathke, supported ousting him and constantly criticized Lewis, claiming she denied them access to financial information and excluded them from important meetings. This faction wanted Lewis to support their takeover of ACORN, which included firing the Kests and all the old-timers. They tried to sabotage every attempt by Lewis to fix ACORN's problems, and even filed an unauthorized lawsuit claiming to speak for the entire board. The suit was needed, they argued, to protect ACORN's financial records from destruction. Most of this faction, including John Jones and Toni McElroy, left to support Lewis, convinced its few remaining members, now calling themselves the ACORN 8, were out to destroy ACORN. One of the leaders of the ACORN 8 attempted to orchestrate a deal with a financial services firm owned by a national fraternity (Kappa Alpha Psi) with which she is affiliated. In presenting her proposal to ACORN's Management Council, she concealed her relationship to the fraternity. None of the ACORN 8 really had the capacity to lead ACORN. While ACORN's leaders downplayed the power and importance of this rogue group along with a few disgruntled employees, one of whom was fired for stealing, the ACORN 8 became the main source of the relentlessly negative reports in the *New York Times* from July until October 21, 2008, and later by Fox News.

Lewis reminded herself and her allies, as well as the funders, that amid the turmoil "I had to keep the trains running on time." Like an injured athlete determined to work through the pain rather than sit on the sidelines, ACORN continued doing what it did best, mobilizing the poor around issues. While Lewis was trying to restore lost funding and resolve differences with Rathke and among the board members, she oversaw an organization that remained a feisty voice for the poor. For example, during just one week in July 2008, ACORN successfully saved 5,881 rental units of working-class housing in Brooklyn, pressured banks in Pittsburgh to end their predatory lending practices, campaigned in Texas to expand health insurance, announced its key role in a new national coalition of unions and consumer and religious groups to fight for universal health care, and continued its ongoing work to rebuild homes in the Lower Ninth Ward. ACORN also pushed Gov. Arnold Schwarzenegger to sign a bill that would help desperate California homeowners avoid foreclosure, counseled homeowners in Connecticut on ways to avoid foreclosure, and pressured local officials in Tucson, Arizona, to adopt a law to prevent unfair lending practices.[26]

ACORN's biggest victory during this period was reported in a *Wall Street Journal* front-page story on July 31, 2008.[27] ACORN, joining other groups, led a lobbying campaign that successfully pressured President Bush to sign a federal affordable housing bill, which provided $5 billion dollars for low-income housing and financial counseling and mortgage restructuring for people and neighborhoods hit hard by the subprime predatory housing crisis. ACORN also launched its campaign to pass the Healthy Families Act. The law would help change the way the United States treats working families by requiring up to seven paid sick days for all workers every year so they can take care of themselves, their sick children, or attend court in cases related to sexual assault or domestic violence.

November 4, Election Day, and New Hope

As Election Day approached, ACORN tried to counter the bad publicity. Its top leaders and staff battled McCain and the Right by holding press conferences, sending e-mails, producing reports, and feeding the media positive stories about ACORN's work. Bertha Lewis kept trying to explain ACORN's strategy to the press. "There are different kinds of power," said Lewis. "There's electoral power. Movie stars have fame. Billionaires have money. Low- and moderate-income people have their numbers, and every great movement for social justice—Nelson Mandela preaching against apartheid, civil rights—have all been led by community organizers who took action and held their elected officials accountable."[28]

Meanwhile, local ACORN organizers continued trying to carry on ACORN's mission to help people help themselves. Typical was Peter Nagy, a twenty-four-year-old University of Utah graduate from Long Island. Nagy met with Hempstead residents worried about safety and services in their buildings and a group of Long Island residents facing foreclosure to generate interest in an anti-eviction plan. Right up until Election Day, November 3, 2008, ACORN's organizers kept knocking on doors and helping people fight predatory lending, support immigration reform, and work on neighborhood improvements, while others worked to get out black, Latino, and poor voters in Ohio, Minnesota, North Carolina, Florida, Colorado, New Mexico, and elsewhere.

On November 3, Bertha Lewis flew to Chicago to meet with several ACORN members and staff. The next day, in Chicago's Grant Park, she stood with thousands of Obama supporters awaiting the election returns to celebrate what they hoped would be a victory. Just after 10:00 pm, when the networks called the race for Obama, Lewis threw her arms in the air and added her voice to the deafening roar from the crowd.

Listening to Obama's victory speech, she heard echoes of Martin Luther King's "I've Been to the Mountaintop" speech. Obama asserted: "Tonight, because of what we did on this day, in this election, at this defining moment, change has come to America"; and "The road ahead will be long, our climb will be steep. We may not get there in one year, or even in one term—but America, I have never been more hopeful than I am tonight that we will get there."

"This is our moment," the president-elect declared. "This is our time—to put our people back to work and open doors of opportunity for our kids; to restore prosperity and promote the cause of peace; to reclaim the American Dream and reaffirm that fundamental truth—that out of many, we are one; that while we breathe, we hope, and where we are met with cynicism, and doubt, and those who tell us that we can't, we will respond with that timeless creed that sums up the spirit of a people: Yes we can." Tears of joy streamed down Lewis's face. Obama's election gave new hope for the values and policies that ACORN had been fighting for since 1970.

A few days later, ACORN's staff and leaders met to strategize about how to take advantage of this historic election—to identify regulatory changes that federal agencies could adopt without legislation, and to develop a wish list of legislative proposals that it wanted the Obama administration to support that would help address the problems of poverty, urban decline, lending, and housing.

The euphoria was real, but now they had to wrestle with the knotty problems of how ACORN would play its inside/outside strategy—direct-action protest and lobbying for legislation—with a friend in the White House. ACORN's leaders had reason to hope that ACORN could make progress on voter rights, foreclosures, and health care with a friendly president and Congress in office, but they believed they needed to keep the heat on to make sure that whatever compromise bills passed, they were the best ones possible.

In February 2009, a family faced the horrible reality of losing a home to foreclosure every thirteen seconds. Credit Suisse was predicting that there would be between eight and nine million foreclosures in the next four years, at a potential cost to the economy of $702 billion. With the epidemic of foreclosures accelerating around the country, the Obama administration planned to announce its new Homeowner Affordability and Stability Plan, a $75 billion effort to help millions of homeowners avoid foreclosure.

To push local and federal officials for something more ambitious, ACORN launched its Home Defenders campaign. On February 17, 2009, the day before Obama announced his plan, the *New York Times* broke a story by Fernanda Santos headlined, "A Bid to Link Arms against Eviction: Effort Takes Shape to Support Families Facing Foreclosure." Santos explained that ACORN would use phone trees, Web pages, and text-messaging networks to "connect families facing eviction with volunteers who will stand at their side as [eviction] officers arrive, even if it means risking arrest." ACORN's direct-action strategy was aimed at getting powerful players—mortgage companies, sheriffs, and politicians—to negotiate with ACORN's members to resolve the political conflict that was generating media attention and public outrage. The following day, February 18, coinciding with Obama's announcement, ACORN released a widely distributed statement praising the president's proposal.

During the months of February and March, ACORN lobbied for a ninety-day moratorium on foreclosures, lifting the ban on allowing bankruptcy-court judges to modify mortgages to help families avoid foreclosure, a move that would help prevent 600,000 foreclosures without further taxing the U.S. Treasury. Local chapters promoted the Philadelphia Foreclosure Diversion Program, a plan ACORN had developed with several city officials, which succeeded in keeping in their homes 78 percent of Philadelphia's families facing foreclosure. ACORN believed the Philadelphia plan, if implemented nationally, could save millions of Americans from suffering the fate of foreclosure. The key to the plan was its mandatory settlement conferences, where lenders and borrowers of subprime loans who were in default on their mortgages would hammer out new terms to keep the borrowers in their homes.

In March 2009, recognizing that if ACORN continued its voter-registration work it would face threats of criminal indictment and media attacks, ACORN's staff began planning a campaign to shift the focus of the media and politicians away from voter-registration fraud and toward government support for enfranchising more voters.[29] ACORN planned to work with Congress to remove unfair barriers to voter registration, ensuring that every eligible citizen is added to the rolls. On March 25, ACORN made some headway when Rep. Zoe Lofgren (D-California) introduced the Voter Registration Modernization Act to update the voter-registration system. ACORN would also follow up its 2008 legal victory based on the National Voter Registration Act. The suit caused Missouri social service agencies to collect a hundred thousand registration applications.

At the same time, ACORN was working on one of America's most serious issues: how to deal with the forty-six million Americans without health-care insurance and the many millions more whose insurance is too expensive or inadequate to address their family needs. Tamecka Pierce, an ACORN national board member from Florida, became one of ACORN's leaders in the national Health Care for America Now (HCAN) campaign. A single mother with three children, she told other board members how ecstatic she was when her new job included employer-provided health insurance. Just after she was accepted into her employer's Blue Cross/Blue Shield program, Pierce had been diagnosed with lupus, an autoimmune disease in which the body slowly eats away at itself. The treatment is complex, ever shifting, and life long, because there is no cure. Blue Cross/Blue Shield spent months trying to deny Pierce coverage.

When Pierce finally won, her problems didn't end. As the sole breadwinner for her family, money was always an issue for her. Because of the deductibles, copays, and cost of medication, at the end of the month she found herself forced to choose between paying health-care bills or the rent. These experiences gave Pierce a firsthand, up-front lesson in what was wrong with the U.S. health-care system and why the country needed universal national health care for her and tens of millions of other Americans. She helped ACORN become part of a sixteen-state HCAN coalition in which ACORN would play the lead role in six states—Florida, Kansas, Arizona, New Mexico, Delaware, and Louisiana. ACORN and HCAN proposed the creation of a health-insurance public option—similar to the popular Medicare program or to the health plan for military vets run by the Veterans Administration—which would create competition with private health insurance companies, reduce costs, and increase the quality of care. The idea was embraced by Obama but faced strong opposition from the insurance industry and its allies in Congress, including moderate Democrats. A major goal of the HCAN campaign was to push those moderate Democrats to support the public option.

While ACORN continued its work in its local chapters and its major campaign initiatives, it faced a budget deficit in the millions that could cripple its future. Many funders, led by Dave Beckwith, the executive director of the Needmor Foundation, viewed the transition as an opportunity to deal with ACORN's weaknesses, and quickly renewed their support for ACORN. Other foundations withheld funding, angered by the embezzlement or old animosities or even Lewis's support for the controversial Brooklyn Atlantic Yards development. With the loss of funding from some foundations and uncertain support from others, Lewis had to close more than two dozen offices and lay off twenty staff. After consulting with several staff, including the Kest brothers, with board members, and with the management, legal, and financial experts, Lewis was ready to present a plan to the April national board meeting, hoping for a workable transition that would bolster ACORN's credibility and effectiveness.

As the April 2009 national board meeting approached, ACORN was at a crossroads. Could Lewis and her team fix what was wrong, keep what was right, unify the board, take advantage of ACORN's growing visibility, and rebuild its reputation so it could go on to make a difference in the lives of the poor? Or would ACORN fall victim to the attacks by right-wingers, its self-inflicted wounds, and what management experts call the "founder's syndrome"—the inability to maintain momentum once the founder leaves?

Chapter 18

The Prostitute and the Assault

The Sahara Hotel and Casino, its arched, domed entrance capped with a minaret, its hallways bedecked with photos of Frank Sinatra's Rat Pack, and its lobby detailed in Moroccan mosaic, seemed a strange place for the ACORN national board to convene. But the fifty-seven-year-old Las Vegas palace had declined so far from its glory days that its motel-bland rooms were now, at forty-five dollars a night, affordable even for community organizers.

For three days in April 2009 in the hotel's nondescript conference hall, within earshot of screaming slot machines, fifty-one board members debated how they should transform ACORN into a more reliable, democratic, and transparent organization. Unlike the acrimonious discussion at the November 2008 board meeting, at which two remaining dissidents who refused to withdraw their unauthorized lawsuit were removed for violating ACORN's bylaws, debate at this meeting was congenial, even when heated. At the November meeting nearly all the board members had agreed with Rev. Gloria Swieringa, a blind preacher from Maryland and foster mother of twenty children. She had emerged as a leading spokesperson for ACORN during the 2008 election. "We found ourselves having filed a lawsuit against ourselves," she said. "Since we didn't know anything about it, and since it was not sanctioned, it's unacceptable for a few angry members who have no interest in reform but just thought they could take over to remain with us." ACORN's lawyer reported that the judge dismissed the suit.

At the April meeting, with ACORN's future in doubt, the board had to take steps to improve staff accountability, financial safeguards, and internal communications. Lewis invited key staff, management experts, CPAs, and lawyers to the meeting so the board could make informed decisions about issues, budget, expansion, political strategy, and staffing. The board adopted the consultants' recommendations. To prevent another embezzlement, and to make sure salaries and payroll taxes were paid on time, the board implemented bookkeeping checks and balances, established an audit committee, hired an independent auditor, and adopted policies to avoid nepotism and encourage whistle blowing. To make ACORN more transparent and to provide reports to the national board, the staff, members, and funders, a new accounting system would accurately track income and expenses for ACORN's complex, multifaceted, multichapter organization.

To build on its strengths, Lewis proposed that ACORN concentrate its organizing work in black and Latino communities, a detour away from Rathke's vision of ACORN as a multiracial group that included whites and people of color. Lewis believed that ACORN could better fight poverty and contribute to a broad progressive movement by concentrating on its base of Puerto Ricans, Mexican Americans, and Caribbean and African Americans, while concurrently building alliances with environmentalists, liberal white churches, and other groups. At the same time, Lewis did not want ACORN to become a civil rights group like the NAACP; rather, she wanted it to continue as a mostly black and brown peoples' group focused on immigration and economic justice issues that could lift the poor into the middle class and improve conditions in urban neighborhoods. While discussing this new strategy, and making it clear that whites were still welcome in ACORN, Lewis turned to one of the few white board members and joked, "You're black, you just have a skin problem." The board, made up of members elected by their state chapters, pledged to pursue new alliances, such as working with unions and other groups as part of a new national health care coalition.

They agreed to beef up fund-raising, and to more than double the membership to one million by 2012. They approved creation of an advisory board that included big names like Kathleen Kennedy Townsend, former lieutenant governor of Maryland; Eric Eve, Citibank's senior vice president of global community relations; and John Podesta, who ran Barack Obama's transition office, served as President Bill Clinton's chief of staff, and founded the liberal think tank Center for American Progress.

Lewis understood that Obama's victory provided new opportunities for ACORN to advance its causes. She urged shifting the central office from New Orleans to Washington. "We have a better chance of making our voices heard behind closed doors, in the corridors of power if we move the central office," Lewis argued. The board agreed. Lewis, though, did not want ACORN to become another inside-the-Beltway lobby group like many public interest groups with offices in D.C. She wanted ACORN to have a voice on national issues, while having its priorities set from the bottom up. The board was determined that ACORN would remain a multi-issue, dues-paying membership association organized in city and neighborhood chapters across the country. ACORN would continue to use a range of tactics including in-your-face, direct-action protests, while staying engaged in elections, lobbying politicians, forging alliances with unions and environmental and other progressive groups, and building partnerships with business. They vowed to remain focused on bread-and-butter issues, combine community action with the delivery of services (like homeownership counseling and tax preparation), and save minority neighborhoods. The board passed resolutions implementing some reforms immediately; others could be implemented only if ACORN could raise the money; and still others—like the goal of one million members—appeared to be more fantasy than reality, unless over the next few years everything tipped in ACORN's favor.

ACORN's leaders recognized that its prospects depended in part on its ability to fight conservative attempts to demonize ACORN, which had damaged its reputation in the mainstream media. Lewis took the unprecedented step for ACORN of hiring a public relations firm, the Advanced Group, to help ACORN repair and polish its image.

Meanwhile, ACORN's basic structure remained unchanged. Unlike the faith-based organizing networks and other antipoverty groups whose local, decentralized structures stifle their ability to mount national campaigns, ACORN would retain its national structure. It would continue to be run by a national board elected by its state and local chapters. The board members recognized that in order for Lewis to execute decisions, she had to have powers similar to Wade Rathke's, but they insisted, and Lewis agreed, that they be given greater access to budget and other information.

During the first half of 2009, Lewis made headway in wooing back ACORN's major funders by cultivating and educating them about ACORN's new internal reforms. Many of the foundations agreed to maintain or restore funding, but with more scrutiny over ACORN's finances. Not everything went smoothly for Lewis, however. The influential Carnegie Foundation remained skeptical and continued to withhold much-needed funds.

Divisions remained among board members over such issues as how to disentangle the organization from Rathke. The New Orleans chapter, Rathke's stronghold, would stay in ACORN, though their delegates angrily left before the April meeting ended because they felt Rathke was being treated unfairly and feared ACORN might neglect New Orleans and the South. The board replaced Paul Satriano, a close ally of Rathke, as ACORN's treasurer, and he soon ended his ACORN membership.

ACORN's future also depended on how its new leaders would manage the balance between local autonomy and national control, and between the powers of the board and the powers of the staff. ACORN had always had the capacity to move quickly, deftly, and cohesively—at the local and national levels—when organizing opportunities emerged. Could it retain that ability while giving the board more decision-making authority? Could Lewis recruit top-flight minority staff and organizers, as she vowed to do at the April board meeting? Would she be able to entice Madeline Talbott and her breakaway Illinois chapter back into the organization? Would ACORN do a better job retaining staff and training leaders? Would it be able to convince foundations and people who believe in the cause of equality and the empowerment of the poor to support it? Would targeting its recruitment efforts on people of color fortify ACORN or weaken it?

ACORN's decision to expand by recruiting primarily people of color raised serious questions. Although the percentage of white membership in ACORN had declined since the 1970s, Rathke's original vision had played out very successfully. Ultimately, ACORN's continued success would depend, as it always had, on whether individuals joined and acted.

Nearly every organization of ACORN's size and stature experiences growing pains; some adapt successfully, others stay alive but stagnate, while still others wilt. Part of ACORN's success over the years has been its pragmatism, including its ability to learn from mistakes. At the April 2009 board meeting, ACORN appeared to be successfully managing the transition from its founder to a new regime, weaning the organization away from Rathke and putting its leadership in new hands.

Yet the future remained uncertain. Two big threats still needed attention. One was the persistent right-wing and Republican attacks that accelerated during the 2008 presidential election but didn't abate after November. These burnished ACORN's reputation as a feisty and effective advocacy group but also made ACORN a political hot potato that some politicians and funders wanted to keep at arm's length. The other threat came from self-inflicted wounds, which disrupted the entire organization and resulted in the need to fix internal oversight and the management of its local chapters as quickly as possible.

While ACORN was learning how to become more democratic and transparent, and shifting from a staff dominated by progressive white males to one led by an African American woman, its leaders had to endure endless conservative attacks on television and in the printed press. Fox News relentlessly repeated negative stories about ACORN, including claims of voter fraud. In one month, between May 18 and June 18, 2009, Fox ran 362 stories about ACORN. Glenn Beck, host of one of Fox's most popular programs, spent more than one week in May attacking ACORN's founders as people inspired by a "strategy" to transform the United States into a "socialist-Marxist state" and arguing that the Obama stimulus package guaranteed ACORN "billions of dollars to buy more votes for the party that helps them the most." He referred to ACORN as "brownshirts" and the SEIU as "their henchmen," and said that both groups might break kneecaps to get what they wanted.[1]

The New ACORN: Building on the Strengths of the Old ACORN

In the spring of 2009, Lewis received news from a poll conducted by Lake Research that could potentially work in ACORN's favor. The media attention on ACORN had not damaged its reputation among its core constituency, African Americans. Among Lake's random sample of 2,034 registered African American voters in several cities, a solid plurality (44 percent) had a positive opinion of ACORN, only 17 percent had an unfavorable opinion, and 38 percent had never heard of or had no opinion about the organization. Among the latter group, the perception of ACORN actually improved once these voters learned more about the organization. This suggested that ACORN had a good opportunity to expand its reach within the black community.[2]

Lewis planned to use the poll as part of a campaign starting in the fall of 2009 to introduce the public to the new, reformed, and better ACORN. Confident that ACORN could recruit members in America's cities and inner suburbs, she needed to convince the opinion shapers within the media, the foundations, and the political world that ACORN could responsibly carry out its mission as an effective voice for change, as well as make them aware of the group's well-documented reputation.

ACORN consistently won plaudits for its efforts to protect and expand affordable housing. Despite the attacks on ACORN by Karl Rove, even Housing and Urban Development (HUD) officials in the George W. Bush administration viewed ACORN's nonprofit housing programs as among the best in the country. Through a competitive process, it had awarded more than $40 million to ACORN for the development of affordable housing as well as a counseling program that helps people to purchase homes. HUD officials transferred a deteriorating 125-unit apartment complex in the South Bronx to the New York ACORN Housing Company, which restored it to health. In a December 2005 news release praising ACORN for rescuing the apartments, Shaun Donovan, New York City mayor Michael Bloomberg's housing development commissioner (later chosen as Barack Obama's secretary of housing and urban development), observed, "These renovations will transform this once-troubled property into a remarkable asset." For five years Donovan worked closely with ACORN on several initiatives, including a successful effort to save Starrett City, the nation's largest federally supported working-class apartment complex, from being sold to a housing speculator. Even officials in the Republican administration of Mayor Rudy Giuliani grew to respect ACORN during the 1990s.[3]

ACORN had long worked on the forefront to protect homebuyers from unjust foreclosures fueled by reckless lending practices and inadequate government regulation. In many cities and states, ACORN pioneered campaigns to prevent unnecessary foreclosures by organizing homeowners and tenants, and pressuring lawmakers to enact laws protecting consumers from foreclosure scams. By the fall of 2009, ACORN and ACORN Housing had helped prevent foreclosures for eight thousand homeowners by obtaining favorable mortgage changes, and was in the process of helping eighteen thousand more save their homes through a loan-modification process. It rescinded sales, restored titles to owners, and negotiated new, affordable mortgages.

In California, ACORN sponsored a bill to protect consumers from rip-offs by mortgage brokers—for example, by prohibiting brokers from steering borrowers toward loans that are most costly rather than loans they qualify for. ACORN worked for two years to ensure the bill's passage in December 2009, despite the opposition of the powerful bankers and brokers.

Even the Catholic Campaign for Human Development, the antipoverty charity of the United States Conference of Catholic Bishops, which cut off ACORN's funding, had issued a statement in 2008 saying, "Local ACORN groups have done impressive work preventing home foreclosures, creating job opportunities, raising wages, addressing crime and improving education."[4]

A Tsunami

As the summer of 2009 drew near, ACORN completed its political plans for the 2010 midterm congressional elections. Concentrating on key swing states, ACORN's voter registration and turnout could tip elections in close Senate and House races toward candidates concerned about the working poor, which could accrue to the benefit of Democrats. ACORN continued its local work as well as a nationwide effort to support a national health care bill.

Then, in July, before all of ACORN's management reforms had been implemented, and unbeknown to Lewis, two conservative activists, twenty-five-year-old James O'Keefe and twenty-year old Hannah Giles, began visiting ACORN's offices with a hidden video camera. O'Keefe, a graduate of Rutgers University, had gotten a grant as a student from Republican activist Morton Blackwell's Leadership Institute to launch the *Rutgers Centurion*, a conservative magazine. After graduation, O'Keefe spent a year with the Leadership Institute in Virginia, which teaches right-wing activists the art of selling conservatism.[5] Giles was a journalism student and the eldest daughter of Doug Giles, minister of the ultraconservative Clash Church near Miami, who had proclaimed that liberals "spit on the Word of God" and complained of what he called the evils of the Obama administration and its alliance with ACORN.[6]

The two activists despised and feared ACORN. O'Keefe saw it as a group engaged in conflict for its own sake and mistakenly believed that ACORN received "billions" in tax money. "[ACORN's] world is a revolutionary, socialistic, atheistic world, where all means are justifiable," said O'Keefe, on a conservative website. "And they create chaos, again, for its own sake." Searching for a scandal to discredit the organization, O'Keefe and Giles devised a scheme to lure ACORN staff into providing questionable, perhaps even illegal, advice on tax evasion, human smuggling, and child prostitution.[7] Over the summer, visiting several ACORN offices, they hit the jackpot. Giles, claiming she was running from a former pimp, coaxed two ACORN workers from Baltimore into giving outrageous advice, and O'Keefe secretly captured it on videotape. On the advice of Andrew Breitbart, one of their conservative advisors, the two waited for an opportune time to go public.[8]

During the first week of September, Lewis met with her staff to discuss when ACORN should roll out its campaign to introduce the new, improved ACORN. On September 9, an address by President Obama to a joint session of Congress on health care reform was broadcast on primetime television. The next day, a carefully edited version of the Baltimore sting operation appeared on Glenn Beck's show on Fox News.

The tape showed that the naive ACORN staffers fell for the ruse, appearing to sympathize with the prostitute's plight. They advised Giles and O'Keefe on how to hide money from the federal government, misreport their prostitution business on tax forms, and buy a place for a brothel. To further sensationalize the tape, O'Keefe, who had worn a dress shirt and khakis and looked like a student while he was secretly videotaping in the ACORN offices, dressed up in cartoonish pimp garb for the bumpers of the tapes shown on television. The outlandish costume aimed to make ACORN's African American intake staff look like buffoons. When reporting the story, most of the media, including the *New York Times*, would be duped into erroneously reporting or suggesting that O'Keefe did dress in the pimp costume while he met with ACORN's staff.

The Baltimore ACORN employees never created client files or bills, filed tax returns, signed or submitted loan documents, or arranged bank loans. But when similar videotapes aired on Fox over the next several days, showing ACORN staff members in four other offices giving advice to the make-believe prostitute, the *New York Post*, CNN, and other mainstream media picked up on the story.

O'Keefe and Giles targeted ACORN not to expose any bad advice being doled out by ACORN staff, but for the same reason that the political right did: to put an end to its massive voter-registration drives that brought out poor African Americans and Latinos to cast ballots against Republicans. "Politicians are getting elected single-handedly due to this organization," he told the press.[9] O'Keefe and Giles timed the release of the video to distract public attention away from Obama's speech.[10] Fox News showed the ACORN tapes around the clock, stirring up public outrage, mostly among conservatives.

Lewis hoped to contain the damage quickly by dismissing the offending employees and launching an independent internal review and audit of the service programs. She scrambled to defend ACORN on television and radio: "We have all been deeply disturbed by what we've seen in some of these videos. . . . We will go to whatever lengths necessary to reestablish the public trust." But her efforts were to no avail. Republican lawmakers looking to hurt and demonize ACORN demanded that the federal government pull any funding from the organization.

The U.S. Census Bureau dismissed ACORN as one of its eighty nonprofit partners after Republican representative Darrell Issa of California, the ranking GOP member of the House oversight committee, objected that ACORN would destroy the 2010 population count. ACORN had been asked to participate in the census to make sure every poor person and minority was counted and properly represented in the next congressional redistricting. Issa, who had been pounding ACORN for months, took credit for the Census Bureau action, bragging to Fox News. Though ACORN had never committed a crime, in July his office had released a report asking whether ACORN was "intentionally structured as a criminal enterprise."[11] On the heels of the Census Bureau action, the IRS decertified the group from conducting taxpayer-assistance programs, despite ACORN's excellent work helping thousands of the working poor obtain their tax benefits.

On September 14, in a rush to judgment, the U.S. Senate voted to strip federal funding from ACORN, blocking HUD from giving it grants. The next day Republican House leader John Boehner publicly urged Obama to cut off all federal money to ACORN. Saddened and outraged by the behavior of the Baltimore staff, Lewis as well as other ACORN supporters like Kathleen Kennedy Townsend thought they could ride out the criticism from the Republican Right. The former Maryland lieutenant governor said she would support ACORN "because they're under an enormous attack by Fox. . . . But ACORN is critical to the well-being of thousands of people across the United States. . . . We have to make sure we're above suspicion, and that we're going to do the right thing."[12]

But no one from the Obama administration, including Donovan and Obama, uttered a word in ACORN's defense, and on September 16, White House press secretary Robert Gibbs called ACORN's employees' behavior "unacceptable." After that, the witch hunt began. Republicans called for a Justice Department investigation. The House voted 345–75 in favor of Defund ACORN, a bill sponsored by Boehner to ban all federal funding for ACORN. Congress had assumed the truth of the Republican allegations against ACORN without troubling to confirm them or even ask ACORN to present its side of the story.

The accusations against ACORN took a bizarre turn when GOP senator David Vitter, who himself was implicated in a real prostitution scandal and never punished by the Senate, conveyed his outrage. Then, on September 29, the Senate adopted, by a voice vote, an amendment by Republican senator Mike Johanns of Nebraska barring any federal funding from going to ACORN in the defense spending bill.

Only seven senators—six Democrats and one Independent—came to ACORN's defense, notably Democratic senator Richard Durbin of Illinois and Independent senator Bernie Sanders of Vermont. Although New York senator Charles Schumer voted against ACORN, he called Bertha Lewis to say he was still a friend. House member Jerrold Nadler of New York branded the Defund ACORN Act a "bill of attainder" and an unfair, punitive act by Congress. Sanders pointed out that Congress had lavishly funded many corporations that unlike ACORN actually committed felonies.

For example, just two weeks before the Senate action, on September 2, drug company giant Pfizer had been hit with the biggest criminal fine in U.S. history as part of a $2.3 billion settlement with federal prosecutors for illegally promoting medicines and for paying kickbacks to doctors. The company was paying $1 billion in civil settlements for Medicare and Medicaid fraud. Blackwater, a company that had five of its employees facing murder charges in a massacre of Iraqi civilians in 2007, had received a $217 million contract to provide security in Iraq. A former Halliburton subsidiary, KBR, had received $80 million in contract bonuses to provide electrical wiring in Iraq, which electrocuted sixteen soldiers and two contractors. Northrop Grumman had to pay a $500 million fine for getting caught nine times committing contract fraud. The Congress that defunded ACORN had also bailed out Goldman Sachs, AIG, J. P. Morgan, and other financial services corporations that lacked transparency, committed unethical or illegal acts, and engaged in practices that led to the crash of our financial system. The political attacks on ACORN revealed an obvious double standard. How else to explain why some members of Congress insisted on defunding ACORN for its errors but failed to seek the same treatment for chronic corporate lawbreakers that receive billions in federal dollars? The hypocrisy was striking.[13]

Why did so many Democrats abandon ACORN? In the frenzied atmosphere created by the media, Democrats (with some notable exceptions) ran to put as much distance as possible between themselves and the "corrupt" outfit portrayed on television. Most members of Congress represent middle class and upscale constituents who had no firsthand knowledge of ACORN and only knew what they heard in the news.[14] For Obama, defending ACORN would play into the Republican strategy of diverting public attention away from his legislative agenda—fixing the economy, regulating the banking industry, passing health care reform, and addressing climate change.

ACORN was unprepared to deal with the relentless, mostly unfounded daily attacks on its credibility by the right-wing media and conservative politicians, and the mainstream media's general acceptance of the right wing's demonizing of ACORN. With almost all its budget dedicated to organizing, research, and services, ACORN never had much money to invest in public relations. In 2009, its salaries started at $27,000 a year, with an extra $1,000 paid to each chapter's head organizer. Its enemies, which included News Corporation, an international media and entertainment conglomerate that owns Fox Broadcasting Company, Fox Cable Networks, the *Wall Street Journal*, and the *New York Post*, overwhelmed ACORN. Most important, ACORN, a poor people's group, could not contribute millions of dollars to both parties, unlike the defense contractors and other corporations who committed crimes and still got federal contracts. Nor did ACORN have the money to hire high-powered lobbyists. If it did, the Defund ACORN bill would never have passed Congress.

"As soon as they see the Democrats are going to roll over on this, all hell breaks loose," ACORN attorney Arthur Schwartz told the press. "It's like all of a sudden, I'm in the middle of a war." Then he corrected himself: "I wouldn't say it's a war, because that's where both sides are shooting at each other. It's more like a tsunami—and one side keeps firing shots."[15]

Many foundations that had praised and funded ACORN's work in the past, fearful that their grant money would be misused or that the controversy would lead to an attack by the organized right wing, either pulled the plug on ACORN or did not renew grants. The foundations included the Ford Foundation and the Annie E. Casey Foundation. It was a triumphal moment for conservative activists, who for over twenty-five years had fought to eliminate foundation funding for groups like ACORN. James O'Keefe and Hannah Giles's sting operation against ACORN was the latest step toward that goal.[16]

Some of the mainstream press, particularly the *Washington Post*, contributed to the feeding frenzy.[17] A September 20 headline blared, "For ACORN, Video Is Only Latest Crisis," which read like an indictment prepared by the Republican Party.[18] Gathering together every rumor and allegation ever made against ACORN, the *Post* made several factual errors. For example, reporters located the attacks by conservatives as beginning in 2008, when the attacks actually went back some twenty-five years. Like CNN and other members of the so-called liberal press, the *Post* failed to explain this long conservative campaign to smear and vilify the group using any means necessary, including lying and exaggeration.[19]

Only a few reporters, such as Kate Linthicum of the *Los Angeles Times* and Christina Hoag of the Associated Press's Los Angeles bureau, actually followed ACORN staff and leaders into their communities to report on what the organization does on a day-to-day basis. *USA Today* reporters Judy Keen and William M. Welch interviewed Kathy Boons, a sixty-year-old ACORN leader in the Watts section of Los Angeles, about her work fighting foreclosures. The story focused on Tommy and Debora Beard, homeowners in Watts for twenty-four years who nearly lost their home to foreclosure in 2009. After hearing about ACORN's assistance on the radio, they had asked for its help, and ACORN organized an anti-foreclosure rally outside their front door. "We had a lot of doors closed in our face," said Tommy Beard. "Except the door at ACORN."[20]

Among philanthropists, some funders stood by ACORN. The California Endowment approved a new $500,000 grant to ACORN to help low-income families access health care and other benefits. Some helped the organization continue to improve its day-to-day management. "A pattern of accusations does not equal a pattern of bad behavior," said Needmor Foundation executive director Dave Beckwith, at a conference. "Needmor should continue to fund the organizing and leadership development work in local ACORN chapters as long as they are governed by their members, hold to a high standard of financial accountability, and provide an effective voice. As for those making false accusations, all it takes is to say to them, 'Go shove it. You're wrong.'" Needmor funded ACORN with grants of about $150,000 a year.

For the working poor, ACORN's dilemma was a tragedy. With a Democratic Congress and the election of Obama, ACORN's modest operation—run out of well-worn offices, using donated computers and torn furniture, paying low salaries for long hours—should have been flexing its muscles to provide a louder voice for the less powerful. Instead, in this hopeful political moment, a flawed but effective group had its capacity to give voice to the poor compromised.[21]

The Fight Back

By November 2009, ACORN was financially on its knees. In October 2009, ACORN's advisory group had engaged Scott Harshbarger, former Massachusetts attorney general and former president of Common Cause, to investigate the videotape incident and, more important, recommend and implement necessary management reforms. ACORN's laudable action contrasted with the stonewalling that regularly occurs by politicians and in the corporate world. One could hardly imagine Pfizer, Goldman Sachs, or AIG hiring an independent investigator to discover what went wrong. Conservative Republicans kept up the attack, however, and some of ACORN's partners in the business community, such as Bank of America, Citibank, and even SEIU, cut off financial support pending Harshbarger's investigation. ACORN's attorney Arthur Schwartz sought help from experts in bankruptcy and reorganization, as well as assistance with broad subpoenas that had been issued in Louisiana, Texas, California, and Pennsylvania, and New York, many instigated by ACORN's political enemies, such as Democratic attorney general Buddy Caldwell.[22]

But while ACORN had been weakened, the war wasn't over. Thousands of its members nationwide continued to pay dues, some more than $120 a year. In addition, some liberals and progressive had quickly come to ACORN's defense. The influential progressive blogs Talking Points Memo and Daily Kos defended ACORN and condemned the congressional vote. Investigative journalist Brad Friedman (Bradblog) and Media Matters for America, an online research and information center, consistently documented conservative anti-ACORN propaganda. Journalists like Harold Meyerson (*Washington Post*) and Joe Conason (Salon.com) accurately reported the facts, giving the ACORN story perspective. Robert Borosage, of the progressive Campaign for America's Future, time and again reminded the public that ACORN was "an organization that has done remarkable work organizing and empowering the poorest Americans."

In several cities, ACORN's supporters organized small rallies, issued statements, and tried to counter the distortions in the media. In September, for example, sixty people met at the House of Prayer Episcopal Church in Philadelphia. Public officials, labor leaders, organizers, and city residents who worked for or had benefited from ACORN's action attended. Speakers praised the organization and told stories of how ACORN helped keep them in their house and obtain health care benefits.[23]

ACORN filed suit against O'Keefe and Giles for violating Maryland's legal requirement of two-party consent to create sound recordings when they visited ACORN's office in Baltimore. The multimillion-dollar suit sought damages from conservative activists including a columnist who posted the videos on his website. On October 1, a progressive coalition that included the NAACP, Leadership Conference on Civil Rights, Center for Community Change, and Alliance for Justice released a statement supporting ACORN. Ben Jealous, president of the NAACP, stated, "We are deeply troubled by the despicable 'railroading' strategy being employed by anti-democratic zealots to bring down [ACORN] and end their invaluable service to poor and disadvantaged communities." But only one newspaper picked up the story.[24]

On October 23, a coalition of two dozen community organizers, labor leaders, and clergy rallied in Watts in support of ACORN. "It's a witch hunt after a segment of the progressive populations," said Paul Zimmerman, director of the California Association of Non-Profit Housing. "I have McCarthy-era déjà vu." The Rev. Richard Estrada, an associate pastor at Our Lady Queen of the Angels/La Placita church, said that the attacks on ACORN had made other community organizers fear that "one day they may come after us." He continued, "Progressive organizations that are being effective and are working to enable the working poor, the immigrant communities and the gay and lesbian communities are being targeted."[25] In November, progressive filmmaker Robert Greenwald's Brave New Films released an online campaign in support of ACORN.

On November 12, the Center for Constitutional Rights filed a lawsuit challenging Congress's defunding of ACORN, charging Congress with violating the bill of attainder provision in the U.S. Constitution and the Fifth Amendment right to due process, and infringing on the First Amendment right to freedom of association by targeting affiliated and allied organizations. For example, the suit claimed that because of budget cutbacks, an ACORN first-time homebuyer class in New York that enrolled one hundred people in September enrolled only seven people in October, after the congressional action.

"It's a classic trial by the Legislature," Jules Lobel, a lawyer with the Center for Constitutional Rights, told the media. "They have essentially determined the guilt of the organization and any organization affiliated or allied with it." The lawsuit sought to prevent the federal government from reallocating funds designated for the organization and its affiliates and to stop Congress from singling out an organization for punishment without proper investigation or due process.[26]

In December 2009, facts exonerating ACORN began to emerge. On December 7 an independent report by Harshbarger cleared ACORN of any illegal conduct.[27] The report stated, "While some of the advice and counsel given by ACORN employees and volunteers was clearly inappropriate and unprofessional, we did not find a pattern of intentional, illegal conduct by ACORN staff; in fact, there is no evidence that action, illegal or otherwise, was taken by any ACORN employee on behalf of the videographers." His report also noted that the videos were doctored and misleading.

"The videos that have been released appear to have been edited, in some cases substantially, including the insertion of a substitute voiceover for significant portions of Mr. O'Keefe's and Ms. Giles's comments, which makes it difficult to determine the questions to which ACORN employees are responding. A comparison of the publicly available transcripts to the released videos confirms that large portions of the original video have been omitted from the released versions."

Although Harshbarger's thorough examination found no evidence of illegal behavior, it attributed the outrageous ACORN staff behavior caught on tape to "ACORN's longstanding management weaknesses, including a lack of training, a lack of procedures, and a lack of on-site supervision." The report also acknowledged that ACORN had already begun to implement many of the reforms urged by Harshbarger. Further, the report reinforced criticism of the mainstream media's handling of the story, including the way CNN played the "prostitution scandal" videotapes over and over again. As Joe Conason reported, "The ACORN videotapes were an exercise in propaganda not journalism."[28]

The mainstream press continued to botch the ACORN story, however. For example, the Associated Press story of the Harshbarger report published in the *Washington Post* didn't mention that the conservative videographers rebuffed attempts by Harshbarger to interview them and refused to permit him to review the unedited tapes so he could compare the raw footage with versions that were released. Most major news outlets did not even mention the report.[29]

Five days after the report was released, on December 12, 2009, federal judge Nina Gershon blocked U.S. officials from enforcing the funding ban on ACORN.[30] She ruled that Congress had violated the Constitution's ban on bills of attainder, legislation that punishes a specific person or group without a fair hearing. ACORN lawyers quoted several Republicans making unsubstantiated accusations about ACORN being a criminal organization that deserved to be punished.

"[ACORN has] been singled out by Congress for punishment that directly and immediately affects their ability to continue to obtain federal funding, in the absence of any judicial, or even administrative, process of adjudicating guilt," Gershon wrote in her decision. Soon after the decision, some of ACORN's projects began receiving federal funds, including between $40,000 and $60,000 for housing assistance.

This decision and the Harshbarger report, which came on the heels of a successful ACORN lawsuit in Ohio that brought the state into compliance with the National Voter Registration Act, brought some hope to ACORN's members that public opinion might shift in ACORN's favor.

Soon after Harshbarger refuted the charges of financial wrongdoing and voter fraud against ACORN, a nonpartisan Congressional Research Service (CRS) report released on December 22 found no evidence of voter fraud associated with ACORN and "no instances in which ACORN violated the terms of federal funding in the last five years."[31] Moreover, the report found that the two conservative activists who secretly videotaped conversations with ACORN workers and distributed those recordings on the Web without their consent violated laws in Maryland and California. CRS also noted that as of October 2009, ACORN had been subjected to at least forty-six federal, state, and local investigations, with only eleven still outstanding. Only one state, Nevada, brought charges against ACORN, under an ambiguous law that prohibited paying staff to register voters.

Despite the fact that the CRS report was a comprehensive source for fact-checking the allegations aimed at ACORN, the *New York Times* buried the story in a short article on page 15, and *USA Today* noted it in a seven-sentence news brief.[32] CNN took just a few seconds to mention the report, again playing a clip of the infamous undercover video. Most of the major news outlets, including the *Wall Street Journal*, ignored the CRS report.[33] *Time* magazine and *U.S. News and World Report* used their end-of-the-year roundup to spin the ACORN story as a scandal. *Time* put ACORN at number 9 in its top 10 scandals of 2009, while *U.S. News* rated ACORN number 4 in its top 10 political scandals of 2009.[34]

ACORN had been defamed, and the positive news failed to undo the damage. Pablo Eisenberg, veteran foundation consultant and senior fellow at Georgetown Public Policy Institute's Center for Public and Nonprofit Leadership, wondered why more people had not come to ACORN's defense. After criticizing ACORN for its past errors and recognizing the leaders' current efforts to correct them, he added, "But the critics have gone much further than ACORN deserved. In the assault on ACORN, no lies have been spared, no accusations tempered by reason, and no acknowledgment has been made of the enormous good ACORN has done over the years. Behind the attacks are a deep hatred of liberals and progressives—especially those in the Obama administration—and a lack of concern and respect for poor and minority constituencies."[35]

The rush to judgment against ACORN continues to threaten its very existence. By any measure, the barrage of subpoenas, investigations, castigations, and hasty official actions of questionable legality were far out of proportion to ACORN's lapses. The onslaught recalls the voter fraud claims against ACORN in Florida and New Mexico in 2004. Only later, in 2007, did the public learn that all charges against ACORN in 2004 had been dropped and that U.S. attorneys had been fired for resisting White House pressure to prosecute ACORN on trumped-up charges of voter fraud.

Katrina vanden Heuvel, editor of the *Nation*, said that what happened to ACORN was "reminiscent of the McCarthy era when individuals and organizations were ruined by allegations that ran as front page news, while later evidence that vindicated them was relegated to the back pages. There was little accountability for the false accusations, little redemption for those whose lives had been shattered."[36]

The Aftermath

For Bertha Lewis and other ACORN leaders, these setbacks against the war on poverty have called for a retreat, not capitulation. In January 2010 the staff and leaders from ACORN's local and state chapters, including its advisory board, began debating how to respond to the ferocious right-wing assault. Seventeen state chapters decided to establish statewide groups separate from ACORN, including the adoption of a new name, each following the recommendations made by the Harshbarger report, such as installing a series of strict financial and oversight controls. These organizations will not conceal that they have emerged from ACORN, but they will emphasize their "newness" and how they will build on ACORN's strengths.

The new community organizations will have blended boards with prominent outsiders as well as outside advisory committees analogous to the national ACORN Advisory Committee. A new national nonprofit, tax-exempt group, tentatively named the Community Action Support Center (CASC), will be established to provide a range of training, technical assistance, and oversight services to the new community organizations. Brian Kettenring will be the CASC interim executive director.

Lewis plans to set up a Black Leadership Institute to engage in several specific projects and issue campaigns with a priority on mobilizing African American support for immigration reform. Steve Kest decided to leave ACORN but will work with the new community groups in a consulting and voluntary capacity. ACORN, Inc., which will have no ties other than history to the new community organizations, will continue to operate with a small budget under the leadership of Lewis, who in her own words is now the "ACORN Lady." Citizen's Consulting, Inc., the entity that provided back office service to ACORN, will close. The emerging community organizations will retain ACORN's commitment to building national power, and are beginning discussions toward a process to federate at some later date, presumably after the 2010 elections or in 2011.

The new groups will emphasize local and state work. The national staff at the CASC will support the continuation of organizing around jobs and low-wage work, bank lending and foreclosures, immigration, state fiscal crises, civic engagement, and green jobs and environmental justice. Given the critical nature of the 2010 elections, ACORN's leaders are putting together a team to employ voter engagement activities. They plan to engage the surge voters of 2008 and turn them into permanent voters in 2010 and beyond.

On January 13, 2010, California ACORN became the first chapter to go independent, calling itself the Alliance of Californians for Community Empowerment. Amy Schur, the former head organizer for California ACORN, will continue in that role. The new group will have the same mission, will be staffed by many of the same employees who worked for ACORN, and will be funded by most of the same donors.

In a bizarre twist to ACORN's destiny, an incident on January 25, 2010, forced some ACORN critics to reevaluate their opinion of the group as well as question the accuracy of the pimp and prostitute videos. In an action reminiscent of the famous Watergate burglary, James O'Keefe, the fake pimp who videotaped ACORN staff, and three other young men were arrested by the FBI and charged with plotting to tamper with phones in the New Orleans office of Senator Mary Landrieu, Democrat of Louisiana. The men planned to embarrass Landrieu to help defeat her in the next election. If convicted, the four would face sentences ranging from a fine to ten years in prison. The episode led former skeptics (like Jon Stewart from *The Daily Show*) to wonder whether their negative views of ACORN were based on accurate information and whether they had been too quick to accept O'Keefe's videos as reflecting the truth about the group.[37]

If the new state groups stay true to the ACORN mission and organizing principles—integrating electoral politics into organizing; working simultaneously at the neighborhood, municipal, state, and national levels; recruiting dues-paying members of all races, colors, and income at the door; encouraging members to control the organization and participate in decision making; and using a variety of tactics and strategies to help the poor help themselves—they will succeed. But if these groups fail to rebuild a national group, the poor will lose a powerful voice.

Epilogue: A Progressive Social Movement

People concerned about poverty in the United States can ill afford to lose ACORN. Few people recognize how hard it is to build membership-based community organizations among the poor—much less an effective one that has lasted four decades. Randy Shaw points out that hundreds of progressive organizers got their start with ACORN. Like the United Farm Workers, ACORN has been a training ground for several generations of organizers who have gone on to work for progressive social change.[1] According to Shaw, "Although Barack Obama's community organizer background was supposed to galvanize young people into following this path, nearly a year after his election there are fewer entry-level community organizing jobs than before. . . . ACORN cutbacks weaken one of the progressive movement's leading organizer training vehicles."

Because ACORN saw organizing low-income families as its mission, it became an entry point for many young people seeking community organizing careers. ACORN's model of training organizers to raise their own salaries through door-to-door canvassing, foundation grants, and local fund-raisers gave a chance to anyone who sought to become a community organizer. Unlike the labor unions or faith-based networks such as PICO, the IAF, and Gamaliel, which rarely hire those without prior experience, ACORN, as Shaw notes, believed that organizing was so hard and complex that "success could not be easily predicted, hence the need to bring in lots of people to find out which could perform." While this led to enormous turnover, it also meant that anyone with enough drive and talent to get through the initial weeks had a chance to become a skilled community organizer.

ACORN's Roots

ACORN's roots trace back to the early 1960s organization Students for a Democratic Society, and even further back to the populists, the interracial Southern Tenants Farmers Union, as well as Jane Addams and the settlement-house movement.[2] Addams, an upper-class college-educated woman, started the nation's first settlement, Hull House, in Chicago in 1889, and the idea soon spread among reformers in cities across the country. Like ACORN, the settlement-house movement worked outside the political system as part of a progressive movement, empowering the poor through education and participation and supporting organized labor. Addams fought for women's suffrage, lobbied to outlaw child labor, and organized against slumlords, causes considered radical in her day. Like ACORN, she and the settlement-house movement mobilized community residents to support playgrounds, garbage collection, and increased police protection. Like ACORN, they were committed not only to empowering individuals but also to strengthening the fabric of neighborhoods.

Out of all the pioneering tactics and strategies ACORN has brought to community organizing, its defining innovation is turning a local community-organizing group into a national association with dues-paying members and the ability to cause substantial improvements for the poor and powerless—as demonstrated by its campaigns against H&R Block and Household Finance and in support of a livable wage and homesteading.

The Hope of Obama

The decline of the Republican Party and the election of Barack Obama provided a unique opportunity for ACORN to achieve more dramatic goals than at any time in its history. That moment has now passed. Like many successful for-profit and nonprofit organizations, ACORN grew too quickly without putting in place suitable administrative oversight. ACORN's leaders also failed to anticipate the capacity of America's right wing. For ACORN to make a comeback, it will have to correct its management weaknesses, concentrate on building up its local chapters, and fight on local issues, such as park rehabilitation and maintenance, predatory lending, and foreclosure prevention.

Its chance of returning to its former strength will also depend on the slender possibility of a large independent, progressive movement that could support ACORN and push Obama to be the kind of transformative president ACORN's base needs. Only such a movement could impel Obama to significantly alter the nation's political landscape around an agenda that includes an increase in jobs that pay a living wage, quality health care, and opportunities for young minority men and women to succeed. Lincoln had the abolitionists; Teddy Roosevelt, the populists and progressives; Johnson, the civil rights activists; and Reagan, the religious and ideological Right and the gun lobby.

The most obvious parallel to ACORN's situation was that facing the labor movement and other grassroots organizations when President Franklin Roosevelt took office as an economic crisis was engulfing the country. FDR had several social movements pushing him and the country's political culture. Huey Long spearheaded a populist movement against the inequalities of wealth and power that accompanied industrialization. Just prior to Roosevelt's election, the Bonus Marchers, a band of jobless veterans, demanded payment of a bonus Congress had promised them for their service in World War I. Tenant organizers protested evictions. Townsend Clubs, advocating for an old-age insurance program, sprouted across the country, representing between two and five million members. Farmers protested against foreclosures, and the labor movement was on the rise, organizing massive strikes and protests throughout the country and garnering the support of political leaders.

Roosevelt recognized that his ability to push New Deal legislation through Congress depended on the pressure generated by these movements. When union leaders urged him to support pro-labor legislation, he allegedly said, "OK, you've convinced me. Now go out, organize, and make me do it." As these movements grew, Roosevelt used his bully pulpit to promote legislation guaranteeing unions a right to organize workers, Social Security, subsidies to house the poor, and policies that encouraged banks to make affordable mortgage loans to boost homeownership. These policies would never have been enacted but for the organized, often disruptive pressure on Roosevelt and other elected officials.

Roosevelt chose a left-of-center pragmatic approach, and with the help of the labor and other populist movements, he revitalized our democracy, saved capitalism from the capitalists, and transformed the way Americans viewed the role of government. ACORN's policy agenda—increasing voter registration among minorities and the poor, making employers pay living wages, promoting responsible homeownership, ending predatory lending, organizing low-wage workers into unions, pushing for national health care, and expanding the Earned Income Tax Credit—is in the populist and New Deal tradition.

Businesses, Conservative Politicians, and Free-Market Ideologues

The attack on ACORN was not really about bogus names on voter registration forms or staff members providing bad advice to a phony prostitute with a video camera. ACORN has long faced harassment from certain businesses, conservative activists, and intellectuals who attack it for ideological reasons, calling the group "socialist," "left-wing," and "opponents of the free market." Businesses that pay low wages have long opposed ACORN's efforts to raise wages for the working poor. Banks, private mortgage companies, and payday lenders have fought ACORN's campaigns to strengthen government regulations on the financial services industry on behalf of consumers. For years conservative politicians have opposed ACORN's success at registering low-income, mostly minority voters, who they fear are more likely to vote for Democrats than GOP candidates. What most Americans know about ACORN is based on recent controversies manufactured by the group's long-term enemies.

The political motivation for the war on ACORN was obvious in September 2008 at the Republican convention in St. Paul, where former New York mayor Rudy Giuliani, former New York governor George Pataki, and newly minted vice presidential candidate Sarah Palin attacked Obama's experience as a community organizer. A month later, on October 15, 2008, in the third and final presidential debate with Obama, John McCain—reflecting the years of groundwork by conservatives and Republicans in demonizing ACORN—charged that ACORN was "on the verge of maybe perpetrating one of the greatest frauds in voter history in this country, maybe destroying the fabric of democracy." At rallies and press events, McCain and Palin repeated this charge and demanded that Obama disclose his ties with ACORN.[3]

These attacks are part of a broader conservative effort to undermine progressive organizations (including unions, environmental groups, and activist religious organizations) and to discredit Obama and divert attention away from the important legislative efforts that many conservatives don't want to succeed: a health care overhaul, stiffer environmental standards, and tougher regulations for financial institutions. Republicans also hoped that destroying ACORN would improve its chances of winning back Congress in 2010.

Is a Twenty-First Century Social Movement Likely?

At the end of the first decade of the twenty-first century, is a new populist progressive movement possible? The powerful financial services sector, the drug and insurance companies, and the energy industry will oppose any reform that diminishes their power and profits. The acquisitive and greedy oppose cutting taxes for the rich to raise revenue, and most of the business community resists labor-law reform. The Right's echo chamber appears to be more skillful in manipulating the media than does the Left.[4] And moderate Democrats in Congress, especially those from swing states and districts tied to business, are wary of Keynesian spending, social programs, and progressive taxation.

To significantly help the poor, ACORN and other community organizing groups need to be part of a movement that includes labor, environmentalists, liberal faith groups, civil rights organizations, and community groups. New and hopeful signs of a progressive movement exist in the ranks of Internet activists such as the Daily Kos and MoveOn.org, the latter a group that according to the *Washington Post* nearly doubled in size, to more than five million members, during the 2008 presidential campaign.[5] These groups are effective fund-raising and mobilizing vehicles but have not yet inspired in their members the kind of passion a movement requires.

Progressive forces do have wealthy supporters, however, such as George Soros, Herb and Marion Sandler, and other participants in the Democracy Alliance, a funding clearinghouse for progressive groups, as well as dozens of think tanks, lawyers, and media groups.[6] And the Millennial Generation may provide the impetus for a progressive movement. For these under-thirty voters, the November 2008 election was a landslide. They gave Obama 66 percent of the vote. Four years earlier, only 54 percent of this age group supported Democratic candidate John Kerry. The 2008 margin reflected the highest share of the youth vote obtained by any candidate since exit polls began reporting results by age in 1976. These under-thirties will add 4.5 million adults to the voting pool every year.

According to polls the American people appear ready for the progressive ideas supported by ACORN. Although we are historically cynical about the capacity of government to act competently, polls indicate that 64 percent of the public favored expanding public investment even if it meant more deficit spending. According to John Halpin and Ruy Teixeira: "More than two-thirds of Americans rate a 'progressive' approach to politics favorably, a 25-point increase in favorability over the last five years, with gains coming primarily from those who were previously unaware of the term. Sixty-seven percent of the public views the term 'progressive' favorably."[7]

More than two in three Americans agree that "government has a responsibility to provide financial support for the poor, the sick, and the elderly," these authors found, while 15 percent are neutral and another 15 percent disagree. Democrats are almost unanimously supportive, and independents lean strongly toward a progressive position. Even a slim majority of Republicans agree.

Polls also indicate that the public is ready for a change from the era of Ronald Reagan and Margaret Thatcher, when the conservative battle cry was that there is no alternative to the untrammeled and unregulated free market. While conservative elites had long held government regulation as an impediment to economic growth, Halpin and Teixeira found that nearly three in four Americans disagree, believing instead that "government regulations are necessary to keep businesses in check and protect workers and consumers."[8] The public want the government to play a strong role in keeping the market economy under control and working for the benefit of all. More than three-quarters (76 percent) of the public say they support stricter federal regulation of the way financial institutions conduct their business.

According to Teixeira: "Fast-growth segments among women like singles and the college-educated favor progressives over conservatives by large margins. And even as progressives improve their performance among the traditional faithful, the growth of religious diversity—especially rapid increases among the unaffiliated—favors progressives. By the election of 2016, it is likely that the United States will no longer be a majority white Christian nation."[9]

As of December 2009, it is unclear whether populist and progressive forces in the United States have the capacity to mount grassroots campaigns to give President Obama the maneuvering room to be a transformational president like FDR, or ACORN the space to grow back. Grover Norquist, a conservative activist, has confidently predicted that progressive groups will fail. Norquist told the *Washington Post* on June 4, 2009, that the Left was made up of "competing parasites" and had too many "contradictions" to coalesce.[10] Indeed, during the past several decades, the unions have fought the environmentalists; the peace movement has opposed liberals who supported America's pro-Israel policy in the Middle East; and even community-organizing groups like ACORN, Gamaliel, and the IAF have rarely worked together and have often competed for foundation funding.

Liberal writer George Packer observed in the *New Yorker* in November 2008 that earlier movements were independent of any president, whereas Obama's movement didn't exist before his candidacy: "Throughout the campaign, Obama spoke of change coming from the bottom up rather than from the top down, but every time I heard him tell a crowd, 'This has never been about me; it's about you,' he seemed to be saying just the opposite. The Obama movement was born in the meeting between a man and a historical moment; if he had died in the middle of the campaign, that movement would have died with him—proof that, whatever passions it has stirred, it remains something less than a durable social force."[11] It is true that Obama's presidential campaign inspired millions of Americans to participate in politics for the first time, but many of the organizations that played a role in Obama's victory—unions, environmental groups, community organizing groups, women's and gay rights groups, and civil rights groups, as well as "netroots" groups like MoveOn—are civically engaged.

Will the newly mobilized Obama supporters join forces with the existing liberal and progressive organizations to forge a stronger movement for change? While many progressive organizations exist, most have not yet built a coherent vision of social justice or come up with ingenious ways to frame issues, find leaders, and otherwise activate people to engage in contentious lobbying and direct action. While they have been somewhat effective in pressing their issues, their work has not provided the kind of energy, passion, certainty, and unity of earlier social movements, such as those organized by the abolitionists; the auto, mine, and other workers of the 1930s; the Student Nonviolent Coordinating Committee (SNCC), Congress of Racial Equality (CORE), and Southern Christian Leadership Conference (SCLC) and the peace movement in the 1960s; Greenpeace, Friends of the Earth, and the environmentalists in the 1970s; and the Christian Right during the 1980s and 1990s.

Some organizing networks that have so much in common—such as the several Hispanic groups involved in immigration reform, the Center for Community Change, and National Peoples Action, as well as ACORN and PICO—including a concise vision and the desire to encourage civic participation, are beginning to coordinate their activities and develop a sense of common history or purpose. The question ACORN and the other groups face is whether the Obama agenda is, as Packer noted, "a list of issues that have different constituencies rather than a single, overarching struggle for freedom or justice."

Is it possible that Obama can build his own large grassroots organization based on the Internet and state field offices, and in cooperation with existing outside-the-party interest groups turn it into a new progressive political coalition? As of December 2009, it appears he has failed to even effectively mobilize his supporters. Called Organizing for America, Obama's post-election group operates out of the Democratic National Committee and is funded with money from Obama backers. If Obama has a policy initiative he wants to push, or a message he chooses to spread, or a gaffe to swat down, Organizing for America unleashes a message machine like the one Obama used during his presidential run, He has used his huge e-mail list to inform his followers about crucial but controversial issues such as his national health care initiative to generate grassroots pressure on members of Congress.

Obama's strategy has discouraged independent action. Just as his presidential campaign centralized messaging and organizing, and discouraged independent expenditures, 527s, and other outside groups from acting separately, Obama has adopted the same strategy for governing. Designed to go over the heads of powerful lobbyists and corporate interest groups, Organizing for America has also corralled all the outside-the-party groups like the Center for American Progress, SEIU, the Health Care for America Now (HCAN) coalition, and USAction, which have the potential to awaken and stir the base. These groups along with dozens of other liberal activist groups sit around the table each month, usually at the Capital Hilton near the White House, with present and former Obama administration aides to debate policy and plot strategy.[12] As these groups did during the presidential campaign, they publicly stay close to the Obama message, afraid of being left out of the action or undermining Obama's ideas. ACORN was asked not to attend the monthly meetings, but fearing further isolation from Obama it mostly keeps its messages in sync with the administration's. However, Obama won not only because of his campaign strategy, but because Bush lost credibility, McCain chose Palin, and the economy tanked. Everything went Obama's way. He can't count on such a smooth path in the future. According to *Esquire*'s Lisa Taddeo, quoting a well-placed Democratic source, "The outside groups are worried about being bulldozed. The question is, is this shortsighted on behalf of Team Obama?"[13]

The campaign around health care reform revealed an ongoing dilemma for progressive activists—a tension between "outsider" and "insider" strategies. For most of 2009, HCAN, of which ACORN was an important part, worked closely with the Obama administration to develop reform legislation that could pass Congress. Staying too close to the Obama message undermined the outside pressure needed to allow his administration room for maneuver. The right-wing rage displayed at the August town meetings almost derailed Obama's plan. In September, however, the health care reform activists changed tactics and helped turn the tide. On October 23, Peter Dreier reported on the use of traditional community organizing tactics instead of polite lobbying, marketing, and hoping for bipartisan compromise: "HCAN and other reform activists regrouped . . . [and] decided to act more like a grassroots movement and less like an interest group. That meant mobilizing voters, focusing attention on the insurance industry, humanizing the battle by giving insurance company victims an opportunity to tell their stories and using creative tactics to generate media attention. In the past month the grassroots movement has focused on the insurance industry's outrageous profits, abuse of consumers and outsized political influence."[14]

But in November 2009, after the Democrats lost the governor's races in New Jersey and Virginia, states that Obama had carried in 2008, the Organizing for America group appeared to have faltered, leaving a grassroots vacuum. African Americans and young people stayed away from the polls in droves.[15] History appears to indicate that without a movement behind him, Obama won't have the power to overcome the opposition to his bold agenda. By the time FDR started his second term, big business and the right wing opposed him every step of the way. Bipartisanship was waning, as it already has for Obama. With the support of the union and other grassroots movements, which he nurtured during his first term, Roosevelt could count on populist attacks against the rich and powerful to sustain his agenda. FDR's second-term acceptance speech at the 1936 Democratic convention attacked the "economic royalists" and "privileged princes" of "economic dynasties" who had "created a new despotism." In that campaign's final speech, Roosevelt said: "I should like to have it said of my first Administration that in it the forces of selfishness and of lust for power met their match. I should like to have it said of my second Administration that in it these forces met their master." FDR used revolutionary rhetoric to voice "anger and resentment," Jonathan Alter writes in *The Defining Moment*, "without destroying the system."[16]

Will a social movement on behalf of the poor and less powerful emerge over the next few years with the kind of clarity and coherence that empowered earlier ones? A testament to ACORN's model is its ability to continue its on-the-ground, day-to-day work across the country, even while its top staff and leaders have been embroiled in the time-consuming distractions of battling attackers, cultivating funders, and reforming internal operations. ACORN is not just any organization. It is an unlikely one—a membership-based community organization among the poor and working class that has proven that activism can improve the lives of the poor and less powerful. Should a powerful inside-outside social movement emerge, ACORN might survive and its successors in the antipoverty movement might grow because of it, and Obama might become a truly transformative president who revitalizes the economy and makes the United States a more humane and democratic society.

Appendix A

Finding and Developing Leaders

An essential part of community organizing is building leadership. Faith-based community organizing groups, such as the Industrial Areas Foundation (IAF) and Pacific Institute for Community Organization (PICO), recruit leaders through churches and other member institutions. ACORN has resisted this approach. Rather, as Wade Rathke says, they "recruit and build leaders 'on the doors' during the initial neighborhood organizing where we are building chapters." ACORN also recruits leaders as it did after Katrina, when people like Dorothy Stukes reached out to the organization after hearing about it through word of mouth, often to get some assistance with finding housing or filling out their tax forms to quality for cash assistance.

Veteran organizers agree that finding and developing indigenous leaders is a tough task. Mike Miller, the former executive director of the San Francisco–based ORGANIZE Training Center, believes that organizers find leaders by discovery and observation—watching leaders in meetings and while working within the group. Steve Max, a longtime staff person at the Midwest Academy, a training school for organizers, says that developing leaders is like teaching singing, acting, or painting. "You can't create talent where none exists, but you can shape and develop what talent there is."

Activist leaders are ACORN's lifeblood. All ACORN head organizers are responsible for recruiting new members, spotting potential leaders, and nurturing them to take an increasingly active role in the group. ACORN is unlike K Street corporate lobby groups, the conservative and liberal think tanks, and even the various liberal advocacy groups, such as the Children's Defense Fund, the National Abortion Rights Action League, or Handgun Control, Inc., that work from their Washington, D.C., offices. Lawyers, lobbyists, and policy experts staff these groups. They seek to influence the government by relying on the courts, regulatory agencies, and congressional subcommittees, as well as by arousing public opinion through the media. Their "members," if they have any, are rarely involved in grassroots advocacy work, but rather are people who pay dues and, in return, get newsletters and e-mails with legislative alerts. Even those who live in the same city are unconnected; they don't hold local meetings or know each other's names. A few professionals do the lobbying, but they don't have a capacity to mobilize their members or those they speak for. These groups don't provide vehicles for broad collective participation. ACORN's leadership development is far from perfect, and its success depends on the local head organizer and dynamics of each local chapter.

Traits of Good Leaders: What ACORN Looks For

To identify potential leaders, ACORN trains its organizers to look for people with certain qualities and characteristics. People who are the first to volunteer, or who have the loudest voices, or who have the strongest opinions aren't necessarily good ACORN leaders. ACORN also tries to avoid "action junkies"—people who are eager to protest without thinking about strategies and tactics, who lack the patience to try different approaches. ACORN also discourages people whose egos would prevent them from respecting others.

For ACORN, leadership involves many different characteristics and skills. The best leaders express their ideas plainly, take responsibility to mobilize others, and help build the organization. Leaders should like people, make friends easily, work hard, be flexible, criticize others constructively, and take criticism without getting defensive. ACORN expects its leaders to be good listeners. Some leaders are good public speakers. Others are most comfortable and effective running a meeting. Some are good at getting people to attend rallies and protests, but don't want to be on stage in front of a large crowd. Some excel at negotiating with politicians and business people. In practice, that means leaders should talk to friends and neighbors, listen to their opinions, encourage them to join, and persuade people to come to events and activities. They also need to have the courage to take risks. Leaders are expected to vote, go to meetings, and demonstrate. As Wade Rathke says, "We look for people who will work, who can lead and hold a base, and who can look you in the eye and hold their own."

Leaders need a wide range of skills, but few leaders possess every possible skill. In ACORN, there are four types of skills to look for in leaders. Technical skills include conducting research, producing a pamphlet, speaking at a rally, and understanding budgets, how to raise money, and use the media. People skills involve engaging in one-on-one conversations with members, encouraging others to become more active, and helping others feel confident about themselves. Procedural skills consist of chairing meetings, encouraging participation at the meetings, bringing decisions to vote, moving along the agenda of a meeting, and understanding the relationship between leaders and organizers. Judgment and strategy skills include planning public actions, making political decisions, weighing alternatives, developing strategies and tactics, understanding the history of people's struggles as well as the history of ACORN, and understanding what issues the group should engage in and how they should wage campaigns that build the organization, recruit new members, and strengthen its political power. One of the hardest lessons for new leaders to learn is that once they become leaders, they represent the organization. When they speak in public about issues, they are supposed to voice the positions agreed upon by the group, not their personal opinions.

Types of Leadership Positions

ACORN has several levels of leadership. Neighborhood chapters, citywide coalitions of neighborhood groups, and state-level umbrella groups all need leaders. And the national organization needs leaders who have been seasoned by their experiences at these other levels. The key to ACORN's success, and its ability to sustain different types of leaders, is its federated structure—its system of neighborhood chapters, citywide groups, and state umbrella organizations, along with its national organization. This allows ACORN to engage in different issue campaigns at the city, state, and national level simultaneously, keeping its members "in motion" and testing its leaders. Neighborhood chapters elect members to local boards, who in turn send delegates to state affiliates, who in turn elect the national board. Each of these boards approves a budget and financial statement at their regular meetings and helps decide what issues ACORN will focus on and what strategies ACORN will employ to win victories for its members.

Like many organizations, ACORN's members elect its leaders. But these elected leaders are not the only people who local organizers train to take a leadership role in the organization. ACORN calls these non-elected leaders "functional" leaders, people who play a leadership role in the group even though they have not been elected and do not have an official title.

Because most people don't have all the characteristics needed to be a good leader, ACORN believes in collective leadership—meaning that leadership roles should be shared. Ella Baker, an African American organizer who trained and inspired many young civil rights activists in the 1950s and 1960s, developed this concept. Organizers are trained to think of small tasks for shy, quiet members to do. They could take minutes at a meeting, attend an action, or help keep people at meetings focused on the agenda. The next time, they may be ready to do more.

Training

Once ACORN organizers identify people with leadership potential, the organizers work hard to develop that potential. According to ACORN's training materials, leadership is "an acquired, learned skill, not something a person is born with." César Chávez, the founder of the United Farm Workers, said that leaders were trained "on the picket line." ACORN's philosophy is similar. ACORN believes that leaders learn by doing, with the support of the paid organizers, who mentor them with people skills and organizational skills (like running meetings and public speaking).

Although ACORN views its real work as being in the streets and in the neighborhoods, some training also takes place in formal settings. Each summer, ACORN brings many of its leaders to an annual weeklong Leadership School. They also sponsor weekend trainings and preboard trainings.

Managing Internal Conflict

Internal organization conflict is inevitable. For example, on April 22, 1979, the headline of the front page of the *Arkansas Democrat* read, "ACORN Official Barred from

Meeting: Leader Resigns." Chairman William Brookerd of Nevada ACORN resigned his position, charging that "if the leadership at any level insists on pursuing their priorities over staff priorities, they are 'democratically' excised from the leadership." He continued: "I have become greatly disappointed in not having the slogan 'The People Shall Rule' materialize for Nevada." Pearl Ford, another board member, made similar charges: "The tactics sound good at first. They come into a neighborhood and ask if you need stop lights and your trash picked up. The next thing you know they get you involved in storming City Hall and other things that I don't approve of."

Conflict is part of ACORN's lifeblood. But for ACORN, conflict means confrontations with people in power—people they call "targets"—including politicians, government agencies, and corporations. Within the organization, however, the staff works to prevent clashes. When staff have disagreements, they are encouraged to talk them through. When leaders and staff disagree about things, they are encouraged to discuss them at meetings, reach consensus, or, if necessary, bring the disputes to a vote. But as in all organizations, conflict inevitably spills out. People, especially those who are passionate about social issues, tend to disagree. Organizers and leaders are taught that serious differences can be avoided if organizers and leaders make sure that as many members as possible are included in the decisions and directions of the group. Attention to detail and understanding how the ACORN structure and vision should work is necessary to successfully deal with internal conflict. When organizers are trained, they are warned that under no circumstances can conflict be ignored in the hope that it will simply go away. It always gets worse, for lack of attention.

Throughout the years, ACORN has spent more and more time and money on resolving internal conflicts and training and nurturing leadership, but the scandals and internal disputes overwhelmed ACORN's attempts to improve training and supervision.

Turnover of Leaders: The Caveat

Like volunteers in any activist organization, leaders of ACORN, like Stukes, get involved because they are angry. They work hard and tackle issues for months (or years), but at some point, some of them leave. Often they are never heard from again. Is it the organizers' fault, or is it just that some people get fed up wish to return to normalcy?

Some leaders see ACORN as their second family, and never leave. Typically, but not always, the leaders who last the longest in ACORN are gregarious people who have fun organizing and going to meetings. Some leaders get involved to solve particular problems and quit as soon as their local problem, such as restoring or razing an abandoned house, is solved. Some lose touch because they move. Some members engage with ACORN because they just want to help. But they quickly get worn out, feeling that they have made their contribution and that it is time for someone else to take on what some organizers call the "struggle." A struggle it is, both internal and external—the kind that most people can endure for only a short period.

ACORN Rethinks Its Leadership Training

ACORN, unlike many antipoverty groups and faith-based nonprofit organizations, relies heavily on a strong national staff for research, strategic planning, and national campaigns. Sometimes inexperienced organizers take on too many responsibilities. Young organizers are enthusiastic, energetic, and committed to righting wrongs. Rather than patiently train leaders, some neophyte organizers do too much themselves. They violate what IAF organizer Ernie Cortes calls the cardinal rule of organizing: "Never do something for someone that they can do for themselves."

ACORN does not invest in "relationship-building" training—the slow, patient work of one-on-one meetings to build trust and ties between organizers and leaders, and between various levels of leaders within an organization, as much as organizing groups like IAF and PICO based in church membership do.

From 2003 to 2007, as ACORN quickly expanded from chapters in fifty cities to over one hundred, ACORN's ability to recruit and train new staff and leaders fell behind its spectacular growth in members. Its membership of about 160,000 grew to over 300,000 members. ACORN's staff realized it needed an ongoing system of leadership training. ACORN embarked on an ambitious effort to expand and deepen its leadership training. In many cities, ACORN chapters began to hold leadership trainings three or four times a year.

For most of its history, its membership was predominantly black. But for grassroots community organizations, demography is destiny. In recent years, ACORN has increased its focus on immigrant leaders. As ACORN recruited more Latino members (the membership is now almost 40 percent Latino), it added Spanish-language training sessions as a regular component of their training programs.

As community organizing has become increasingly complex, dealing with such problems as education reform, job retention, community reinvestment, predatory lending, slum housing, and regional development, ACORN has also put more emphasis on training its staff and leaders not only about organizing skills but also about policy issues.

Appendix B

Running Voter-Registration Campaigns

Running a large-scale voter registration campaign that reaches poor and minority citizens is a complicated, people-intensive process. It's hard to find volunteers or temporary employees to do the work. When ACORN ramps up its periodic voter registration campaigns it has to hire, retain, and supervise thousands of temporary staff. Every new employee and volunteer requires training and supervision. Disputes inevitably erupt between the new staff and their supervisors over the number of hours worked, getting paid on time, and salaries. Because voter registration is expensive, ACORN needs to raise hundreds of thousands of dollars from donors and foundations. Other difficulties the organization must handle include keeping track of registered voters, cash-flow problems, and computer photocopier glitches.

After recruiting staff at college campuses, low-income housing projects, and unemployment offices, as well as through media ads and Internet sites, the campaign needs to locate unregistered voters. To do this, canvassers go to places where people eat, pay bills, pray, play, and buy clothes. They visit courthouses, hospitals, check-cashing outfits, bus stops, grocery stores, Wal-Marts, and movie lines. To encourage enthusiasm for the difficult work, almost every morning for months, organizers, canvassers, and new trainees will meet for office pep rallies. ACORN needs leaders to inspire and remind recruits of their mission to raise the minimum wage and register poor people and minorities.

For the 2004 election, ACORN was determined to hire thousands of staff and register over 1 million voters. ACORN knew that using thousands of volunteers and temporary workers in its drive had the potential for mistakes and duplication in the registration process. This is one of the consequences of essentially "outsourcing" voter registration to the private sector rather than placing the burden of registration on the government as is done in most democracies. If voter registration were mandatory like paying taxes, voter registration drives would not be necessary.

To avoid any hint of fraud, ACORN instituted Project Vote's quality control procedures to make sure that all voter registration cards were handled properly. ACORN's organizers knew foul-ups would occur, but ACORN's procedures minimized any fraud and ensured that the organization flagged these problems itself before delivering completed cards to elections officials. Using experienced staff from Project Vote, ACORN provided training and support for staff and volunteers. It paid its employees by the hour. Most supervisors checked the quality of the voter registration work to catch and correct any problems. As registration cards flowed into local offices en masse, staff visually reviewed them to identify oddities such as signatures that looked like they were written by the same person or just taken from a phone book. At the end of each day, most quality control teams took a random selection of at least 20 percent of collected registrations and called them to confirm that he or she had met a person from ACORN that day and filled out a registration card. (By the time of its 2008 drive, ACORN and Project Vote had increased quality control staffing and called nearly all registrants—making at least three attempts to reach the person listed on each of the more than one million cards collected before turning them in.)

In the course of ACORN's voter registration drives, Brian Mellor, an ACORN attorney who worked on voter registration oversight, liaised with Board of Elections officials to review the quality of its work, and to establish a cooperative relationship. When Mellor turned in registration cards, he agreed to flag incomplete or potentially invalid cards for follow-up by the Board of Elections. Ironically, ACORN's opponents would use the results of ACORN's careful quality control program to attack the organization's work. Despite the fact that most of the time the process worked smoothly, the complexity of the voter registration process always leads to many difficulties. Supervisors, however, emphasized that ACORN had a zero-tolerance policy against fraud. Suspected violators were terminated.

Acknowledgments

During the years I worked on this book, many people helped me. While I was a Revson Fellow at Columbia University in 2004, I took Sam Freedman's book writing course in the journalism school. Freedman, an inspiring teacher, taught me a great deal about narrative nonfiction, some of which may have seeped into this book. When I test-drove some chapters in his class, he took unruly drafts and guided me toward a coherent narrative. For several months at Columbia, weekly conversations with Herbert Gans enlightened my thinking about how to analyze an organization.

John Paine reduced an encyclopedic first draft and made it more readable, especially by removing unnecessary adverbs and needless rhetorical flourishes. Special thanks to writers, friends, and journalists Eric Levin, Alyssa Katz, Christina Baker-Kline, Kevin Pyle, Janice Fine, and Joe Fine, who commented on various chapters. I am very grateful to Bill Lee, who critiqued chapters and was generous with his time.

To produce an accurate portrait of ACORN, many people gave me useful information, including scores of community organizers; former and present ACORN staff, leaders, and members; and accountants, consultants, and lawyers who provided services and advice to ACORN. Dozens are mentioned in the notes for each chapter, and others include Sunday Alabi, Heather Appel, Kate Atkins, Steve Bachman, Tanisha Brady-Christie, Matt Brennan, Alison Brim, Fred Brooks, Valarie Coffin, Joe Cox, Clair Crawford, Tom Dawes, Aaron Dorfman, Darrel Durham, Judith Freeman, Andrea Gabbidon-Leven, Malhotra Garima, Karyn Gillette, Lewis Goldberg, Becky Gomer, James Gray, Rebekah Green, Brennan Griffin, Gia Hamilton, Chester Hartman, Richard Hayes, Kedra Hills, Marie Hurt, Charles Jackson, John R. Jones, Jeff Karlson, Stuart Katzenberg, Omer Khwaja, Austin King, Beth Kingsley, Mitch Klein, Scott Klinger, Peter Kuhns, Scott Levenson, Stephanie Luce, Rachel Mann, Jilnar Mansour, Warren J. Matthew, Pat McCoy, Michael McDunnah, Tim McFeeley, Sonja Merchant-Jones, Sonya Murphy, Jeff Ordower, Tamecka Pierce, Cate Poe, Miles Rapoport, Mary Rickard, Craig Robbins, Tom Santilli, Arthur Schwartz, Ed Schwartz, Ralph Scott, Neil Sealy, Christina Spach, Nadya Stevens, Josh Stuart, Ann Sullivan, Amanda Thorson, Andrew Weltchek, Liz Wolfe, and Gerard M. Zack. Thanks also to Kevin Whelan and Nathan Henderson-James, who always made themselves available.

I want to thank all the wonderful past and present staff and board members at Citizen Action and the New Jersey Tenant Organization, who informed my notions of civic engagement and whose organizing talents have made New Jersey a better place to live. Thanks also to the past and present staff, especially Harold Simon, and board members at the National Housing Institute, the publisher of *Shelterforce*, for their ideas and assistance. I have been involved with NHI since 1976. This book is part of an NHI project to better understand how we can reduce poverty, create affordable housing, and sustain thriving communities.

I feel a special debt to Dave Beckwith, Heidi Swarts, and Robert Fisher. Each read the entire book and made useful comments. A special thanks goes to my friend Cris Doby for her support and belief in the project. Thanks also goes to John Judis, one of the most perceptive political observers in America, who read parts of the book and always gave me unexpected, insightful ideas. Thanks to my young-at-heart and indefatigable literary agent Frances Goldin and her colleagues Ellen Geiger and Sam Stoloff. I am grateful to all those who work at Vanderbilt University Press, particularly director Michael Ames, managing editor Jessie Hunnicutt, and Sue Havlish, Bobbe Needham, and Dariel Mayer.

I could not have written this book without the serious and humorous conversations I had with my crony Neil Mullin. After telling him I was writing about a group called ACORN, he said, "That's crazy, I've never heard of them. Who's going to read a book about an obscure organization?" For the next four years he read many chapters, radiated enthusiasm, made numerous thoughtful comments and useful edits, and instilled faith in me that I could complete the book.

Through years of collaborative work writing articles and working at the National Housing Institute, I have learned immensely from my good friend Peter Dreier, who spent many hours nurturing the manuscript and made numerous useful suggestions. I could not have begun or finished the book without his ideas, inspiration, and support. He was a virtual co-author.

My brother Ron offered me sharp and wise advice all his life, and he continued to influence me even after his untimely death. The love and patience of my family is essential to everything I do. I am lucky to have two great children, Reuben and Becky Atlas, whose intelligence and curiosity expand my world, allowing me to understand it better. My children and I also share the agony and ecstasy of being New York Giants fans. Bonnie Friedman, my wife, anchor, and best friend, took many of the photographs that appear in the book, tracked down others, read many drafts, and made countless helpful comments and corrections. Her movie *The Flashettes* is the best community organizing film ever made. We have been married for thirty-one years, and this book like everything I have accomplished since we met is due to her love and encouragement.

Notes

Preface

1. I collaborated with the Working Group on Human Needs and Faith-Based Community Initiatives, and the Council on Civil Society, which identified ways to recover community, character, and public morality in the United States. See Council on Civil Society and the Institute for American Values, "A Call to Civil Society: Why Democracy Needs Moral Truths," May 27, 1998, *www.americanvalues.org/html/r-call_to_civil_society.html*; Working Group on Human Needs and Faith-Based Community Initiatives, *Harnessing Civic and Faith-Based Power to Fight Poverty* (Washington, DC: Search for Common Ground, 2003).

Introduction

1. Elizabeth MacBride, "A Believer Fights the Good Fight," Crain's New York Business, 2007, *mycrains.crainsnewyork.com/100women/view/64*; "The Influentials: Politics," *New York* magazine, May 8, 2006, *nymag.com/news/features/influentials/16927/index1.html*.
2. Jess Henig, "ACORN Accusations: McCain Makes Exaggerated Claims of 'Voter Fraud': Obama Soft-Pedals His Connections," *Newsweek*, October 18, 2008, *www.newsweek.com/id/164722*.
3. Fred Brooks, Robert Fisher, and Daniel Russell, "ACORN's Accelerated Income Redistribution Project: A Program Evaluation," *Research on Social Work Practice*, 2006. In author's possession. The researchers looked at New Orleans, San Antonio, and Miami, where ACORN was piloting its tax service model. The data was from the IRS reports of electronically filed tax returns.
4. Lisa Ranghelli, "The Monetary Impact of ACORN Campaigns: A Ten-Year Retrospective, 1995–2000," November 2006, *www.acorn.org/fileadmin/ACORN_Reports/2007/ACORN_Wins_Report.pdf*.
5. Sol Stern, "ACORN's Nutty Regime for Cities," *City Journal*, Spring 2003, *www.cityjournal.org/html/13_2_acorns_nutty_regime.html*.
6. Lara Jakes Jordan, "Officials: FBI Investigates ACORN for Voter Fraud," Associated Press, October 16, 2008, *abcnews.go.com/Politics/wireStory?id=6049549*.
7. Susan Jones, "De-Fund ACORN, Republican Leader Insists," CNS News, October 10, 2008, *www.cnsnews.com/public/content/article.aspx?RsrcID=37232*.
8. "Re-Seeding the Housing Mess," *Wall Street Journal*, September 27, 2008, *online.wsj.com/article/SB122247015469280723.html*; "Obama and ACORN: Community Organizers, Phony Voters, and Your Tax Dollars," *Wall Street Journal*, October 14, 2008, *online.wsj.com/article/SB122394051071230749.html*.
9. Stanley Kurtz, "Obama's Radical-Left Ties Broad and Deep," National Review On Line, June 2, 2008, *www.cbsnews.com/stories/2008/06/02/opinion/main4145761.shtml*.
10. "Report: Conservative Media Consistently Scapegoat Undocumented Immigrants, ACORN," Media Matters for America, April 7, 2009, *mediamatters.org/reports/200904070005*.

11. "CNN Reports Leave Out Relevant Facts on ACORN Voter Registration Allegations," Media Matters for America, October 16, 2008, *mediamatters.org/research/200810160020.*
12. Barack Obama, *Dreams from My Father* (New York: Three Rivers Press, 1994).
13. Alec MacGillis, "Obama Seeks to Transfer Campaign's Spirit to Challenges Ahead," *Washington Post*, January 21, 2009, *www.washingtonpost.com/wp-dyn/content/article/2009/01/20/AR2009012004083.html.* See also Peter Dreier, "The History of Hope," *Nation*, February 19, 2008, *www.thenation.com/doc/20080303/dreier.*
14. Ibid.

Chapter 1
Wade Rathke and the Roots of ACORN

Some of the information for this chapter comes from my in-person and telephone interviews, as well as e-mail exchanges with Wade Rathke, numerous ACORN staff, Rathke's friends and acquaintances, ACORN staffer Carolyn Carr, Daniel Russell, Ken Wade, and Maya Wiley. I spent dozens of hours following Rathke while he worked, hanging out drinking coffee, talking on the phone, and exchanging e-mails. The chapter is also based on information from *ACORN News* and memos from Rathke to the ACORN staff.

1. At this meeting, Bernadine Dohrn, a law student who would soon lead the Weatherman faction of SDS, instantly dominated everyone's attention and led the debate against a coterie of students from the Progressive Labor Party, a rigid, militant, sectarian group. The Progressive Labor faction rejected the sexual and drug excesses of the countercultural movements in favor of a Marxist-Leninist popular front movement similar to the pre-1950 Communist USA strategies.
2. Rathke wanted the energy and enthusiasm of some antiwar activists to transfer to the welfare rights movement. His vision was informed by Martin Luther King's 1967 Riverside Church speech that linked the money spent in Vietnam to the shortage of funds to rebuild U.S. cities—a speech that made a big difference in making this connection.
3. Interview with Wade Rathke. See also Nick A. Kotz and Mary L. Kotz, *Passion for Equality: George Wiley and the Movement* (New York: W. W. Norton, 1977).
4. Pastreich's strategy refined the methods of Alinsky, who would start organizing by getting the support of a priest or pastor who could mobilize his congregation. Pastreich's hero was Fred Ross, an Alinsky protégée; the farmworkers César Chávez organized around individual membership was his model. Welfare recipients would not rely on a church or a labor union but would form their own chapters and cohere through the excitement of picketing and sit-ins and the immediate gratification from the increases in welfare money. How NWRO would last over time was never clear.
5. One of NWRO's many influences on ACORN's culture was the expectation that an organizer's work was a mission, a job description that worked well with a young, mobile, white middle-class staff, less well with organizers drawn from ACORN's neighborhoods. ACORN's organizational culture would confront this difference when it greatly increased its hiring of organizers of color.
6. Coincidently or perhaps prophetically, the city had been the wellspring of one of America's earliest community-organizing efforts. In the 1780s, the Springfield area suffered from bad harvests, economic depression, and high taxes. Daniel Shays, a former captain in the Continental army, organized hundreds of farmers unable to pay their mortgages and loans to stop state and local courts from seizing their lands and furniture. Shays witnessed a sick woman unable to pay her debts have her bed taken from under her. He organized parades and demonstrations that closed down courthouses and stopped foreclosures, frightening the country's early political leaders, who crushed the movement within two years. Wade Rathke, aware of Shays' Rebellion, appeared in Springfield 184 years later to try to organize an uprising of the urban poor, with better results.

7. When Rathke decided a high school policy that prohibited partisan political debates was folly, he facilitated a debate on the presidential election and was called down to the principal's office. "You should have known better," the principal said, and then suspended him. In a civics class in Rathke's junior year, his teacher talked about the role of elections, then asked him what he thought. Rathke responded, "That was the most asinine opinion I ever heard." He was suspended again.
8. The story of this event is based on interviews with some of the participants, as well as on accounts in the *Springfield Daily News*. I thank Professor Daniel M. Russell, who teaches at Springfield Community College where the events took place, for giving me copies of the articles.
9. Madeleine Adamson and Seth Borgos, *This Mighty Dream* (New York: Routledge, 1984).

Chapter 2
Stepping onto a Larger Stage

Some of the information for this chapter comes from my in-person and telephone interviews and e-mail exchanges with Wade Rathke, Gary Delgado, Carolyn Carr, and Mary Lassen.

1. From the 1930s through the early 1960s, although Alinsky's local community organizing work was successful, it was marginal to American's New Deal "social contract." The New Deal coalition was primarily urban political machines, organized labor, immigrants and their children, African Americans, white southern small farmers, middle-class reformers (i.e., planners, intellectuals, journalists, social workers), and liberals within the business community. The New Deal adopted Social Security, the minimum wage, the right to unionize, government-subsidized housing for the working class, the TVA, and other progressive policies. It wasn't until the mid-1960s Great Society era that Alinsky-style community organizing around urban renewal, job training, and other antipoverty issues began to play an important part in the liberal-progressive coalition; Alinsky helped lay the groundwork for the emergence of black power in the cities.
2. In the 1970s, New Leftists such as Todd Gitlin and the populist Christopher Lasch criticized Alinsky for espousing no ideology. Alinsky celebrated citizen participation based on self-interest as an end in itself. "Having exalted process over objectives, [Alinsky] was free to define 'participation' itself as the objective of community organization—of politics in general," wrote Lasch in the *New York Review of Books*. Alinsky's ideology was akin to interest-group liberalism, Lasch argued, in which "self-interest" guides everything—as if principles were irrelevant. See Lasch, "Can the Left Rise Again?" *New York Review of Books*, October 21, 1971. In the 1980s, Alinsky's Industrial Areas Foundation would evolve into an organizing network that emphasized community values and the importance of moving beyond protest to the rebuilding of human relationships. The IAF groups gained strong support in Christian churches; because the churches' spiritual traditions, rich in symbolism and meaning, fed motivation and solidarity, the connection helped the groups form powerful networks.
3. In Alinsky's view, only by "rubbing raw the sores of discontent" could one inspire a depressed community to act on its own behalf. In 1964 when Chicago's mayor Richard Daley started to back out of a commitment he made to the Woodlawn group, the members threatened to ridicule him by tying up all the bathrooms at Chicago's O'Hare Airport. The first "shit in," Alinsky called it.
4. Ross also differed with Alinsky regarding the building of statewide and national groups to lobby for the interests of neighborhood people. Alinsky feared the budding "fascism" of large organizations and sought to build only local organizations. His successful efforts at creating local groups in Chicago, Buffalo, and Providence lacked the long-term potential for making the kind of social change that would shift the country's priorities enough to significantly reduce poverty.
5. At another session with the governor, in the middle of an argument over furniture for the poor, Rathke nodded at Rockefeller's monogrammed cowboy boots and commented,

"Since we have the same initials, maybe we should trade boots." Rockefeller wasn't amused.

6. *Houston Post* quoted in Gary Delgado, *Organizing the Movement: The Roots and Growth of ACORN* (Philadelphia: Temple University Press, 1986).
7. Hampton quoted in ibid.

Chapter 3
ACORN's Model T

This chapter is partly based on my in-person or telephone interviews or e-mail exchanges, and sometime all three, with present and former ACORN staffers John Beam, Carolyn Carr, Allison Conyers, Steve Kest, Wade Rathke, and Mike Shea. It also draws from Gary Delgado, *Organizing the Movement: The Roots and Growth of ACORN* (Philadelphia: Temple University Press, 1986), the *ACORN News*, memos from Wade Rathke to the ACORN staff, and the ACORN Archives. The chapter partly relies on articles published in the *Harvard Crimson* between November 7, 1973, and June 13, 1974.

1. Quotes are from Delgado, *Organizing the Movement*, 95.
2. I use the term "ACORN's assembly line" for ACORN's model because, while it has served the group well, in its quest for efficiency the model left some former staff and leaders feeling like interchangeable parts; one disillusioned organizer complained, "ACORN basically uses people as fodder." I and other researchers have found former organizers who criticized workshops at the annual year-end staff meeting for sometimes engaging in ruthless criticism and encouraging cookie-cutter thinking that appeared to ignore local conditions. ACORN's culture of confrontation, used thoughtlessly, can encourage oppositional tactics when a local chapter could have accomplished its goals by cooperation. Improperly applied, the model sometimes neglected to incorporate cooperation, which can be just as empowering as confrontation and less likely to alienate possible allies (for a recent example of the problem, see Jason Pulliam, "Pioneer Park Group Severs ACORN Ties, New Association Cites Aggressive Tone toward Police," *Des Moines Register*, May 24, 2007). An assembly line can also sacrifice the individual attention to leadership development that is typical of the faith-based organizing models, such as the Industrial Areas Foundation. In some local chapters, inexperienced organizers in ACORN ignored the local political context. On balance, however, the deficits of the assembly-line model counted less than its benefit to a national organization that depends on hiring numerous organizers, namely, replicability—it is a model that is easy to teach.
3. *Christian Science Monitor*, November 11, 1978, ACORN archives.
4. Delgado, *Organizing the Movement*, 58.
5. In 1973, the staff salaries seemed sufficient. Organizers for ACORN were paid a living wage (although many ex-organizers would say it was barely that). The low pay was partly due to lack of funds, and partly because Rathke looked for smart, confident but humble organizers accountable to the people they organized. It was also due to Rathke's commitment to expansion, a strategy some head organizers believed caused too much turnover and undermined ACORN's depth and the quality of the work. Several organizers could afford to work for ACORN only because their parents subsidized them.
6. Saul Alinsky, *Rules for Radicals* (New York: Random House, 1975). As a local organizer in Mountain Pine, Arkansas, Steve Holt, another Harvard graduate, chose the chapter's first two issues via the Alinsky art of manipulation. When it was time for the group to elect officers, he made sure that the person he thought was the best leader was elected chair. He was more concerned that the group had good leadership at the start than whether he had manipulated the result.

Chapter 4
The Innovation of Electoral Politics

This chapter relies heavily on Gary Delgado, *Organizing the Movement: The Roots and Growth of ACORN* (Philadelphia: Temple University Press, 1986) and my in-person interviews and e-mails with Wade Rathke, Carolyn Carr, Allison Conyers, John Beam, Zach Polett, and Daniel L. Russell.

1. See Delgado, *Organizing the Movement*, 98; and *www.acorn.org/index.php?id=12447.*
2. Secrecy was a problem with a few of ACORN's members. Bill Brookerd, former chair of Nevada ACORN, complained that in spite of his responsibilities he did not have sufficient financial numbers or the playbook for the group's organizing strategies. Similarly, an Arkansas alderman and former ACORN member fought with the staff to obtain access to membership lists and dues receipts. Both felt manipulated by ACORN's white, college-educated staff members, who they believed tended to dominate decision making.
3. Speculating about the future, Rathke wrote in an ACORN Training Handbook: "The leadership and membership of ACORN dream of the day when ACORN might elect someone to the mayor's chair, the governor's seat, and the White House. They also dream of the day when ACORN members might break the income and other barriers and find themselves in those offices. At this point it seems less important which dream will prevail, because the dream itself is a powerful one, though still years from reality, if it will ever be achieved." Wade Rathke, "ACORN Update: More of a Movement, More of a People's Machine," in Institute for Social Justice, *ACORN Community Organizing Handbook #2* (Little Rock, Ark.: Institute for Social Justice, 1977).
4. Rathke and Falwell both believed they were building a new majority coalition. Among groups that organized the poor, Rathke pioneered the idea of a "majority constituency," meaning all the low- and moderate-income "people who are shut out of power." ACORN's issues were bread-and-butter economic ones; Falwell's were prohibiting abortion, homosexuality, and pornography and pushing for more generous federal grants to parochial and Christian schools. Rathke was the first antipoverty organizer to mix politics and community organizing; Falwell popularized the mixing of religion and politics on the right. In the mid-'70s, Falwell's strategy had much more influence than Rathke's. During Bill Clinton's first statewide campaign for attorney general in Arkansas, he recounts in his autobiography, he lost votes because of the influence of Falwell's Moral Majority. Bill Clinton, *My Life* (New York: Knopf, 2004), 239.
5. Falwell also used this strategy. With the help of conservative political activists, Falwell mastered the complexities of campaign techniques. He used these techniques plus the liberalized financing rules to help create a powerful, independent grassroots force. In 1980, he would claim credit for electing President Ronald Reagan.
6. Fear of red-baiting had a long history in community organizing. To fortify his bonds with the Catholic Church and certain labor unions *and* to insulate his groups from any identification with the Communist Party, Saul Alinsky avoided "ideology." I suspect many leaders of community-organizing groups followed his example by claiming they were promoting "democracy" or "fairness" rather than a broader ideological perspective, for fear of being branded "red."
7. Delgado, *Organizing the Movement.*
8. With great enthusiasm, after the 20/80 memo Rathke wrote another one to the staff in 1976 predicting that "ACORN will expand and organize in more cities and towns . . . perhaps leading to governmental takeovers similar to the Quorum Court. . . . Perhaps ACORN would even up the ante at other levels of government, leading the organization even further past the bounds of what one would normally expect of a community organization." The statement was misleading: the Quorum Court victory was far from a government takeover. ACORN didn't control any government entity anywhere in sight. It would be a mistake, however, to write off the memo as deliberately misleading or naive; it demonstrated Rathke's boldness, his dreams, and his attempts to inspire his staff.

Opposition forces on the Left included neoliberalism, identity politics, the "rights" revolution, and the liberal civic and public interest organizations that operated outside the Democratic Party but inside the Washington, D.C., beltway.

9. Nelson Lichtenstein, *The Most Dangerous Man in Detroit: Walter Reuther and the Fate of American Labor* (Urbana: University of Illinois Press, 1995). Reuther argued that a full employment program would dramatically address the nation's poverty population, create job opportunities for blacks, and rebuild the nation's troubled cities without being as politically divisive as a federal program identified primarily as serving poor blacks. Had Reuther's ideas been adopted, they might have paved the way for Rathke's class-based organizing.
10. For example, even at the peak of the War on Poverty, welfare benefit levels (including food-stamp benefits) never brought families to the official poverty threshold. Medicaid, which began in 1965, was a means-tested health insurance entitlement for the poor. Further, both welfare and Medicaid benefits varied by state. Housing subsidies, not an entitlement at all, would never reach more than one-third of the families eligible for them.
11. Some date the beginning of this offensive to an early 1970s confidential memo to U.S. business leaders from Lewis F. Powell, a leader of the American Bar Association and a future Supreme Court justice. See for example, Bill Bradley, "A Party Inverted," *New York Times*, March 30, 2005. Powerful liberals threatened America's future, Powell warned: "Survival of what we call the free enterprise system [lies in] careful long-range planning and implementation, in consistency of action over an indefinite period of years, in the scale of financing available only through joint effort, and in the political power available only though united action and national organizations." Lewis F. Powell Jr., "Attack of American Free Enterprise System," Confidential Memorandum to the United States Chamber of Commerce, August 23, 1971.
12. One organizer spent days getting suggestions from his members so they could have a say in the platform. He asked questions such as: "Should a percentage of all people who sit on governmental regulatory boards be low income? How should they be chosen?" But he also complained: "This platform stuff is a waste of time. It takes away from my time on the streets, and it won't do a goddamn thing to move the Democrats in this state."
13. Delgado, *Organizing the Movement*. Reflecting the growing number of leftists following ACORN's progress, Delgado thought ACORN should adopt something closer to a socialist ideology.
14. On deindustrialization, see Michael B. Katz, *The Undeserving Poor: From the War on Poverty to the War on Welfare* (New York: Pantheon, 1989).

Chapter 5
Organizing a Union in the 'Hood

This chapter draws on Victor Livingston, "Whose Renaissance?" *Detroit News Magazine*, July 27, 1980, 12; and Keith Kelleher, "From ACORN to ULU to SEIU: Building a Homecare Workers' Movement in the New Economy; The Illinois Model/Experience, 1983–2003," as well as my in-person interviews and e-mail exchanges with Danny Cantor, Keith Kelleher, Madeline Talbott, and Wade Rathke.

1. Wyndham Mortimer, *Organize! My Life as a Union Man* (Boston: Beacon Press, 1971). Two books by the preeminent labor historian Irving Bernstein, *The Lean Years: A History of the American Worker, 1920–1933* (Baltimore: Penguin Books, 1972) and *The Turbulent Years: A History of the American Worker, 1933–1941* (Boston: Houghton-Mifflin, 1970) also influenced Rathke. Bernstein's books showed how New Deal labor policy empowered workers and helped build unions, and how unions helped preserve democracy and capitalism at a time—before and after World War II—when the survival of both was tenuous.
2. Rathke thought funding union organizing would appeal to liberal foundations, one of whose criteria for funding nonprofits was that they frequently initiate new programs. But

he could raise only a small amount of money from a welfare rights spin-off run by Burt DeLeeuw. Any new organizing would have to depend on dues.

3. Like her mother, Madeline was independent and feisty. In high school, she joined in antiwar events with her friends, even though her father was serving in Vietnam. In her senior year of high school, 1968, she read Betty Friedan's *Feminine Mystique* and continued to be active with her teen social action group. While she did not consider herself a leftist or a radical, events during the winter and spring of 1968 began to shape her worldview. She received an acceptance letter from Radcliffe College about the time Martin Luther King was assassinated. She was aware of the militants who paralyzed France with a general strike and nearly toppled the government of Charles de Gaulle. In the United States, Robert F. Kennedy was assassinated the same day Madeline gave her senior class valedictory speech. Madeline's older brother filed a conscientious objector petition with the draft board and then traveled to Chicago to protest the war at the 1968 Democratic National Convention. Madeline watched in horror and then anger as TV coverage of the convention showed protesters clashing with police in the streets of Chicago and was relieved when her brother escaped unscathed.
4. Another experience that influenced Talbott, she said, was attending "a speech by a well-known doctor who had a clinic in the inner city of Boston. It cared for children who were victims of lead poisoning that caused brain damage, hyperactivity, slow growth, hearing problems, and even death. I remember him saying that after he had treated these kids, they'd get sick again. They would return to their apartments, where the children would eat the sweet smelling, peeling, lead paint, and inhale lead infused dust particles." The frustration and hopelessness of the doctor's task reminded her of the Sisyphus myth.
5. Victor Livingston, "Whose Renaissance?" *Detroit News Magazine*, July 27, 1980.
6. The *Detroit Free Press* reported the fight to unionize as a face-off between "a neophyte union led by four young men who have backgrounds in community organization, a large amount of enthusiasm and drive, staffed by a growing population of workers who can't find much good to say about their employers." "Having It Their Way: Fast Food Union Wins Burger King Vote," *Detroit Free Press*, March 16, 1980.
7. A ten-year-old ACORN organizing manual, based on Rathke's experience, that instructed organizers in the South to mobilize white neighborhoods before recruiting black people was passed out at the meeting. When questioned by the press, Talbott said the manual has been revised.
8. Ira Katznelson, *City Trenches: Urban Politics and the Patterning of Class in the United States* (New York: Pantheon Books, 1981).
9. Madeleine Adamson and Seth Borgos, *This Mighty Dream* (New York: Routledge, 1984).

Chapter 6
Partnering with the Enemy

Some of the information in this chapter comes from my in-person and telephone interviews and e-mail exchanges with Wade Rathke; former ACORN staffers Madeline Adamson and Mary Lassen; ACORN Housing staffers Bruce Dorpalen, Michael Shea, and Marty Shaloo; ACORN president Maude Hurd; and Peter Dreier.

1. In May 1976, Missouri ACORN became affiliated with the Missouri Tax Reform Group, the organization responsible for coordinating the statewide initiative petition. ACORN had long been involved in tax reform, an issue in states where ACORN organized along with health care, insurance redlining, mortgage redlining, utility rate increases, and the allocation of Community Block Grant funds. For example, one of its statewide campaigns in Arkansas addressed the tax on intangible property—stocks and bonds. Tax reform would become so integral to ACORN's early work that it became part of its national People's Platform, first rolled out at ACORN's second national convention, in St. Louis in 1979.

2. The term "banks" in this chapter includes savings and loans, which were limited by law to making loans to homeowners.
3. Mary Lassen and Madeline Adamson, "Erasing the Red-Line: The St. Louis Anti-redlining Campaign," in Institute for Social Justice, *Actions & Campaigns: Community Organizing Handbook #3* (New Orleans: Institute for Social Justice, 1979), 22. In three and a half years, nineteen neighborhood chapters would be established, with 1,500 dues-paying families.
4. The best ACORN campaigns were designed not only to help ACORN members, but also to increase ACORN's power by building the organization through media exposure, gaining new allies, and recruiting more members. A bigger organization with more members brought in more money. More money meant that ACORN could hire more organizers. And so on. Of course, many ACORN campaigns that looked good on paper fizzled out. In 1977, for example, Missouri ACORN won a hard-fought bill in the state legislature that banned redlining by insurance companies. After the bill went into effect, though, ACORN continued to receive complaints from members. Its own studies demonstrated that insurance companies failed to follow the new regulations.
5. See Jim Campen, "The Community Reinvestment Act: A Law That Works," *Dollars and Sense*, November–December 1977, *www.dollarsandsense.org/archives/1997/1197campen.html.*
6. Frances Moore Lappe, *Democracy's Edge: Choosing to Save Our Country by Bringing Democracy to Life* (San Francisco: Jossey Bass, 2006).
7. Sol Stern, "ACORN's Nutty Regime for Cities," *City Journal*, Spring 2003, *www.city-journal.org/html/13_2_acorns_nutty_regime.html.*
8. Woodson quoted in ibid.
9. For up-to-date information regarding contemporary racial discrimination, see the websites of the Center for Responsible Lending and National Community Reinvestment Coalition. See also studies by the Joint Center for Political and Economic Studies, *www.jointcenter.org/publications_recent_publications/economics_business*, and Stephen Ross and John Yinger, *The Color of Credit: What Is Known about Discrimination in Mortgage Lending* (Cambridge, Mass.: MIT Press, 2002). Attempts to blame the subprime crisis on the CRA turned out to be absurd. See John Atlas and Peter Dreier, "The GOP's Blame-ACORN Game," *Nation*, October 22, 2008, *www.thenation.com/doc/20081110/dreier_atlas.*
10. Paul Grogan and Tony Proscio, *Comeback Cities* (Boulder, Colo.: Westview Press, 2000).
11. Brad Lender, "Cities Revive, but What About the People?" *Shelterforce*, November–December 2000, *www.shelterforce.org/online/issues/114/bookreview.html.*
12. See John Atlas and Ellen Shoshkes, *Saving Affordable Housing: What Community Groups Can Do and What Government Should Do* (New York: National Housing Institute and Ford Foundation, 1997).
13. Lisa Ranghelli, "The Monetary Impact of ACORN Campaigns: A Ten-Year Retrospective, 1995–2004," November 2006, *www.acorn.org/fileadmin/ACORN_Reports/2007/ACORN_Wins_Report.pdf.*
14. ACORN was not alone in forcing banks to change their lending practices. Dozens of other local and state groups, usually with the support of national networks such as the Center for Community Change, National Peoples Action, and the National Community Reinvestment Coalition helped move $1 trillion in bank lending back into inner cities. Major national lenders provided philanthropic funding support for home-ownership counseling and home-building programs, and worked with these groups to provide more affordable mortgage loans. ACORN was able to build on its CRA success and move on to other issues besides lending, addressing problems such as education, crime, voter registration, political campaign finance law, and living wages. It was the only group to move beyond its CRA accomplishments in a way that would increase organizational funding and its constituency base and build its national political clout. Most of the groups engaged in the battles with banks focused with single-minded dedication on issues of unfair lending. ACORN, however, wasn't born as a bank watchdog and didn't intend to limit its focus. It was, as organizers say, a multi-issue organization committed to improv-

ing people's living conditions. ACORN's campaign around bank lending helped build its organization by recruiting new members, generating funding support for its staff, and attracting media attention for its research reports and its confrontational tactics. ACORN Housing Corporation was founded in 1986 and as of August 2005 the AHC website lists offices in forty-two cities. See *www.acornhousing.org/index.php* (accessed August 10, 2005).

15. Fred Brooks, "The Evolution of Community Organizing Campaigns at ACORN, 1970–2006," paper presented at the annual meeting of the American Sociological Association, New York City, August 11, 2007 (author files).

Chapter 7
Urban Homesteading

Some of the information in this chapter is based on my interviews with Peter Dreier, Seth Borgos, Jon Kest, Steve Kest, Wade Rathke, and former ACORN staffer Frances Streich.

1. According to Robert Neuwirth, in *Shadow Cities: A Billion Squatters, A New Urban World* (New York: Routledge, 2004), about one of every six people on the planet are squatters, that is, they occupy their homes illegally—a billion people; by 2050, perhaps one in three. In the early 1970s, seeking to repair the growing inventory of vacant, federally owned houses created by wide-scale foreclosures, U.S. big-city mayors successfully pressured Congress to enact a federal homesteading bill, passed in 1974, but only a handful of the vacant buildings were occupied and repaired, most of them by middle-income families. These programs barely made a dent in the growing problem of housing abandonment in older U.S. cities that were losing population as the middle class fled to suburbia. For a history of squatting, see Neuwirth.
2. This decline was partly because the proportion of Americans who owned their own homes had reached 64 percent, and the number of homes without indoor plumbing, electricity, or other basics had plummeted. By 1970, most experts believed that serious housing problems were confined to the poor—apartments that were in slum condition or seriously overcrowded, or that cost more than families could afford (one-third of their income, by the government's rule of thumb).
3. Paul Nussbaum, "A Long, Strange Trip for Milton Street," *Philadelphia Inquirer*, September 27, 2008. Milton Street's biggest supporter and his attorney, his younger brother, John, became Philadelphia's mayor less than two decades later.
4. The squatting campaign catapulted Street into the public eye. He used the mass media to create a larger-than-life public image and in 1980 won a seat in the state legislature representing North Philadelphia. He continued to be a controversial figure but forsook his work with squatters. Unlike Kest, he was not interested in building an organization.
5. A Republican moderate, Stewart McKinney from Connecticut, was the strongest sponsor of homesteading reform in the House of Representatives. Seth Borgos, ACORN's research director, was so inspired by the passage of the National Homesteading Act that he saw the squatter's movement as a step toward changing national housing policy, influencing federal property disposition policies, the tax foreclosure process, housing speculation, redevelopment plans, and code enforcement. Writing in *Critical Perspectives on Housing*, he said the campaign "disseminated new approaches to home rehabilitation financing, . . . [and] went beyond policy demands of the squatters; it was a blatant challenge to the assumptions and values on which U.S. housing policy is founded. The desperation of the squatters mocked the assumption that Americans are well housed; their eagerness to tear down the boards asserted the primacy of housing needs over property rights." The squatters certainly drew attention to housing issues, made a dent in the housing shortage caused by widespread abandonment, beefed up the National Housing Act, and helped build ACORN.
6. ACORN clearly differentiated itself from Citizen Action, another national left-leaning community activist organization with its roots in both the student movement of the 1960s and Alinsky organizing. Instead of organizing individual members among poor

and working-class city dwellers, it organized statewide coalitions with unions, seniors, environmental groups, and churches. It would become one of the most effective grass-roots lobbying groups on behalf of the poor and middle class, especially in the areas of health care and protecting Social Security, primarily using a professional canvassing operation, the electoral process, and coalition building with progressive unions. Although the groups were involved in similar issues, attempts at merger that might have made both groups stronger failed to materialize.

7. Dues and the takings from a door-to-door canvass in middle-class neighborhoods, raffles, bake sales, and community fairs accounted for 62 percent of the budget. Each organizer raised on average about $5,000 per year. Most members paid $18 a year in dues.

Chapter 8
Political Ground Shifts

1. Lawrence Goodwyn, *The Populist Moment: A Short History of the Agrarian Revolt in America* (New York: Oxford University Press, 1978). Traveling was not a problem for Rathke. He had the soul of a migrant, cultivated by his father's job that required him to move the family often. By the age of seven, Wade had lived in seven cities or towns.
2. William Julius Wilson, *The Truly Disadvantaged: The Inner City, the Underclass, and Public Policy* (Chicago: University of Chicago Press, 1987).
3. Paul Krugman, *The Conscience of a Liberal* (New York: W. W. Norton, 2009).
4. See Robert Putnam, *Bowling Alone: The Collapse and Revival of American Community* (New York: Simon and Schuster, 2000).
5. I have drawn in the next three paragraphs on Theda Skocpol, *Diminished Democracy: From Membership to Management in American Civic Life* (Norman: University of Oklahoma Press, 2003). Although ACORN's founders and leaders never drew upon the civic associations of the pre-1960s, the organizational model Rathke developed for ACORN resembled groups like the American Legion. The Legion, like ACORN, provided a vehicle through which the middle, working and lower classes spoke with one voice. When the American Legion drafted and lobbied for GI bill, because it was a cross-class group, it insisted the GI bill be a universal program and apply to all veterans. Although it initially discriminated against blacks, the GI Bill became one of the most expansive and inclusive federal assistance programs ever enacted.
6. Ibid.
7. Hayden's Campaign for Economic Democracy is praised in the influential book by Robert N. Bellah, Richard Madsen, William M. Sullivan, Ann Swidler, and Steven M. Tipton, *Habits of the Heart: Individualism and Commitment in American Life* (Berkeley: University of California Press, 1986).
8. See Thomas Byrne Edsall and Mary D. Edsall, *Chain Reaction: The Impact of Race, Rights, and Taxes on American Politics* (New York: W. W. Norton, 1992).
9. See Lisa McGirr, *Suburban Warriors: The Origins of the New American Right* (Princeton, N.J.: Princeton University Press, 2001); Rick Perlstein, *Before the Storm: Barry Goldwater and the Unmaking of the American Consensus* (New York: Hill and Wang, 2001). In the late 1950s, conservatives appeared to have run out of gas. McCarthyism had been discredited. Pearlstein documents how they created a network of right-wing publications and talk-radio stations, recruited college students and funded their campus organizations, and identified, cultivated, and trained potential political candidates. McGirr shows that while the 1960s media focused on student activists fighting for student rights and civil rights and against poverty, behind the headlines a new conservative movement was incubating.
10. One goal of the Reagan Administration was to redistribute wealth upward, from the have-nots to the have-a-lots. Americans were mobilized to worry about "family values" or to "look out for Number One." To liberals, the Reagan philosophy amounted to one in which God helps those whom God has already helped. The country had swung to the right and the concerns of low- and moderate-income people drifted off the public's radar.

See also Nina Easton, *Gang of Five: Leaders at the Center of the Conservative Ascendancy* (New York: Simon and Schuster, 2002).

11. On Norquist, see John Cassidy, "The Ringleader," *New Yorker*, August 1, 2005; Todd Gitlin, *The Bulldozer and the Big Tent* (San Francisco: Wiley, 2007).

Chapter 9
New York: A New Model

Most of the information in this chapter comes from my interviews with Jon Kest, Bertha Lewis, Wade Rathke, Frances Streich, and Ron Shiffman. The quotes in this chapter were reported to me or documented in Steven Erlanger, "For a New Homesteader, Struggle Leads to Success," *New York Times*, October 12, 1987; Steven Erlanger, "New York Turns Squatters into Homeowners," *New York Times*, October 12, 1987; William R. Greer, "Squatters and City Battle for Abandoned Buildings," *New York Times*, August 2, 1985; and Walter Thabit's *How East New York Became a Ghetto* (New York: New York University Press, 2003).

1. Fred Siegel, *The Future Once Happened Here* (New York: Free Press, 1997). The city would soon become embroiled in corruption; see Jack Newfield and Wayne Barrett, *City for Sale* (New York: Harper and Row, 1988).
2. White quoted in Jim Sleeper, *The Closest of Strangers: Liberalism and the Politics of Race in New York* (New York: W. W. Norton, 1990).
3. John Mollenkopf, *Phoenix in the Ashes: The Rise and Fall of the Koch Coalition in New York City Politics* (Princeton, N.J.: Princeton University Press, 1992).
4. During the 1990s, ACORN, as well as several housing and tenant groups, helped stabilize neighborhoods through their management and rehabilitation of abandoned buildings. As real estate prices in Manhattan bounced back, owners and speculators began to realize the potential value of the abutting neighborhoods these groups helped to revive. As a result, the process of abandonment ceased almost entirely. In some neighborhoods such as the fashionable East Village, tenants faced a new threat: speculators anxious to remove poor and working-class occupants in order to convert their buildings for upscale tenants.
5. By this time New York ACORN had won several important victories in areas other than housing. The New York chapter's budget grew from under $50,000 in 1982 to over $3.5 million in 2006, its membership from 3,000 to nearly 35,000, and its staff from four to fifty. ACORN created the High School for Social Justice, by a resolution of the Board of Education one of three high schools sponsored by ACORN. Students could engage in a comprehensive academic program and participate in citywide campaigns dealing with issues of social injustice that affect Brooklyn. ACORN then fought a bitter battle against Mayor Giuliani when in 2001 he tried to let for-profit Edison Schools Incorporated take over five failing public schools. After that battle, ACORN and its labor and community-based allies in the Brooklyn Educational Collaborative pushed for better science education in the borough's middle schools and won initial funding of $200,000 to open fully stocked science labs. In 2001, after organizing for NYC ACORN for twenty years, Streich had become the parent outreach coordinator for the United Federation of Teachers; in 2005 she became the UFT director of a joint organizing campaign with ACORN to unionize family child-care providers. Louise Stanley, the former chair of ACORN, remains an ACORN member in Arizona. Jon Kest became the head organizer for New York State ACORN.

Chapter 10
A Living Wage

The section of this chapter on the Chicago Living Wage campaign is partly based on my in-person or telephone interviews and e-mail exchanges with ACORN organizers, leaders, and staff, including Steve Andrews, Toni Foulkes, Jen Kern, Keith Kelleher, Brian Kettenring, Laura Wede Kai, Katy Gall, Maude Hurd, Frank Houston, Rev. Robin Hood, Beatrice Jackson,

Mahaley Summerville, and Madeline Talbott; and with Tim Drea, political director of the United Food and Commercial Workers; John Henley, Florida campaign director for the Service Employees International Union; John Donahue, executive director of the Chicago Coalition of the Homeless; Paul K. Sonn from the Brennan Center for Justice at NYU School of Law; and writer David Moberg.

The reporting on the Florida minimum wage campaign is partly based on my in-person and telephone interviews and e-mail exchanges with ACORN's Brian Kettenring; in-person interviews with John Myle and numerous ACORN canvassers and staff; a telephone interview with state senator Tony Hill; in-person interviews with Florida residents and with Rick McAllister from the Florida Retail Federation, John Henley from the Service Employees International Union, Ellen Roggemann, a student researcher, and the Carlton College Council Minutes 1991, 1992. I also spent two weeks in Florida observing the campaign and writing about it for *Shelterforce* magazine and *Commonweal*; see John Atlas, "In Red State Florida, Victory for Working People," *Shelterforce*, January–February 2005; John Atlas, Peter Dreier, and Kelly Candaele, "Florida Gets It Right: Raising the Minimum Wage," *Commonweal*, June 3, 2005; John Atlas and Peter Dreier, "Voters Gave Big Thumbs Up to Minimum Wage Boost," *(Bergen County, N.J.) Record*, November 26, 2006.

1. Keith thought old-time labor leaders resembled those in the skilled trade unions whose arrogance and chauvinism led to a split labor movement over the issue of organizing workers by industry instead of by skilled craft. When it came to organizing home-care workers, Keith saw the glass as half full, even though the glass was nearly empty.
2. Like New York ACORN, ACORN Chicago was also involved in several other issues, including school reform. In 1993, Illinois ACORN developed a relationship with the University of Illinois Small Schools Collaborative and worked to establish two public schools. When the state passed a charter law, Chicago ACORN started running a charter high school in Little Village, a Latino community without a high school.
3. Hank De Zutter, "What Makes Obama Run?" *Chicago Reader*, December 8, 1995.
4. Judy Keen, "Obama Comes Out Swinging in IOWA," *USA Today*, February 12, 2007.
5. In 1995, in the midst of this campaign and other living- and minimum-wage campaigns, Wade Rathke authorized a lawsuit in California seeking to exempt ACORN from the state's minimum wage of $4.25 per hour. ACORN alleged in its complaint that minimum-wage laws "were unconstitutional as applied to it, because they restricted its ability to engage in political advocacy by forcing it to hire fewer workers, and that its workers, if paid the minimum wage, would be less empathetic with its low- and moderate-income constituency and would therefore be less effective advocates." ACORN withdrew from similar litigation, realizing it contradicted ACORN's living-wage campaigns around the country. The suit did not slow down ACORN's minimum-wage action, but it would later be used by right-wing opponents to prove ACORN was antiworker.
6. Keith, in New Jersey at a union meeting, got a call: Come home, pick up your kids, and bail your wife out of jail. "What the hell," Keith said. He called a friend who picked up the kids and gave them to another friend to watch until Madeline got out of jail early the next morning. Keith took the first plane he could get and flew back.
7. The mayor and his allies had mobilized against Thomas, mailing out several impressive glossy pieces in the final ten days urging voters to support Ted's opponent. On Election Day, buses and city vehicles crisscrossed the ward, dropping off more than four hundred well-paid veteran patronage workers and last-minute hires from the mayor's allies in the surrounding wards. On election night, the first returns for Thomas looked bleak. One volunteer started writing a concession speech; a few others went to break the bad news to Thomas in private. On their way, a campaign worker interrupted them. The tide had started to turn.
8. David Moberg, "Martha Jernegons's New Shoes," *American Prospect*, June 19 and July 3, 2000.
9. Like the Christian Right's effort to increase conservative and Republican turnout by putting measures against gay marriage on the ballot in swing states, ACORN's minimum-

wage campaign was not directly tied to the Democratic Party or specific candidates. But the funding for this grassroots effort (almost $2 million) came from many of the sources—wealthy liberals, unions, and others—that back Democrats.

10. The one thing that surprised ACORN's staff was the extent to which Florida's Republican Party and its allies went to suppress voter turnout. *New York Times* columnist Bob Herbert reported that the Florida Department of Law Enforcement sent armed troopers into the homes of elderly voters in Orlando. Secretary of State Glenda Hood, a Republican, refused to accept voter registration applications that didn't include a check mark affirming citizenship—even though a signature at the bottom of the application provided an oath of citizenship. Hood also ruled that provisional ballots cast in precincts other than the voter's own would be thrown out, a blow to ACORN's get-out-the-vote efforts. In Fort Lauderdale, an ACORN member was not allowed to vote because he was on the inactive-voter list—even though the law clearly stated that could be rectified at the polling place. It would take about two years for ACORN to understand that the White House was behind this effort. Meanwhile, the organizers did the best they could to contend with the onslaught.
11. Robert Pollin, Mark Brenner, and Jeannette Wicks-Lim, *Economic Analysis of the Florida Minimum Wage Proposal* (Washington, D.C.: Center for American Progress, September 2004), *www.americanprogress.org/atf/cf/percent7BE9percent20E03 percent7D/minimumwage-layout8.pdf.*
12. Changing the practices of one of America's most powerful corporations seemed like a daunting task, if not outright folly. The group's efforts got a boost when the Brennan Center for Justice at NYU School of Law agreed to advise the City Council in designing the proposed law and served as counsel to ACORN's group in support of the legislation.
13. In Missouri, Democrat Claire McCaskill defeated the incumbent, Republican Jim Talent, by less than 2 percentage points in one of the nation's most closely contested Senate races. McCaskill acknowledged that the grassroots get-out-the-vote effort mounted by ACORN and its labor union allies on behalf of the minimum wage initiative helped put her over the top. She enthusiastically supported the wage hike, while Talent took no official position. In Ohio, ACORN's increased voter turnout for the minimum-wage measure, engineered by Katy Gall, helped Rep. Sherrod Brown defeat incumbent senator Mike DeWine, and Democrat Ted Strickland beat Republican Ken Blackwell for governor.
14. Wade Rathke, *Citizen Wealth* (San Francisco: Barrett Koehler, 2009).

Chapter 11
Never Borrow Money Needlessly

Some of the information in this chapter is based on my in-person interviews and emails with Jordan Ash, Alton Bennett, Carolyn Carr, Lisa Donner, Julie Goodridge, Steve Kest, Keith Kelleher, Scott Klinger, Paul Satriano, Mike Shea, Robert Trigaux, and Kevin Whalen. I read dozens of newspaper reports, the most important of which are listed in the bibliography. I found the HSBC website useful; it is one of the largest banking and financial services organizations in the world and the parent company of Household Finance until it merged that company into Household International, *www.hsbcusa.com/ourcompany/hiarchive/hi2004/hipr_press_release240.html.*

1. Neither the Democrats nor the Republicans mentioned housing or predatory lending in their 2000 presidential campaigns, although Green Party candidate Ralph Nader made affordable housing an issue, linking housing to raising the minimum wage, blasting the hundreds of billions in corporate welfare going to developers to build $500,000 homes in the suburbs, and calling for a crackdown on predatory lenders. Gramlich had a PhD in economics from Yale and in the late 1990s, as chair of a federally chartered redevelopment agency, had urged Congress to better protect consumers against predatory lending practices and toughen regulations of mortgage lenders and banks. He called the mortgage process "confusing, costly and far less than optimal."

2. Within ACORN, the idea of taking on HFC was not controversial. Steve Kest, Donner's supervisor; Ash; O'Brien, the national field organizer; Rathke; and Shea considered HFC an attractive national symbol of predatory lending and a potential target for action. They hoped if ACORN could change HFC's practices, it would make a difference in the industry as a whole. Because HFC was in every state, most local chapters could be involved. But HFC's size also insured that it would be a formidable adversary.
3. Household Finance Corporation. *Financing the American Family*, video (Chicago Film Laboratory, ca. 1935, *www.archive.org/details/Financin1935*.
4. Steve Brand, "Targeting Abusive Lending Practices; ACORN to Help Home Buyers," *Minneapolis Star Tribune*, June 15, 2001.
5. ACORN's Minnesota bill would have created a new category of high-cost loans. New restrictions would be placed on such loans to limit prepayment penalties, bar financing credit insurance through the loan, and block loans without a financial benefit to the borrower. It also would put a lid on points and fees, require loan counseling for borrowers, and beef up legal remedies for borrowers in cases where the law had been broken.
6. The top 20 percent of U.S. households earned 56 percent of the nation's income. In nearly two decades the number of millionaires had doubled, to 4.8 million, and the number of "deca-millionaires"—those worth at least $10 million—had more than tripled, from 66,500 to 239,400. The bottom 40 percent of Americans earned just 10 percent of the nation's income and owned less than 1 percent of the nation's wealth. The bottom 60 percent did only marginally better, accounting for about 23 percent of income and less than 5 percent of wealth. The contrast between the middle and top was equally dramatic. A household in the middle—the median household—has wealth of about $62,000; in the top 1 percent, $12.5 million. The racial gaps were even more disheartening. The typical African American household had fifty-four cents of income and twelve cents of wealth for every dollar in the typical white household. Hispanics had sixty-two cents of income and four cents of wealth.
7. Klinger was a former corporate manager and financial analyst. United for a Fair Economy and the Coalition for Responsible Wealth (RW) was founded by Chuck Collins, an heir to the Oscar Mayer fortune. Members were rich business leaders and several other wealthy heirs—only people in the wealthiest 5 percent of Americans. At first Donner was leery; ACORN was trying to build a cross-class majoritarian group and had never considered millionaires to be part of its constituency. But Klinger convinced Donner he had a good strategy.
8. After graduating from Harvard, Goodridge had been an ACORN organizer and thought it was a great group. Now forty-four, she had recently made headlines as one of the lead plaintiffs in the landmark Massachusetts gay marriage case that extended marital rights to same-sex couples in that state.
9. ACORN issued a News Advisory on May 7: Household International, parent company of two of the country's biggest predatory lenders, Household Finance and Beneficial, is holding its annual shareholders' meeting on May 8, 2001 in the Tampa, Fla., area. As part of ACORN's ongoing campaign to urge Household to change its predatory lending practices, more than 50 ACORN members and victims of Household plan to protest outside the gathering. Events are also scheduled for the May 8th and 9th in: Albuquerque, Boston, St. Louis, Hempstead (NY), Minneapolis and St. Paul (MN), Little Rock, Hartford, Denver, San Diego, and Los Angeles. ACORN members and allied elected officials will announce a drive to urge cities.
10. Robert Trigaux, "Florida Newest Turf in Lending Hostilities," *St. Petersburg Times*, May 9, 2001, *www.acorn.org/acorn10/household/press/newfla.htm*.
11. Household made the change in its loan structure after consulting with the National Community Reinvestment Coalition, which like ACORN worked for capital flow into underserved areas.
12. ACORN's aggressive practices were not well received by every AG. In April 2002, ACORN led twenty HFC customers in a protest at Huey's office in Washington State. Huey understood the importance of protest and did not take offense, but his more con-

servative colleagues didn't want to see their picture in the paper or be linked to ACORN. One assistant AG referred to ACORN as "less rational . . . on the fringes, prone to do things like showing up at offices, chanting with signs."

13. Peter Eavis, "Lawsuits and Regulators Shadow Big Lender's Future," *New York Times*, August 17, 2002; Bernard Condon, "Home Wrecker," *Forbes*, September 2, 2002. Donner had supplied details to several reporters, including one from the *New York Times* and another from *Forbes*, but had difficulty getting reporters to understand the central role that ACORN played. She was becoming frustrated because the media would call her about HFC, predatory lending, and the names of victims, but not about ACORN.
14. Iowa Attorney General's Office, "Miller: Iowa's Share of Household Settlement Could Reach about $1.3 Million—States Settle with Household Finance: Up to $484 Million for Consumers," press release, October 11, 2002, *www.state.ia.us/government/ag/latest_news/*.
15. On August 15, 2003, the AGs' offices in every state mailed letters to hundreds of thousands of eligible recipients informing them of the record-breaking settlement. The press, the attorneys general, and bank regulators heralded the settlement as a "blueprint for national standards" in the mortgage lending industry. The thousands of dollars of relief allowed borrowers to refinance into a better loan. The ACORN FAP program channeled funds to borrowers who were most in need and who otherwise would lose their homes. Interest rates were lowered and second mortgages completely forgiven. For a single mother with two children, for instance, HFC forgave a $10,000 second mortgage and reduced the interest rate of her first mortgage from over 10 percent to 6 percent. Her payment decreased from $1,825 to $881, saving her nearly $1,000 per month and $169,920 over the life of the loan. For another couple, the wife permanently disabled and the husband working three jobs, HFC reduced their interest rate from 10.5 to 3.9 percent. HFC reduced mortgage payments from $1,270 to $647, a savings of $112,140 over the life of the loan. In February 2004, a few months after the settlement, a single parent called ACORN Housing. Her home was scheduled for a sheriff's sale because of payment problems due in part to a family crisis. Through the ACORN program, the sheriff stopped the sale of her home and ACORN got the interest rate on the loan reduced to 4.9 percent, lowering her monthly payment from $585 to $325.
16. Despite Satriano's uncertain future, his commitment to ACORN deepened; he would soon be elected treasurer of the national ACORN board. Washington attorney general David Huey, whose report made headlines and helped spur the settlement, was honored with the prestigious Marvin Award from the National Association of Attorneys Generals (NAAG) for his work on the Household case. Donner would soon leave ACORN's financial justice organizing for a job with New York's Working Families Party.
17. The National Community Reinvestment Coalition (NCRC) set up a foreclosure-prevention program that has saved thousands of homeowners from losing their homes by pressuring lenders to change adjustable-rate mortgages into fixed-rate loans. Of all the banks slammed by the subprime crisis, there was one beacon of sanity that moved aggressively to minimize the pain to itself and customers: HSBC, the world's second-largest bank by assets and the one that took over HFC. Having learned the hard way, it staved off a wave of potential foreclosures. Faced with numerous borrowers behind on payments and with delinquencies climbing, in October 2007, it assigned about 640 employees to work with troubled borrowers twenty-four hours a day, seven days a week, to modify their mortgages so they didn't lose their homes. To prevent the crisis from getting worse and to avoid future crises, ACORN in the summer of 2008 lobbied Congress and, despite strong opposition from the White House and its congressional allies, with other housing groups made sure the 2008 housing bill that helps victims of the subprime crisis included money for a new $600 million affordable-housing trust fund and $4 billion in grants to restore housing in ravaged neighborhoods.
18. See Elizabeth Williamson and Brody Mullins, "Democratic Ally Mobilizes in Housing Crunch; Acorn Leads Drive to Register Voters Likely to Back Obama," *Wall Street Journal*, July 31, 2008.

Chapter 12
ACORN's Family Party

Some of the information for this chapter comes from my in-person and telephone interviews, as well as e-mail exchanges, with the following staffers of ACORN and the Working Families Party: Eva Bonime, Dan Cantor, Steve Kest, Jon Kest, Bertha Lewis, and Zach Polett. I also interviewed members of the WFP and journalist Errol Lewis.

1. In 1988, Cantor, then thirty-three, went to work for Jesse Jackson's presidential campaign within the Democratic Party primary system, a campaign supported by ACORN. Cantor and ACORN made important connections that would help build ACORN, but it still did not produce an enduring organizational afterlife.
2. *The Oyez Project, Timmons v. Twin Cities Area New Party,* 520 U.S. 351 (1997), *oyez.org/cases/1990-1999/1996/1996_95_1608.*
3. Josh Benson, "It's Mean Mark Green: Former Front Runner Jostles Freddy Ferrer," *New York Observer*, October 14, 2001.
4. Another example of the risk of this kind of mix occurred when members of a local WFP chapter got angry with Cantor, Master, and other WFP leaders for rejecting their chapter's candidate endorsement decisions. The local chapter activists, who were dues-paying members, accused the WFP leadership of being heavy handed and undemocratic. In fact, the ruckus was caused by a few Republicans activists who had cleverly infiltrated and hijacked the WFP chapter in Suffolk County. Some legitimate members felt that the structure of the party gave the unions what amounted to veto power. Also when the WFP endorsed several Republican state senate candidates who agreed to help pass a statewide minimum-wage increase, friendly Democratic Party and African American leaders angrily criticized the WFP. "At times their focus on particular issues has put them in conflict with the Democratic Party, and even with progressive goals in general," said one Democrat. In an August 2005 decision, Judge Thomas Whelan took the Executive Committee of the New York State Working Families Party to task for subverting election law through its attempts to prevent formation of county committees and to deny county committee members control of nominations. See *Martin v. Alverez et al.* Index No. 05-15985, *Matter of New York Working Families Party v. Berman*, 11 AD3d 646,764 NYS2d 557 (2d Dept 2004).

Chapter 13
Atlantic Yards, the Nets, and the Battle of Brooklyn

Some of the information for this chapter comes from my in-person and telephone interviews, as well as e-mail exchanges, with ACORN staff and members, including Jon Kest, Bertha Lewis, Ismane Speliotis, Tunisha W. Walker, and Pat Boone; and family, friends, and acquaintances of Bertha Lewis. I interviewed many people, including opponents, living in the area of Atlantic Yards, including Tom Angotti, Steve Ettlinger, Cris Owens, and Ron Shiffman. The thorough online Atlantic Yards Report by the anti–Atlantic Yards reporter Norman Oder was helpful. I also interviewed several members of Ratner's staff, including Lupè Todd and Joe DePlasco, as well as the project's architect, Frank Gehry. Some information comes from my interviews with Errol Lewis; Gene Russianoff, senior attorney, NYPIRG Straphangers Campaign; and Nicole Marwell, assistant professor at Columbia University Department of Sociology. I spent dozens of hours with Bertha Lewis while she worked and traveled, made speeches, and ran meetings. I tape-recorded many of our conversations. The chapter is also based on information from *ACORN United* and internal ACORN memos to and from Lewis. I was also able to observe many of the events I describe here.

1. Nicolai Ouroussoff, "Seeking First to Reinvent the Sports Arena, and Then Brooklyn," *New York Times*, July 5, 2005. See also Nicolai Ouroussoff, "Outgrowing Jane Jacobs and Her New York," *New York Times*, April 30, 2006.

2. Herbert Muschamp, "Courtside Seats to an Urban Garden," *New York Times*, December 11, 2003. For additional information on this struggle over low-income housing in Brooklyn, see John Atlas, "The Battle in Brooklyn," *Shelterforce*, Spring 2006, as well as the websites of Brooklyn United for Local Development, *www.buildbrooklyn.org*; Develop Don't Destroy Brooklyn, *www.developdontdestroy.com*; and Forest City Ratner, *www.fcrc.com*.
3. Tom Angotti, "Atlantic Yards: Through the Looking Glass," *Gotham Gazette*, November 15, 2005, *www.gothamgazette.com*.
4. Encouraging its members to participate in decision making makes ACORN quite different from many left-wing activist organizations, antipoverty agencies, and community groups. If these groups have members at all, they are rarely low-income people. The few poor people on the boards of such advocacy groups seldom have a strong constituency base that they can mobilize to change public policy; the staff usually leads. ACORN members not only elect a democratically run group but also pay dues, march, and vote. Critics such as Mark Winston Griffith, a prominent journalist and community development professional, have described New York ACORN as a top-down group manipulated by the staff (M. W. Griffith, "Calling the Question of ACORN," DMI Blog: Politics, Policy and the American Dream, December 30, 2005, *www.dmiblog.net/archives/2005/12/calling_the_question_of_acorn.html*). It is not easy for outsiders to fully understand how the group works, since there have been few studies that document how ACORN makes decisions. Kest, Lewis, and most of the organizers and leaders claim ACORN is a bottom-up group, with all major decisions driven by members.

   ACORN's Atlantic Yards campaign would reveal a complex process in which the staff and grassroots leaders shared decision making. Heidi Swarts's study of ACORN's St. Louis and San Jose chapters characterizes their authority structure as "fluid and frequently negotiated." (Heidi Swarts, *Organizing Urban America* [Minneapolis: University of Minnesota Press, 2008]). This preeminence of participation is so deeply ingrained in most ACORN staff that it engenders a culture of respect—a byproduct of the organizing culture. This culture enhances the staff's ability to provide effective services, recruit members, mobilize them, and get them to pay dues. ACORN's genius lies in collaboration. Sometimes staff lead; sometimes members lead. The synergy between staff and leaders, feeding off each other's expertise and savvy, brings results.

   At training sessions for new organizers, Lewis emphasizes: "In the end, the members call the shots. They vote with their feet, they vote with their level of participation and support for the organization. If you have some deep, hidden issues with poor people, if you are patronizing or really don't like poor people, then it will come out. The members will sense it, and this is not the job for you."

   Bertha Lewis and the other New York staff genuinely like the members and care deeply about their concerns. "The members are the bosses. This is organizing culture!" asserts Lewis. "If the staff comes up with a plan that is not supported by the members, the members won't volunteer, vote, demonstrate or in any other way support ACORN's action."

   ACORN's notion of decision making is more like representative government than the direct deliberation of the ancient Athens agora or the New Left's notion of participatory democracy, where everybody speaks their piece, consensus is the goal, and leadership and hierarchy are unwelcome. Like Saul Alinsky's organizations, ACORN focuses on solving problems and securing the active participation of its members and neighbors, but it also has a formal decision-making process. In the tradition of Alinsky's approach, ACORN's emphasizes strong leadership and centralized decision making by the leaders. It has bylaws and a hierarchy within the staff and leadership office holders.
5. Siegel quoted in Christopher Montgomery, "Cleveland Is Home, but Is That Enough? Urban Revival: Forest City's Rise," *Plain Dealer*, December 1, 2005.
6. On March 15, 2004, the New York ACORN board members gathered at headquarters in Brooklyn. The board included two members from each neighborhood group representing Flatbush, East Flatbush, Bushwick, Brownsville, the Bronx, and Manhattan. It also

included four members from neighborhood groups representing Crown Heights, East New York, and Long Island; two members from the ACORN political action committee (PAC); and ten from ACORN'S housing development arm, the ACORN Mutual Housing Association of New York (MHANY). The board unanimously approved an organizing campaign to make a deal with Ratner.

7. Shumer quoted in Greg Sargent, "First among Thirds," *American Prospect*, April 16, 2006.
8. The UFT and DC 37 were just two on a long list of organizations determined to propel affordable housing to the top of the city's political agenda in 2005, an election year. "We have a special window of opportunity," Lewis said, pointing to Atlantic Yards and other projects proposed for the city and the fact that 2005 was a mayoral election year. "History can be made here. No longer will development in the city leave out its working families." One after another, others at the rally, speakers and members of the crowd alike, echoed these demands. "The mayor and City Council have the power, right now, to make sure that homeless people living with AIDS have safe, permanent housing and don't languish for months in dangerous, expensive welfare hotels," said Amos Hough, a formerly homeless member of the New York City AIDS Housing Network.
9. Bertha Lewis, "Supporting Atlantic Yards: Simply Not Enough Housing in Brooklyn," *City Limits Weekly*, July 31, 2006.
10. The other signatories were the All-Faith Council of Brooklyn, the First Atlantic Terminal Housing Committee, the Downtown Brooklyn Education Consortium, the Public Housing Communities, the New York State Association of Minority Contractors, and BUILD. At the urging of Assemblyman Roger Green, the Downtown Brooklyn Educational Consortium was added to the mix at the last minute, several months after ACORN began negotiations. Its chair, Freddie Hamilton, was the vice chair of the Brooklyn Democratic Party and the executive director of a nonprofit child-welfare agency. In 1993, after her youngest son was shot and killed by another youth in the community, Hamilton, an African American, channeled her grief into activism. Her new organization would also try to create a charter school devoted to technology. The *New York Sun* editorialized on June 6, 2005, under the headline "Brooklyn Fairy Tale": "New York's housing market certainly needs many things, but an extra 2,250 units of market-distorting, dependence-inducing housing on a prime spot in the heart of Brooklyn isn't on the list."
11. See DDDB's website *www.developdontdestroy.com*; also see *www.americancity.org/print_version.php#*.
12. See DDDB's website *www.developdontdestroy.com*.
13. See DDDB's website *dddb.net/php/reading/shiffman.php*. The opposition also insisted that the project was too massive for this community. A young architect who lived near the proposed building site said: "Office towers, high-rise towers, sports arenas, that's not a community. Brooklyn doesn't want to be Manhattan. If we wanted Manhattan, we'd live there." City councilman Charles Barron, a former Black Panther, joined his colleague Letitia James in opposing the project. He complained that rents would be too high and that too many of the below-market units would go to households with high incomes.
14. In the midst of the battle over Atlantic Yards, on July 23, 2005, the U.S. Supreme Court ruled that local governments may force property owners to sell to make way for private economic development when city officials decide it would benefit the public, even if the property is not blighted and the new project's success is not guaranteed. The five-to-four ruling gave state and local governments wide latitude for using eminent domain for urban revitalization. As a result, condo owners and others facing displacement were not likely to prevail if they sued Ratner and the city.
15. Goldstein quoted in Justin Rocket Silverman, "The War for Brooklyn Battleground: Atlantic Yards," *Time Out New York*, July 27–August 2, 2006.
16. Norman Kelley, "Pastor of the People," *Brooklyn Rail*, April 2005, *www.brooklynrail.org/2005/04/local/pastor-of-the-people-david-dyson*.
17. Other celebrities included Jennifer Egan, Jonathan Safran Foer, Nicole Krauss, Peter Galassi, and Jonathan Lethem.

18. Paul Goldberger, "Gehry-Rigged," *New Yorker*, October 16, 2006; Cynthia Carr, "Voices of the Fading Community in the Shadow of the Atlantic Yards," *Village Voice*, July 25, 2006.
19. See Nicholas Confessore, "Perspectives on the Atlantic Yards Development through the Prism of Race," *New York Times*, November, 12, 2006.
20. Lander quoted in ibid. The number of units with gross monthly rents between $1,000 and $1,499 went up by 17 percent, and those costing $1,500 or more rose by 20.6 percent.
21. Lander quoted in Alan Feuer, "Affordable Apartments a New York Luxury," *New York Times*, February 11, 2006.
22. New York ACORN, "Sweetheart Development: Gentrification and Resegregation in Downtown Brooklyn," March 16, 2006, *www.acorn.org/fileadmin/Afforable_Housing/03.16.06_sweetheartdevelopment.doc.*
23. Byrd quoted in TimesRatnerReport blog, *timesratnerreport.blogspot.com/2005/12/more-on-observers-roger-green-story.html.*
24. Blankinship quoted in Jarrett Murphy, "The Battle of Brooklyn: Grassroots Groups Split on Whether Arena Plan Scores for Borough," *Village Voice*, July 19, 2004.
25. Errol Louis, "A Groundbreaking Coalition," *New York Daily News*, December 22, 2006.
26. In the midst of the Atlantic Yard controversy, New York ACORN was using its clout to save Starrett City, a 5,881-unit complex near Jamaica Bay in Brooklyn, the nation's largest federally subsidized apartment complex. In 2007, after a long-running dispute, ACORN helped the working-class Starrett City residents block a sale of the complex to a real estate investor who would evict them in favor of higher-paying residents in order to make an enormous profit. On July 29, 2009, New York's governor David Paterson signed legislation guaranteeing that Starrett City will remain affordable to its current tenants and the next generation of poor and working-class families. "When this began, they said we couldn't win . . . ," said Pat Boone, president of New York ACORN, in an e-mail statement. "But we fought and fought, and residents pushed the owners into accepting that they had to do business with us—and that we needed a plan to keep Starrett affordable." See The Brooklyn Rail, "The Battle of Starrett City," *www.brooklynrail.org/2007/4/local/the-battle-of-starrett-city*; *www.savestarrettcity.org/*; Charles V. Bagli, "In New Sale, Starrett City Would Stay Affordable," *www.nytimes.com/2008/06/02/nyregion/02starrett.html?_r=1&scp=1&sq=starrett%20city&st=cse.*
27. Stalled by the recession and lawsuits, construction work on the twenty-two-acre Atlantic Yards site was halted in December 2008. Ratner sought federal stimulus money to revive the project, scrapped Frank Gehry's plan and replaced it with one that would shave millions off the cost of the arena, and in a most surprising turn, Russian billionaire Mikhail Prokhorov agreed to buy an 80 percent stake in the Nets from Forest City. Prokhorov, a six-foot-nine basketball fan, will become the first foreign majority owner in National Basketball Association history who is not Canadian. In an interview with the *New York Times*, Ratner said: "He planned to start the first residential tower, which would contain a large percentage of units for low-, moderate- and middle-income families, about six months after work begins on the arena." On October 14, 2009, New York's highest court, the Court of Appeals, planned to hear a legal challenge over the use of eminent domain to seize private land for the Atlantic Yards project. While Forest City Ratner had won lower-court rulings in the case, a victory by opponents here could doom the project. See Charles V. Bagli, "Developer Drops Gehry's Design for Brooklyn Arena," *New York Times*, June 4, 2009.

Chapter 14
Then, Overnight, It Is Washed Away

Much of the information for this chapter came from my in-person and telephone interviews and e-mail exchanges: with ACORN staff and members and former members, including Wade Rathke, Stephen Bradberry, Beth Butler, Darryl Durham, Ginny Goldman, Tanya Harris, Marie Hurt, Steve Kest, Dennis Livingston, Tony McElroy, Mike Shea, Amy Schur, Marty Shaloo, Joe Stafford, and Dorothy Stukes; also with Ron Shiffman from the Pratt Institute;

Chester Hartman, founder of the Planners Network, which specialized in supporting community planning; and Ken Reardon, chair of the Regional and Local Planning Department at Cornell University. From November 2005 to 2008, I read the excellent reporting of the *Times-Picayune* every day. I visited New Orleans on five occasions and witnessed many of the events reported in this chapter and Chapter 15.

1. Bruce Alpert, "FEMA Chief Dawdled," *New Orleans Times-Picayune*, November 3, 2005. By June 26, 2006, the public would learn that the incompetence of Bush's FEMA and the Red Cross combined with lack of congressional oversight had led to scams, schemes, and stupefying bureaucratic bungles that cost taxpayers up to $2 billion—"nearly 11 percent of the $19 billion spent by FEMA on Hurricanes Katrina and Rita as of mid-June, or about 6 percent of total money that has been obligated," according to Eric Lipton, "'Breathtaking' Waste and Fraud in Hurricane Aid," *New York Times*, June 27, 2006.
2. New Orleans ACORN, like the New York and Illinois chapters, exemplified the best of ACORN's inside-outside strategy, because its roots were deep and its organizers ensconced in these places for a least a decade. While it agitated on the outside, it also supported established politicians on the inside. In addition to the events in this and the next chapter, another example occurred on July 30, 2005. ACORN applied to the city for approval to expand its office. An attorney from a neighboring business, Gene's Po-boys, objected. ACORN, he claimed, should not be allowed to cram its large operation into a historic residential neighborhood adjacent to the French Quarter. When he suggested that it look elsewhere, councilwoman Cynthia Willard-Lewis attacked him yelling, "ACORN has every right to be in Faubourg Marigny." The council president, Oliver Thomas, said ACORN's presence in the neighborhood raises property values and spurs other investment. Councilwoman Jacquelyn Brechtel Clarkson, whose district includes Marigny, called ACORN "a great cause." The city council unanimously approved the expansion.
3. Peter Dreier, "Katrina: A Political Disaster," *Shelterforce*, Spring 2006.
4. Roberta Brandes Gratz, "In New Orleans' Mud, a Ward Determined Not to Slip Away: "The Lower Ninth wants to rebuild," November 7, 2005, *www.commondreams.org/views05/1107-28.htm*. A shotgun blast fired through the front door of a "shotgun" home could reach the back wall of the narrow house without hitting anything.
5. Between 1994 and 2004, the number of jobs in New Orleans grew by only 4.3 percent compared to 23.1 percent for Houston. For decades the power brokers of New Orleans had concentrated on an elite-driven agenda that contributed to its poverty and slums. Nearly half of all full-time New Orleans hotel workers—like Dorothy's friend Adam—could not earn enough to keep a family above the poverty line. See Joel Kotkin with David Friedman, "Katrina and Urban Liberalism Left Behind," *New Republic*, September 13, 2005.
6. ACORN has local and state chapters, members who know each other, act together, and along with ACORN staff drive the organization. The effectiveness of this process varies substantially from chapter to chapter, depending on the talent of the local organizers and how effective they are in finding and educating leaders. Goldman was one of ACORN's most accomplished.
7. One of the flyers landed in the hands of New Orleans ACORN member Irma Williams. She'd had to evacuate her New Orleans three-story home bought with assistance from ACORN's Housing program. After being trapped in her house by over fourteen feet of water, Williams chopped a hole in her roof to signal for help. Four days later, the Williams family was rescued by helicopter and taken to an Interstate 10 interchange, only to endure more hardships: lack of food and water, filthy living conditions, and hot and miserable weather. Finally, FEMA transported them to the airport and eventually to a shelter in Corpus Christi, Texas, where she called her uncle from Houston. He picked her up and brought her back to Houston to stay with him. Williams's cousin in Houston, who was involved in helping hurricane survivors, went to the gathering with Williams.
8. Peter Dreier and John Atlas, "Katrina, the Missing Story," *Tikkun*, January–February 2007.
9. Based on reports from members and staff and personal observations, Wade Rathke would

later contrast Houston's mayor White with Mayor Kip Holden of East Baton Rouge Parish. "Hardly a week had passed since Katrina made landfall when Mayor White stood in front of a crowd, prepared with specific proposals and resources to address the immediate demands he knew he would hear including housing and food cards for host families. Throughout the crisis, White seemed to bend over backward to accommodate every demand and *keep* the Katrina survivors in his city. In daily 8:00 am meetings that included ACORN, business leaders, and other civic authorities, White would crack the whip to move goods and services to evacuees, with speed and efficiency being the first premium ahead of equity. Without waiting for FEMA, the City of Houston stood behind one-year rental commitments to fill the city's backlog of vacancies through the apartment association, where 9,000 units had stood open before the hurricane. On the other hand, Baton Rouge, which had even more refugees than Houston, seemed virtually to resent the intrusion, the traffic, and everything but the sudden income from so many additional residents. There was no reachout or welcome or real assistance. The location of the first FEMA trailer park on the outskirts of the parish in the old Klan stronghold in Baker said it all.

10. The program emphasized living-wage jobs and first-source hiring for survivors and residents, affordable housing and right of return for those dislocated, and public services that would allow families to live in safer communities. On September 16 ACORN members appeared on the nationally syndicated Travis Smiley radio show to reach out to others around the country on the issues of mortgage and credit. On September 19 in San Francisco ACORN members had joined Roseanne Barr, the comedian and television personality, in meetings and benefits to support ACORN's Katrina campaign. But by the end of September, the failure of federal relief and rebuilding efforts had become clear. President Bush's post-2004 election fixation with privatizing Social Security had already failed. The Iraq war continued to deteriorate. The census Bureau's annual report, released in the midst of the Gulf disaster, found that an additional 4.1 million Americans had slipped into poverty between 2001 and 2004. Any positive feelings about Bush were all but lost in the heaving waters of New Orleans. Most Americans no longer believed in Bush's ability to lead.
11. Peter Dreier, "Katrina and Power in America," *Urban Affairs Review* 41, 1 (March 2006): 1–21.
12. M. A. Fletcher and S. S. Hsu, "Storms Alter Louisiana Politics; Population Loss Likely to Reduce Influence of Black Voters," *Washington Post*, October 14, 2005; J. Havemann, "A Shattered Gulf Coast; New Orleans' Racial Future Hotly Argued; The U.S. Housing Chief Expresses Doubts About Rebuilding, and Draws Anger and Concern," *Los Angeles Times*, October 1, 2005.
13. Countering the administration's idea, Gene Dewey, a former career assistant secretary of state for population, refugees, and migration, proposed a bold recovery plan. He had told the *New York Times* that Bush should pay returnees to build roads, plant trees, and restore schools, a program that would provide dignity as well as money: "This is a time when you need that kind of Franklin Roosevelt thinking." James Dao, "No Fixed Address," *New York Times*, September 11, 2005.
14. The enormity of the task required a centralized coordinated plan. Two weeks after the storm, ACORN president Maude Hurd, based in Boston, set up a conference call of ACORN national board members and leaders from cities active in the hurricane rescue efforts. (Global Crossing, the international communications company, provided ACORN with free conference calls.) Rathke and other national staffers answered the many questions about the status of the New Orleans situation, the devastation of Katrina, the state of the membership and office, and the initiatives being taken to locate members. New Orleans was still quarantined and neither Rathke nor anyone else knew the situation there, since they were unable to enter the city. The most important news that Toni McElroy, the president of Texas ACORN, reported was its intention to form a survivors association. She warned that such a group would be extremely difficult to build: "We don't have organizers, we're having trouble with the dues thing or lots of folk are apa-

thetic—just too overwhelmed trying to pull their personal lives together." Hurd's conferences would continue weekly for the next three months as ACORN's leadership tried to assess what they saw on television and figure out a way to ameliorate the situation somehow, someway. On September 15, a few days after the first phone conference, Bush went on TV, standing in front of Jackson Square in New Orleans, to assure the nation that "we have a duty to confront [New Orleans's] poverty with bold action. . . . We will do what it takes, we will stay as long as it takes to help citizens rebuild their communities and their lives." Rathke looked closely to see if there was any life in Jackson Square. He saw none. It was surreal. He dashed off an op-ed to the *New York Times* that ended with an elegant plea (the essay never saw print): "If the government could not hear our peoples' screams above the water as the waves rose or in the din of the Superdome crowd, perhaps they could call this a "bought lesson," as we say in New Orleans, and listen now . . . Let's have a real experiment in democracy right now on the floodplains of New Orleans and let our people have a real voice, not just the corporations bidding to make us Falluja on the Mississippi. We may be working people and poorer and blacker than the rest of America, but we are Americans nonetheless with the right to have our special place and our separate dreams. We know some things that other people do not know. We know coffee is better with chicory. We know to eat red beans and rice on Mondays and fish on Fridays. We know that Mardi Gras still has something to do with Lent. We know the difference between a shotgun and a camelback house. We definitely know enough to have a real say in the future of our city. Let's hope this time our voice is heard."

15. At staff meetings the dilemma was approached this way: Should ACORN revitalize the New Orleans chapter, even though its members lived in Baton Rouge, Houston, Dallas, and elsewhere? Or should ACORN put its resources into organizing the evacuees into ACORN locals like the Houston chapter? Or should ACORN put its money into building the Katrina Survivors Association, and if so, what would that be?
16. The Shaw Group and Halliburton had hired the lobbyist Joe Allbaugh, a former FEMA director and Bush's 2000 campaign director, to secure the federal contracts. Allbaugh had no disaster-management experience when he took the job, and he didn't seem interested in learning. He had told Congress in May 2001 that FEMA might have evolved into an "oversized entitlement program" and that expectations for FEMA "may have ballooned beyond what is an appropriate level." The not-so-implicit suggestion of the new FEMA director was that perhaps FEMA could be cut back, and Congress followed his lead.
17. They issued a press release and held a press conference. Just a few reporters showed up and it went unreported in the press, which was focused on individual catastrophes, small acts of heroism, and the government's bungled response. Schur, Bradbury, Goldman, O'Brien, and Harris supported building the AKSA. While organizing to address urgent local problems, the AKSA met by phone and drafted a united platform, which they announced in late October to the national press via teleconference. Stories appeared in newspapers across the country, but ACORN staff and leaders were upset that some of them failed to refer to ACORN. Rathke always wanted to project the ACORN brand to gain name recognition, which in turn helped to build the organization, wield influence, and raise money from foundations. Soon after the teleconference, they brought their platform to elected officials in Washington, D.C., and around the country through various media events, lobbying meetings, and rallies. AKSA hoped to put public pressure on government at all levels and negotiate with FEMA to provide housing assistance to displaced survivors as well as other disaster relief. On October 28 ACORN along with its allies sponsored a rally of a thousand people on the capitol steps in Baton Rouge to demand that the state coordinate its response to Katrina with New Orleans and FEMA. None of the events seemed to budge the governor, the state legislators, or members of Congress.
18. James Dao, "Study Says 80% of New Orleans Blacks May Not Return," *New York Times*, January 27, 2006.

19. Miriam Axel-Lute, "Picking Up the Pieces," *Shelterforce*, Spring 2006, *www.nhi.org/online/issues/145/pickinguppieces.html.*
20. Several of the religious organizations faced especially difficult challenges. The priests, nuns, or ministers ran their congregations. When the churches were washed away, the clerics went with them. Sixty Methodists pastors in New Orleans were left churchless. Rev. Fred Luther, pastor of the seven-thousand-member Franklin Avenue Baptist Church, the largest African American congregation in the Southern Baptist denomination, relocated to Birmingham and preached throughout the South while the doors of his New Orleans church remained shuttered—until after Thanksgiving 2005. At a meeting of Katrina survivors in New York City, Rathke ran into a Muslim Imam whose mosque was located several blocks from the New Orleans ACORN office, who told Rathke that he would remain in New York for quite a long time. The dues paid to faith-based community organizations such as the PICO and IAF affiliates in the New Orleans area came from congregations. When these institutions did not exist, neither did the membership base under them. Rathke's strategy of building an organization of individual dues payers was perhaps looking better and smarter.
21. Christopher Cooper, "Old-Line Families Escape Worst of Flood and Plot the Future," *Wall Street Journal*, September 8, 2005.
22. Associated Press, "Harsh Urban Renewal in New Orleans: Poor, Black Residents Cannot Afford to Return, Worry City Will Exclude Them," October 12, 2005.
23. The poor and working class of New Orleans needed a large-scale federal public program similar to a Truman-like Marshall Plan or a New Deal Civilian Conservation Corps that could build the category five levees, renovate and build affordable housing, employ evacuees, and restore the city's economy. New Orleans could not rely on the market. Economists such as Robert Reich correctly pointed out that there was no incentive for the private market to move back or reopen a business or invest, "because no one can be sure there will be enough other people moving back, reopening and investing to make it worthwhile." Robert B. Reich, "Chickens and Eggs in New Orleans: How a Republican Congressman from Louisiana Plans to Rebuild New Orleans," *American Prospect*, February 16, 2006.
24. The lawsuit charged that the city wanted to raze houses without properly notifying the owners or allowing them the opportunity to appeal. After that confrontation, city officials agreed to a legal settlement binding them to a fairer notification process for homes on the teardown list. "Our first priority is to secure and ensure the safety of all people," Mayor C. Ray Nagin said in a press release, after the settlement. January 19, 2006, *www.cityofno.com/pg-1-66-press-releases.aspx?pressid=3397.*
25. Rathke liked to think the location of the office, 1024 Elysian Fields, symbolized ACORN's future prospects. Elysian Fields in Greek mythology is the final resting place of the heroic and the virtuous. Elysian Fields is also the street on which Tennessee Williams's play *A Streetcar Named Desire* is set and symbolized the déclassé netherworld for Blanche Dubois and Stanley and Stella Kowalski.

Chapter 15
A Rich Gumbo

In addition to sources noted at the beginning of the notes to Chapter 14, much of the information for this chapter came from my in-person or telephone interviews and e-mail exchanges with ACORN staff and members and former members. During the period covered in this chapter I consulted many websites, including the Metropolitan Organization, *www.tmohouston.net*; the Jeremiah Group, *jeremiahgroupNO@yahoo.com*; PICO Louisiana Interfaiths Together, *www.piconetwork.org/index-1.html*; ACORN Katrina Relief, *www.acorn.org/index.php?id=9704*; New Orleans Network, *www.neworleansnetwork.org*; Greater New Orleans Community Data Center, *www.gnocdc.org/index.html*; National Housing Institute, *www.nhi.org/resources/katrina/*; and People's Hurricane Relief Fund and Oversight Coalition, *www.communitylaborunited.net*. All these groups made important efforts in helping to save New Orleans for the residents who were forced to evacuate.

1. Brinkley quoted in Deborah Sontag, "Delery Street: Keepers of the Culture; When the Lower Ninth Posed Proudly," *New York Times*, February 9, 2006; Ebbert quoted in Dan Baum, "The Lost Year: Behind the Failure to Rebuild," *New Yorker*, August 21, 2006. Public officials repeated the falsity that the Lower Ninth was the "lowest-lying area." After the storm, Lakeview, an upscale white neighborhood, had lain under deeper water than had the Ninth.
2. James Dao, "Study Says 80% of New Orleans Blacks May Not Return," *New York Times*, January 27, 2006. Dao quotes Elliott B. Stonecipher, a political consultant and demographer from Shreveport, who predicted people wouldn't return: "Unless New Orleans built housing in flood-protected areas for low-income residents, and also provided support for poor people to relocate, chances were good that many low-income blacks would not return." If they didn't have enough resources to get out before the storm, Stonecipher said, "how can we expect them to have the wherewithal to return?"
3. Homeowners whose neighborhood was turned into a park or wetland would get 60 percent of the equity on their house from the money coming from the federal legislation introduced by Louisiana congressman Richard Baker, whose bill was still pending in Congress; the other 40 percent would come from funds controlled by the Louisiana governor. Howard, dissenting from her own BNOB group, was enraged for a reason opposite ACORN's. She opposed any compromise to the ULI's plan. "If you let people go back and rebuild wherever they want, you just—it's an invitation to just terrible blight." Sean Reilly, one of the Louisiana Recovery Authority members, emphasized on a radio interview on NPR that New Orleans leaders had to make some difficult decisions and they had to make them now, not wait for a year: "The people in New Orleans, the victims, are looking for guidance, they are looking for leadership, they are looking for elected officials that will stand up, paint a realistic future, and make decisions based upon it. I know that's where I would be if I were a flood victim down in New Orleans. I would like to know: 'What are my options? What can I do now?' You know, that will take some leadership." Reilly wanted the state to withhold from anyplace that was very low-lying the $6.2 billion dollars for housing that the state just received from the federal government. *All Things Considered*, NPR, January 10, 2006.
4. Douglas Brinkley, in *The Great Deluge: Hurricane Katrina, New Orleans, and the Mississippi Gulf Coast* (New York: William Morrow, 2006), assailed Nagin for his lack of response to Hurricane Katrina.
5. Dan Baum, "The Lost Year," *New Yorker*, August, 21, 2006; Gerard Shields, "Recovery Plan 'Dead,'" *Advocate*, January, 25, 2006, *www.2theadvocate.com/news/2228001.html*.
6. Linton Weeks, "The Big Easy? Now It's Limbo Land," *Washington Post*, February 9, 2006.
7. Petula Dvorak, "Hurricane Victims Demand More Help: Survivors Say Federal Government Not Doing Enough to Aid Rebuilding," *Washington Post*, February 9, 2006.
8. Cathy Booth Thomas, "New Orleans Mayor's Newest Foe," *Time*, February 1, 2006.
9. Most of the ACORN staff and its longtime leaders had no use for Nagin. Beth Butler called him the "dandy of the elites" because of his close ties to the white business establishment. Nagin didn't oppose ACORN and sometimes supported its campaigns. But Nagin was anti-union and an unreliable ally in ACORN's efforts to reduce poverty and promote equality. ACORN, working in coalition with labor, including its sister organization SEIU Local 100, prevented Nagin's three-year attempt to privatize the city's water supply. In a close vote, the Sewer and Water Board rejected bids from private companies to manage the city's water. According to the public interest research group Public Citizen, water privatization would have fostered corruption and resulted in rate hikes, inadequate customer service, and a loss of local control and accountability. See Public Citizen, "New Orleans Water Privatization Bids Defeated, Consumer Advocacy Groups Laud Board's Decision," October 16, 2002, *www.citizen.org/pressroom/release.cfm?ID=1241*.
10. One polling location on Eastover Drive in New Orleans East, a predominantly black

neighborhood, was the bare skeleton of a building, with exposed wiring and no walls. Several buildings couldn't accommodate the disabled, including one with a zigzagging set of fifteen stairs. According to one civil rights attorney, a majority of the seventy-six polling sites did not meet the requirements of the Americans with Disabilities Act due to uneven sidewalks, absence of wheelchair ramps, and inadequate parking. The most important election in New Orleans's history was coming, and public officials were reluctant to do everything to ensure a big turnout by displaced voters.

11. ACORN had affiliated tax-exempt corporations, such as the Institute for Social Justice and ACORN Housing.
12. Some observers saw ten thousand as a positive sign. See Brian Thevenot, "Absentee Voters' Interest Is Brisk; But How Many Cast Ballot Is Big Question," *New Orleans Times-Picayune*, April 3, 2006; see also Salatheia Bryant, "Evacuees Make Road Trip to Vote, Two Buses Take about 110 People from Houston to Polls in Louisiana," *Houston Chronicle*, April 11, 2007.
13. Tracy Clark-Flory, "Deficient Polling Places and Confusing Absentee Ballots Could Shut Thousands of Black Residents out of the City's Mayoral Election," *Salon*, April 15, 2006, *salon.com/news/feature/2006/04/15/neworleans_vote/index.html*.
14. Kim Cobb and Kristen Mack, "New Orleans Mayoral Election, Black Voters Made Their Presence Felt: Predictions of Large Racial Shift in City Politics Prove Unfounded," *Houston Chronicle*, April 24, 2006.
15. Ibid.
16. Juan A. Lozano, "Evacuee Voters Caravan to New Orleans for Mayoral Election," Associated Press, May 11, 2006.
17. Susan Saulny, "A Legacy of the Storm: Depression and Suicide," *New York Times*, June 21, 2006, *www.nytimes.com/2006/06/21/us/21depress.html?ex=1159675200&en=830c4ffbca c022fc&ei=5070*; Susan Saulny, "After Long Stress, Newsman in New Orleans Unravels," *New York Times*, August 10, 2006. New Orleans residents suffered from persistent feelings of sadness, hopelessness, and stress-related illnesses. Mental health care for survivors was nearly nonexistent.
18. Jesse Muhammad, "Post-Katrina Survival: The Struggle Continues," *FinalCall.com News*, *www.finalcall.com/artman/publish/article_2819.shtml*; see also C. C. Campbell-Rock and Hazel Trice Edney, "Nagin Re-elected but City Faces Serious Problems," *Carolina Peacemaker*, May 23, 2006.
19. Governor Kathleen Blanco and the Louisiana Recovery Authority (LRA), convinced that the city's efforts were insufficient, persuaded the Rockefeller Foundation to provide a $3.5 million grant to pay for a new planning process.
20. NOCSF said ACORN had "exceptional capacity" for planning. ACORN was also one of just five teams that were selected to work at both the neighborhood and larger district planning level.
21. Nicolai Ouroussoff, "In New Orleans, Each Resident Is Master of Plan to Rebuild," *New York Times*, August 8, 2006.
22. Ibid.
23. ACORN member Bo Fields pleaded: "August 29 should be a day for remembering our loved ones lost to the disasters following Hurricane Katrina, not a date for worrying about whether or not you have a house to return to. Show some compassion." The City Council tried to tone down the opposition by pointing to its new Good Neighbor Plan, which sought to educate owners of blighted properties on their options: gut, remediate and board up; renovate or rebuild; or demolish. Part of the plan involved an electronic database through its website on which residents and civic groups could post the addresses of buildings that appeared to be potential public nuisances or in imminent danger of collapse. The city then would verify the condition of the properties and, if warranted, notify the owners to take action.
24. Nicolai Ouroussoff, "High Noon in New Orleans: The Bulldozers Are Ready," *New York Times*, January 19, 2007.
25. In a news release, Lee said: "We regret having to make this decision as we were looking

forward to working with ACORN and their team of experienced consultants. However, even a perceived conflict of interest is not acceptable in a situation where so many community concerns have been raised." Author files.

26. Amy S. Clark, "Judge: FEMA Must Resume Katrina Payments: Agency Abruptly Ended 18-Month Housing Program in August," *Associated Press*, November 29, 2006.
27. "Senate Studies Katrina Rebuilding," Associated Press, January 29, 2007.
28. Even Adam Nossiter of the *New York Times*, who mostly ignored ACORN's work, covered the event. See Nossiter, "In New Orleans, Progress at Last in the Lower Ninth Ward," *New York Times*, February 23, 2007. See also Wade Rathke, *The Battle for the Lower 9th: ACORN and the Rebuilding of New Orleans* (London: Verso, in press).
29. Nossiter, "In New Orleans, Progress at Last."
30. See for example, Richard Morin and Lisa Rein, "Some of the Uprooted Won't Go Home Again," *Washington Post*, September 16, 2005.
31. Rathke, *The Battle for the Lower 9th.*
32. Ibid.
33. Adam Nossiter, "Steering New Orleans's Recovery with a Clinical Eye," *New York Times*, April 10, 2007.
34. Michelle Krupa and Frank Donze, "Leaders Stand United Behind Recovery Plan: Blueprint Addresses Fears of Abandonment," *New Orleans Times-Picayune*, March 30, 2007.

Chapter 16
The Right to Vote

The information for this chapter is partly based on my in-person and telephone interviews and e-mail exchanges with ACORN staff, including Mathew Henderson, Nathan Henderson-James, Brian Kettenring, and Kevin Whelan, as well as with numerous members and canvassers, Mike Slater from Project Vote, and Ellen Roggemann, a student at Occidental College, who was a participant in the Florida voter registration campaign. Some information comes from my telephone and in-person interviews with ACORN staffer Carolyn Carr, who has been with ACORN from the early 1970s. I also interviewed Lorraine C. Minnite, an assistant professor at Barnard College, Columbia University, an expert on voter fraud. The chapter is also based on information from several lawyers involved in the litigation against ACORN, including Brian Mellor, senior counsel of Project Vote; Faith Gay of White and Case; and John Boyd. The chapter also relies on David Iglesias's book, *In Justice: An Insider's Account of the War on Law and Truth in the Executive Branch* (San Francisco: Wiley, 2008), and documents released on August 11, 2009, by the House judiciary committee. The committee released over five thousand pages of White House and Republican National Committee e-mails, with transcripts of closed-door testimony by political advisor Karl Rove and counsel Harriet Miers. See U.S. House of Representatives, Committee on the Judiciary, "House Judiciary Committee Releases Rove and Miers Interview Transcripts and Over 5,400 Pages of Bush White House Documents," press release, August 11, 2009, *judiciary.house.gov/news/090811.html*; Carrie Johnson, "Miers Told House Panel of 'Agitated' Rove: Bush White House Counsel Said Adviser Called U.S. Attorney a 'Serious Problem, *Washington Post*, August 12, 2009.

1. The following sources deal with the Republican Party's voter suppression tactics: Donna Brazile, "New U.S. Attorneys Seem to Have Partisan Records," *Roll Call*, April 17, 2007; Greg Gorden, "Gonzales Should Answer Questions on Voter Fraud," *McClatchy Washington Bureau*, March 23, 2007; Greg Gordon, Margaret Talev, and Marisa Taylor, "Justice's New U.S. Attorneys Have Partisan Records," *McClatchy Newspapers*, March 23, 2007; Greg Gordon, "Restricting Turnout to Help GOP Has Been Federal Goal, Officials, Documents Show," *McClatchy Washington Bureau*, April 19, 2007; Joseph D. Rich, "Bush's Long History of Tilting Justice: The Administration Began Skewing Federal Law Enforcement before the Current U.S. Attorney Scandal," *Los Angeles Times*,

March 29, 2007 (Rich was chief of the voting section in the Justice Department's Civil Rights Division from 1999 to 2005); Steven Rosenfeld, "Project Vote Report Accuses GOP of Decades of Voter Suppression," *AlterNet*, September 27, 2007, *www.alternet.org/rights/63574/*; Steven Rosenfeld, "Turning Back the Clock on Voting Rights," *Social Policy*, Fall 2007, *www.socialpolicy.org/fileadmin/SocialPolicy/images/voting_rights_article.pdf.*

2. Absentee balloting also differs from state to state. See Teresa James, "Your Ballot's in the Mail: Vote by Mail and Absentee Voting," Project Vote, July 9, 2007, *www.electionreformproject.org/Resources/adb77fd9-cf1f-46f9-a6f2-e6c8aa5c4d0e/r1/Detail.aspx.* A partisan challenger at the polls can dispute the eligibility of a voter, and the rules for such challenges are even more irregular across states than the rules for absentee balloting. The complicated rules and the delegation of authority to states prevent people from voting and increase the likelihood of an unintentional illegal vote.
3. For details regarding the burdens facing citizens seeking to register to vote, see National Election Commission, *Report of the Task Force on the Federal Election System*, chapter 2, "Voter Registration," July 2001, *www.tcf.org/Publications/ election reform/ncfer/hansen_chap2_voter.pdf.* The National Voter Registration Act (the Motor Voter law) requires each state to provide individuals with the opportunity to register to vote when they visit government agencies and when they apply for a driver's license or seek to renew one; but some states have not complied with federal law and where states have complied, the forms are often not available.
4. Donald P. Green, "Mobilizing African-Americans Using Direct Mail and Commercial Phone Banks: A Field Experiment," *Political Research Quarterly* 57, 2 (2004): 245–55; Donald P. Green, Alan S. Gerber, and David W. Nickerson, "Getting Out the Vote in Local Elections: Results from Six Door-to-Door Canvassing Experiments," *Journal of Politics* 65, 4 (2003): 1083–96; Julia Azari and Ebonya Washington, "Results from a 2004 Leafleting Field Experiment in Miami-Dade and Duval Counties, Florida," Institution for Social and Policy Studies, Yale University, 2006, author files.
5. This account of what happened in Florida is partly based on the following newspaper accounts and news releases, as well as the complaints, answers, affirmative defenses, counterclaims, depositions, and court orders of the following court cases: *Charles Rousseau et al. v. Acorn*, U.S. District Court, Southern District of Florida, Miami Division, Case No. 04-61636-civ (2004); *Mac Stuart v. Acorn*, U.S. District Court, Southern District of Florida, Miami Division, Case No. 04-2276-civ (2004); deposition of Mac Stuart, January 12 and 13, 2005; American Center for Voting Rights, "Vote Fraud, Intimidation and Suppression in the 2004 Presidential Election," *ACVR Legislative Fund Report*, August 2, 2005, 41–44, *www.ac4vr.com/reports/072005/080205report.pdf*; Brendan Farrington, "Accusations of Fraud, Wrongdoing Abound Ahead of Nov. 2 Election," Associated Press, October 10, 2004; Fox News, *Fox News Special Report with Brit Hume*, "Democrat Voter Fraud Watch: Former ACORN Employee on Questionable Voter Registrations," October 27, 2004; Meghan Clyne, "Acorn and the Money Tree," *National Review Online*, October 31, 2004; Joni James, "Voter Fraud Charges Collapse, Judges' Rulings Negate a Fired Worker's Claims That the Grass Roots Group ACORN Mishandled Voter Registrations," *St. Petersburg Times*, December 15, 2005; Lucy Morgan, "Group Faces Accusations of Broken Voting Laws," *St. Petersburg Times*, October 22, 2004; Jeremy Milarsky, "Ex-Worker Sues Activist Group," *South Florida Sun-Sentinel*, October 21, 2004; ACORN, "ACORN Defeats Anti-Voter Legal Attacks: Group's Voter Registration Efforts Vindicated as Baseless Lawsuits Collapse," press release, December 14, 2005; Project Vote, "One Year Later: Results of 2004 Voter Fraud Investigations Give Vote Groups a Clean Slate, Community Group Vindicated as Baseless Lawsuits, Investigations Collapse," press release, December 15, 2005; Florida Department of Law Enforcement, "FDLE Investigates Statewide Voter Fraud," press release, October 21, 2004; Ellen Roggemann, "Tale of Two Organizers," December 29, 2004, unpublished paper in author's possession; Jerry Seper and Donald Lambro, "Anti-Bush Registration Drive Stirs Fraud Concerns: Party Memo Urges 'Pre-emptive Strikes' on GOP," *Washington Times*, October 15, 2004; Terrence Scanlon, "Democratic Deception; Acorn's Fraud Could Taint Elections, *Washington*

Times, October 19, 2004; Paige St. John, "Rumors of Vote Fraud Rampant," *Florida Today*, October 2, 2004); Brittany Wallman and Alva James-Johnson, "Filled-In Voter Forms Surface," *South Florida Sun-Sentinel*, October 27, 2004; Brittany Wallman, "Group Sued over Alleged Disenfranchisement of Felons," *South Florida Sun-Sentinel*, October 29, 2004; Brittany Wallman, "Voter Registration Drive a Subterfuge, Lawsuit Claims," *South Florida Sun-Sentinel*, October 30, 2004; Tom Zucco, "Activist Group Blamed for Voter Roll Goofs," *St. Petersburg Times*, October 4, 2004.

6. Ford Fessenden, "A Big Increase of New Voters in Swing States," *New York Times*, September 26, 2004.
7. Florida Department of Law Enforcement, "FDLE Investigates Statewide Voter Fraud," press release, October 21, 2004.
8. Terrence Scanlon, "Democratic Deception; Acorn's Fraud Could Taint Elections," *Washington Times*, October 19, 2004.
9. Fox News, *Fox News Special Report with Brit Hume*, "Democrat Voter Fraud Watch: Former ACORN Employee on Questionable Voter Registrations," Fox News transcript, October 27, 2004.
10. Robert Trigaux, "Ten Who Made a Splash," *St. Petersburg Times*, December 13, 2004.
11. *Mac Stuart v. Acorn*, U.S. District Court, Southern District of Florida, Miami Division, Case No. 04-2276-civ (2004). Deposition of Mac Stuart, January 12 and 13, 2005.
12. This account of what happened in New Mexico is partly based on the following newspaper accounts, news releases, and court records: *Larry Larranaga et al. v. Mary E. Herrera, Bernalillo County Clerk, and Rebecca Vigil-Giron, New Mexico Secretary of State*, Second Judicial District Court, Bernalillo County, New Mexico, District Court No. CV-2004-05391, September 8, 2004; ACORN, "ACORN Denounces Republican Party Deceit," press release, September 29, 2004; Shea Andersen, "More Glare on Voter Sign-Ups," *Albuquerque Tribune*, August 25, 2004; Shea Andersen, "Mischief Reports Justify Probes," *Albuquerque Tribune*, September 9, 2004; Shea Andersen, "Group Stands Firm in Bid for Sign-Ups," *Albuquerque Tribune*, September 10, 2004; Ed Asher, "Task Force Will Eye Voter Fraud," *Albuquerque Tribune*, September 8, 2004; Associated Press, "Court Orders Inspection of Voter Registrations," September 30, 2004; Jo Becker and Dan Eggen, "Voter Probes Raise Partisan Suspicions: Democrats, Allies See Politics Affecting Justice Department's Anti-Fraud Efforts," *Washington Post*, September 20, 2004; Michael Coleman, "Gripes about Iglesias Not New: E-Mails Show Long History of Complaints," *Albuquerque Journal*, March 15, 2007; Christopher Drew and Eric Lipton, "G.O.P. Anger in Swing State Eased Attorney's Exit," *New York Times*, March 18, 2007; "Phony Fraud Charges," editorial, *New York Times*, March 16, 2007; Michael Gisick, "GOP VIPs Ponder David Iglesias Fallout," *Albuquerque Tribune*, March 3, 2007; Sue Major Holmes, "Voter ID Case Heads to Court, Could Affect Thousands," Associated Press, September 2, 2004; Andy Lenderman, "3 GOP Candidates Want Voter Records," *Albuquerque Journal*, September 15, 2004; Andy Lenderman, "Court Gets Voter Registration Lawsuit," *Albuquerque Journal*, September 30, 2004; Andy Lenderman, "Fight over Voter ID Heats Up," *Albuquerque Journal*, September 19, 2004; Dan McKay, "Bernalillo Thinks Forms May Be Fake: Sheriff Wants Voter Card Probe," *Albuquerque Journal*, August 6, 2004; Dan McKay, "Too Young to Vote," *Albuquerque Journal*, August 20, 2004; Dan McKay, "'Dad of Voter' Joins Suit to Require IDs," *Albuquerque Journal*, August 25, 2004; Dan McKay, "Election 'Mischief' under Scrutiny," *Albuquerque Journal*, September 10, 2004; Dan McKay and Andy Lenderman, "County's Early-Polling Places 'Slammed' with Voters, Calls," *Albuquerque Journal*, October 19, 2004; Margaret Talev, "Bush, Gonzales Reportedly Discussed Fired Prosecutor," *McClatchy Newspapers*, April 17, 2007; Adrian Vigil, "Voter ID Hearing Was Nothing More Than a Ruse," *Las Cruces Sun-News*, August 8, 2006.
13. Dan McKay, "Bernalillo Thinks Forms May Be Fake; Sheriff Wants Voter Card Probe," *Albuquerque Journal*, August 6, 2004.
14. Dan McKay, "'Dad of Voter' Joins Suit to Require IDs," *Albuquerque Journal*, August 25, 2004.

15. One woman had told an ACORN canvasser that she might already be registered. She testified that the canvasser replied, "If you're not sure, register, and if there were duplicates only one would be recorded." It turned out that she had in fact registered previously. No fraud was intended. Another instance involved a couple who had registered but had not received their cards. Worried that their applications had been lost, the husband returned to a street-corner registration table, filled out two new forms. and signed his wife's name, with her permission. Robert Kennedy and Greg Palast went through the names the GOP asserted were "obviously, undeniably and clearly fraudulent" voter registrations. Among these was that of Melissa Tais, whom the GOP claimed was a dubious ACORN registrant; the reporters' conclusion: "Her two voter registration forms show, admittedly, suspiciously different signatures. Republicans suggested Melissa was part of a massive fraud to allow Democrats to vote twice. They were wrong. Ms. Tais, a Cerrillos, New Mexico, waitress, told us she had signed one form on a table and one form holding the paper in her hand. Hence, a second, wobbly signature. Then there was Patricia White, who Republicans claimed was a fictitious voter. When we filmed her at home in Albuquerque, she seemed real enough." See Robert Kennedy and Greg Palast, "Drinking the ACORN Kool-Aid: How Cries of Voter Fraud Cover Up GOP Elections Theft," *Huffington Post*, October 28, 2008.
16. ACORN, "ACORN Denounces Republican Party Deceit," press release, September 29, 2004.
17. "We took over 100 complaints" from the GOP, Iglesias told Robert Kennedy and Greg Palast of the *Huffington Post*. "We investigated for almost 2 years, I didn't find one prosecutable voter fraud case in the entire state of New Mexico." Iglesias, a John McCain supporter, also told Kennedy and Palast that despite finding none of the voters guilty, the White House nevertheless ordered him to illegally prosecute baseless cases against innocent citizens, just to gin up voter-fraud publicity. His refusal, he said, cost him his job. "They were looking for politicized—for improperly politicized US attorneys to file bogus voter fraud cases." See Kennedy and Palast, "Drinking the ACORN Kool-Aid." For more information, see SourceWatch, "Bush Administration's U.S. Attorney Firings Controversy," *www.sourcewatch.org/index.php?title=Bush_administration_phony_%27voter_fraud%27*.
18. Lorraine Minnite, "The Politics of Voter Fraud," report to Project Vote, March 2007, *www.projectvote.org*; "Phony Fraud Charges," editorial, *New York Times*, March 16, 2007.
19. False allegations of voter fraud were recycled in conservative and Republican Internet sites, plus conservative periodicals and news organizations like Fox News, the *National Review*, the *American Spectator*, and the op-ed pages of the *Wall Street Journal*. As Peter Dreier and Christopher Martin document in their report *Manipulating the Public Agenda: Why ACORN Was in the News, and What the News Got Wrong*," September 23, 2009, *www.uepi.oxy.edu/acornstudy*, this concerted action is the classic modus operandi of an "echo chamber." Here are a few examples. The conservative public relations outfit Berman and Company through the website *LaborPains.org* had a March 19, 2007, posting titled "Prosecutors Eye Union-Backed ACORN (Again)": "We've discussed before the union-backed group ACORN, which has been tied to voter fraud in more than a dozen states in recent years. . . . News from this weekend suggests that systematic voter fraud is fact, not myth. The [*New York*] *Times* reports that one of the federal prosecutors mired in a political mess failed to investigate ACORN in a meaningful way for its repeated (and galling) shenanigans in New Mexico." In fact the posting misinterpreted the *New York Times* story it referenced. The *Times* story was about David Iglesias, the federal prosecutor in New Mexico who didn't find merit in charges of voter fraud against ACORN despite the urgings of his state's Republican Party officials, and he was one of the federal attorneys fired. "I thought I was insulated from politics," Iglesias said. "But now I find out that main Justice was up to its eyeballs in partisan political maneuvering." See Christopher Drew and Eric Lipton, "G.O.P. Anger in Swing State Eased Attorney's Exit," *New York Times*, March 18, 2007. The effect of the LaborPains posting was to keep repeating misinformation about ACORN to make a controversy seem legitimate. Later

in 2007, *Investor's Business Daily*, a conservative business newspaper, repeated more misrepresentations: "ACORN has been accused of voter fraud in 13 states since 2004 and was convicted of falsifying signatures in a voter registration drive last July, drawing a fine of $25,000 in Washington state," stated an editorial that was often repeated around the conservative blogosphere as evidence of evil at ACORN. See "George Soros: The Man, the Mind, and the Money behind MoveOn," editorial, *Investor's Business Daily*, September 20, 2007. But accusations don't amount to wrongdoing and, as the *Seattle Times* reported, it was rogue ACORN employees who falsified voter registrations: The defendants "concocted the scheme as an easy way to get paid, not as an attempt to influence the outcome of elections, King County Prosecuting Attorney Dan Satterberg said." ACORN agreed to pay $25,000 to King County for investigative costs. See Keith Ervin, "Felony Charges Filed against 7 in State's Biggest Case of Voter-Registration Fraud," *Seattle Times*, July 26, 2007, *seattletimes.nwsource.com/html/localnews/2003806904_webvotefraud26m.html.* Conservative publicist and Republican strategist David Horowitz added to the efforts to stigmatize ACORN with his "DiscoverTheNetworks.org: A Guide to the Political Left" website that he launched in early 2005. The profile for ACORN included this deceptive and misleading description: "Was implicated in numerous reports of fraudulent voter registration, vote-rigging, voter intimidation, and vote-for-pay scams during recent election cycles." DiscoverTheNetworks.org: A Guide to the Political Left, "Association of Community Organizations for Reform Now," *www.discoverthenetworks.org/groupProfile.asp?grpid=6968* (accessed June 20, 2009).

20. In 1981, New Jersey civil rights groups protested the Republican Party's use of armed guards to challenge Hispanic and African American voters and exposed a plan to disqualify voters using mass mailings of outdated voter lists. The federal courts stopped the practice, calling it an illegal attempt to suppress voter participation based on race. Six years later, similar "ballot security" schemes were launched against minority voters in Louisiana, Georgia, Missouri, Pennsylvania, Michigan, and Indiana. Republican National Committee documents bragged that a Louisiana plan would "eliminate at least 60-80,000 [black] folks from the rolls." See Chandler Davidson, *Race and Class in Texas Politics* (Princeton, N.J.: Princeton University Press, 1992). Three years later, in North Carolina, the state Republican Party and the Helms for Senate Committee sent postcards to 120,000 African American voters, lying about voter eligibility and threatening them with criminal penalties for voter fraud. See also People for the American Way Foundation, "Voter Intimidation and Suppression in America Today: The Long Shadow of Jim Crow," People for the American Way (*www.pfaw.org*) and NAACP (*www.naacp.org*), *site.pfaw.org/site/PageServer?pagename=report_the_long_shadow_of_jim_crow*.
21. Despite Indiana's officials conceding that only one individual was guilty of in-person voter fraud in the last hundred years, on April 28, 2008, the U.S. Supreme Court in *Crawford v. Marion County Election Board* upheld Indiana's restrictive voter-ID law, which "threatens to impose nontrivial burdens on the voting rights of tens of thousands of the state's citizens," according to the dissenting opinion of Justice Souter. See Steven Rosenfeld, "Voter Purging: A Legal Way for Republicans to Swing Elections?" *AlterNet*, September 11, 2007. Purging voters rather than registering them became the official policy of Bush's Department of Justice, whose Voting Section chief, John Tanner, in the spring of 2007 pressured ten states to purge their voter rolls before the 2008 election, which disqualified thousands of voters. In Florida and Missouri in 2000, 100,000 legal voters were wrongly removed. In Cleveland in 2004, voter purges caused long lines, and people left without voting. In 2006 the Maryland Republican Party gave activists a manual with false information about voters' rights, and based on that information told them to challenge voters and warn poll workers and election judges they could face jail time if a challenge is ignored. The GOP hype has had its intended effect. Nearly thirty states have passed voter ID or proof-of-citizenship laws or are considering them. A recent University of Washington study estimates that more than 20 percent of the state's black voters lack required ID, compared to 15.8 percent of white voters. See Wendy Weiser, "Recent Voter Suppression Incidents," Brennan Center for Social Justice, October 22, 2008, *brennan.3cdn.net/a9dfd09c356bb55d6b_fnm6bnf57.pdf.*

22. Various polls have shown that election outcomes change dramatically depending on how many minority voters cast ballots. For example, in the 2006 gubernatorial race in Maryland a *Washington Post* poll, taken just before the election measured black turnout at 25 percent. It showed Baltimore mayor Martin O'Malley (D) with a lead of 10 percentage points over Gov. Robert L. Ehrlich Jr. (R). Another poll published just before the election by the *Baltimore Sun* that assumed a smaller black turnout—19 percent—showed the race as a statistical dead heat. Matthew Mosk, "Md. Democrats Say GOP Plans to Block Voters," *Washington Post*, November 2, 2006. See also Donald P. Green and Melissa R Michelson, "ACORN Experiments in Minority Voter Mobilization," in *The People Shall Rule: ACORN, Community Organizing, and the Struggle for Economic Justice*, ed. Robert Fisher (Nashville: Vanderbilt University Press, 2009). According to Green and Michelson: "Historically underrepresented minority groups are therefore often underrepresented at the city and state level, both in terms of descriptive representation and policy preferences" (235). See also Z. Hajnal and J. Trounstine, "Turnout Matters: Voter Turnout and City Spending Priorities." Paper presented at the annual meeting of the Midwest Political Science Association, Chicago, April 15–18, 2004.
23. Clinton, *Giving: How Each of Us Can Change the World* (New York: Knopf 2007). Referring to New Orleans after Katrina, Clinton writes: "About the same time, in the Lower Ninth Ward, which was virtually wiped out by Katrina, volunteers turned the first new homes over to residents. Built of pine, elevated five feet, and designed to resist hurricane winds, the houses cost only $125,000 each. The project was organized by ACORN (Association of Community Organizations for Reform Now), which also provided the financing with support from a California bank. ACORN works to empower low-and-moderate income people through the grassroots activism of more than 200,000 members in one hundred communities all over America" (51). Later in the book: "After Katrina hit the Gulf Coast, Operation HOPE joined my foundation and ACORN, an NGO of grassroots activists committed to empowering poor people, to assist eligible survivors to claim the earned income tax credit. Together HOPE and ACORN helped people secure more than $10 million to which they were entitled but for which they had to apply" (79).
24. As Fred Brooks points out: "The issue of providing individual services historically has been a major dilemma for social action, Alinsky-style community organizations." Prominent organizing strategists Kim Bobo, Jacky Kendall, and Steve Max even argued that because an organization needs a clear mission, it should never combine services and organizing. Action organizations that provide services invariably lose their direct action and power-building path. For over two decades ACORN was able to incorporate the provision of individual services such as tax preparation, welfare advocacy, and homeownership counseling into its model without sacrificing its ability to mobilize low- and moderate-income people to build power and win issues by challenging government and business. See Fred Brooks, "Resolving the Dilemma between Organizing and Services: Los Angeles ACORN's Welfare Advocacy," *Social Work*, July 1, 2005; and K. Bobo, J. Kendall, and S. Max, *Organizing for Social Change: Midwest Academy Manual for Activists* (Santa Ana, Calif.: Seven Locks Press, 2001).
25. Hajnal and Trounstine, "Turnout Matters."

Chapter 17
Growing Pains

Some of the information for this chapter comes from my in-person and telephone interviews, as well as e-mail exchanges, with dozens of ACORN board members, funders, staff, former staff, Pablo Eisenberg, and Rick Cohen.

1. Sam Graham-Felsen, "ACORN Political Action Committee Endorses Obama," Organizing for America Community Blogs, February 21, 2008, *my.barackobama.com/page/community/post/samgrahamfelsen/gGC7zm*.
2. See, for example, *Association of Community Organizations for Reform Now v. Department of Industrial Relations*, 41 Cal. App. 4th 298, 301 (Cal. Ct. App. 1995).

3. Fred Brooks, "Racial Diversity on ACORN's Organizing Staff, 1970–2003," *Administration in Social Work* 31, 1 (2007).
4. Garry Wills, *Certain Trumpets: The Call of Leaders* (New York: Simon and Schuster, 1994.)
5. Along with Soros and billionaire Peter Lewis, the Sandlers fund some of the most important players of the progressive Left. Prior to 2003, Golden West was voted the nation's most admired savings institution seven times in Fortune magazine's annual list of the nation's most admired companies. The Sandlers were named "2004 CEOs of the Year" by Morningstar, Inc., which called their bank a "paragon of corporate governance." See also Joe Nocera, "Self-Made Philanthropists," *New York Times Magazine, www.nytimes.com/2008/03/09/magazine/09Sandlers-t.html?ref=magazine.*
6. Eric Eckholm, "City by City, an Antipoverty Group Plants Seeds of Change," *New York Times*, June 26, 2006.
7. Erik Eckholm, "Chicago Orders 'Big Box' Stores to Raise Wage," *New York Times*, July 27, 2006.
8. Stephanie Strom, "Funds Misappropriated at 2 Nonprofit Groups," *New York Times*, July 9, 2008.
9. Pablo Eisenberg, "After an Embezzlement, an Advocacy Group Seeks to Regain Trust," *Chronicle of Philanthropy*, October 2, 2008.
10. Rebecca Mowbray, "Lawsuit over ACORN Filed in New Orleans Court," *New Orleans Times-Picayune*, October 1, 2008.
11. John Fund, "Obama's Liberal Shock Troops," *Wall Street Journal*, July 12, 2008. Fund's accusation is misleading because right-wing activists created a public outrage and scandal by making false accusations against ACORN for committing voter fraud.
12. Consumer Rights League, "CRL Supports Senator Ensign's Call to Suspend Federal ACORN Payments in Light of Voter Fraud Raid," *www.consumersrightsleague.org/News/DocumentSingle.aspx?DocumentID=23826*. See also Sourcewatch, "Consumer Rights League," *www.sourcewatch.org/index.php/Consumers_Rights_League.*
13. Reuters, "ACORN Embezzlement Scandal Is the Latest Controversy in Group's Long, Corrupt History Says Employment Policies Institute," July 9, 2008, *www.reuters.com/article/pressRelease/idUS221224+09-Jul-2008+PRN20080709.*
14. SourceWatch, Employment Policies Institute, *www.sourcewatch.org/index.php?title=Employment_Policies_Institute.*
15. Wikipedia, "Richard Berman," *en.wikipedia.org/wiki/Richard_Berman.*
16. Thousands of additional staff were hired to call each new registrant for verification; Mellor distributed standardized coversheets for each batch of registrations and flew to meet personally with elections officials around the country to let them know exactly how the drive would proceed and that ACORN would seek their help in prosecuting any misconduct it discovered. A manager's manual distinguished how to supervise staff to reasonable levels of productivity without imposing hard and fast quotas or paying per card, which was prohibited in some states. Each canvasser had to sign a statement acknowledging that he or she would be dismissed and prosecuted for turning in any false information. In the spring of 2008 the media were invited to tour the offices and view the voter registration and quality-control system in action but showed little interest. ACORN's quality-control procedures included phone-verifying every card, flagging problematic cards, and identifying offending workers for local officials.
17. Sorting Out Fact and Fiction in the Presidential Candidates' Final Debate," *Annenberg Public Policy Center of the University of Pennsylvania*, FactChecking Debate No. 3, October 17, 2008, *www.factcheck.org/elections-2008/factchecking_debate_no_3.html; www.factcheck.org/elections-2008/acorn_accusations.html.* FactCheck.org is a project of the Annenberg Public Policy Center of the University of Pennsylvania. Established by publisher and philanthropist Walter Annenberg in 1994 to create a community of scholars within the University of Pennsylvania, APPC addresses public policy issues at the local, state, and federal levels. According to FactCheck: "There's no evidence of any such democracy-destroying fraud. Here's what is true: In recent years, ACORN employees

have been investigated multiple times for voter *registration* fraud. ACORN workers have been convicted of submitting false voter registration forms in Colorado Springs in 2005, Kansas City, Mo., in 2006 and King County, Wash., in 2007. ACORN's Las Vegas office was raided by a state criminal investigator on Oct. 7, 2008. ACORN workers were also the subjects of ongoing investigations in Wisconsin, Missouri, Ohio, Pennsylvania, and Indiana. No evidence has yet surfaced to show that the ACORN employees who submitted fraudulent registration forms intended to pave the way for illegal *voting*. Rather, they were trying to get paid by ACORN for doing no work. Dan Satterberg, the Republican prosecuting attorney in King County, Wash., where the largest ACORN case to date was prosecuted, said that the indicted ACORN employees were shirking responsibility, not plotting election fraud.

"Satterberg: '[A] joint federal and state investigation has determined that this scheme was not intended to permit illegal voting. Instead, the defendants cheated their employer, the Association of Community Organizations for Reform Now (or ACORN), to get paid for work they did not actually perform. ACORN's lax oversight of their own voter registration drive permitted this to happen. . . . It was hardly a sophisticated plan: The defendants simply realized that making up names was easier than actually canvassing the streets looking for unregistered voters. . . . [It] appears that the employees of ACORN were not performing the work that they were being paid for, and to some extent, ACORN is a victim of employee theft. The $8-an-hour employees were charged with providing false information on voter registration forms, and in one case with making a false statement to a public official. Five of the seven who were charged pleaded guilty. ACORN was fined for exercising insufficient oversight, but it was not charged with masterminding any kind of deliberate fraud.' "

18. Steven A. Holmes and Mary Pat Flaherty, "GOP Officials Assail Community Group, McCain Campaign Accuses ACORN of Voter Fraud, Highlights Ties to Obama," *Washington Post*, October 14, 2008.
19. Greg Gordo, "Death Threat, Vandalism Hit Acorn after McCain Comments," *McClatchy News*, October 17, 2008.
20. "Manipulating the Public Agenda: Why ACORN Was in the News, and What the News Got Wrong," *departments.oxy.edu/uepi/acornstudy*.
21. For example, a number of news reports made much of a voter registration card turned in to election officials in Lake County, Indiana, with the name "Jimmie Johns"—a local sandwich shop. Many of the news stories failed to report that ACORN's quality-control staff had attached a "problematic card report coversheet" that stated this very fact.
22. Lorraine Minnite, "The Politics of Voter Fraud," report to Project Vote, March 2007, *www.projectvote.org*.
23. Think Project, *thinkprogress.org/2008/10/18/cnn-acornfact-check/*; The American Prospect, *www.prospect.org/cs/articles?article=are_the_republicans_right_about_acorn*.
24. The details refuting this absurd allegation in the next five paragraphs can be found in Peter Dreier and John Atlas, "The GOP's Blame-ACORN Game," *Nation*, October 22, 2008.
25. Center on Budget and Policy Priorities, "Testimony of Robert Greenstein, Executive Director, Center on Budget and Policy Priorities," April 24, 2008, *www.cbpp.org/4-24-08climate-testimony.pdf*. About 32 percent of the U.S. population is made up of low- and moderate-income citizens. See Urban Institute, "A Profile of Americans in Low-Income Working Families," October 1, 2000, *www.urban.org/publications/309710.html*. See also Jack Newfield, "How the Other Half Still Live," *Nation*, March 17, 2003.
26. John Atlas and Peter Dreier, "ACORN under the Microscope," *Huffington Post*, July 14, 2008, *www.huffingtonpost.com/john-atlas/acorn-under-the-microscop_b_112503.html*.
27. Elizabeth Williamson and Brody Mullins, "Democratic Ally Mobilizes in Housing Crunch, Acorn Leads Drive to Register Voters Likely to Back Obama; New Federal Funds," *Wall Street Journal*, July 31, 2008, *online.wsj.com/article/SB121745181676698197.html*.

28. Peter Applebome, "Feeling the Sting of Republican Barbs," *New York Times*, September 6, 2006.
29. As noted earlier, in nearly all other democracies, the government accepts responsibility for compiling and maintaining voter-registration lists. The United States is the only major democracy that places the burden of registration almost entirely on the individual.

Chapter 18
The Prostitute and the Assault

1. See relevant clips on the website Media Matters: *mediamatters.org/mmtv/200905070034*, *mediamatters.org/mmtv/200905120032*. Beck also suggested ACORN may kill him: *mediamatters.org/mmtv/200905120032*. See also John Cook, "Glenn Beck Says ACORN Ninjas Are Trying to Kill Him," *Gawker*, May 13, 2009, *gawker.com/5252723/glenn-beck-says-acorn-ninjas-are-trying-to-kill-him*.
2. Memorandum from Celinda Lake et al., Lake Research Partners, to Bertha Lewis and Jeff Robinson, ACORN, "ACORN's Image among African American Voters," 2009. Memo is in author's possession.
3. Jim Rutenberg, "Acorn's Woes Strain Its Ties to Democrats," *New York Times*, October 15, 2009. Rutenberg looked at ACORN's substantial role in the political ecology of New York, the ability of the organization to deliver in the arena of affordable housing, and the political phenomenon of Democrats running for cover. "ACORN's housing wing was a well-established partner with the city in rehabilitating its affordable housing stock," Rutenberg writes.
4. United States Conference of Catholic Bishops, "Catholic Campaign for Human Development Ends All Funding to ACORN," press release, November 13, 2008, *www.usccb.org/comm/archives/2008/08-175.shtml*.
5. Mike Stark, "All You Need to Know about the ACORN Scandal and Who Is Behind It," *Huffington Post*, October 22, 2009, *www.huffingtonpost.com/mike-stark/all-you-need-to-know-abou_b_330643.html*; Michael Rispoli, "ACORN Sting 'Pimp' Is N.J. Man Who Attended Rutgers University," *Star Ledger*, September 17, 2009.
6. Darryl Fears, "ACORN to Review Incidents," *Washington Post*, September, 17, 2009; Kate Linthicum, "Young Conservative Activist Hannah Giles Speaks in Santa Barbara," *Los Angeles Times*, November 15, 2009.
7. James O'Keefe, "Chaos for Glory: My Time with ACORN," *Big Government*, *biggovernment.com/2009/09/10/chaos-for-glory/*.
8. James Taranto, "Taking on the 'Democrat-Media Complex': The Conservative Internet Entrepreneur on Bringing Down ACORN, Hollywood Liberals, and Embarrassing the Mainstream Media," *Wall Street Journal*, October 16, 2009.
9. "'Pimp' in ACORN Video Shares Story," *Los Angeles Times*, September 19, 2009. *www.latimes.com/news/nationworld/nation/la-na-acorn-student19-2009sep19,0,686603.story*.
10. Taranto, "Taking on the 'Democrat-Media Complex.'"
11. "Census Bureau Severs Ties With ACORN," *FoxNews.com*, September 11, 2009, *www.foxnews.com/politics/2009/09/11/census-bureau-severs-ties-acorn/*.
12. Darryl Fears, "ACORN to Review Incidents, White House Joins Criticism over Hidden-Camera Videos," *Washington Post*, September 17, 2009.
13. See the website ContractorMisconduct.org, as well as the following sources: Corporate Fraud Task Force, Report to the President, 2008, *www.justice.gov/dag/cftf/corporate-fraud2008.pdf*; Jeremy Scahill, "Pentagon Instructs Officials to Cancel Contracts with ACORN: The Problem: They Don't Exist," CommonDreams.org, *www.commondreams.org/headline/2009/10/21-9*; Mary Williams Walsh, "J. P. Morgan Settles Alabama Bribery Case," *New York Times*, November 4, 2009; Christopher Hayes, "ACORN and Accountability," *Nation*, October 12, 2009.
14. Dennis Cauchon, "In Major Flip, House Dems Now Represent Richest Regions," *USA Today*, October 14, 2009.

15. Lincoln Anderson, "Right Has ACORN on Ropes, but Fight Isn't Over: Attorney," *Villager*, October 21–27, 2009, *www.thevillager.com/villager_338/righthas.html.*
16. Murial Kane, "The Right Isn't Only Trying to Take Down ACORN, It's Got a 25-Year Project to 'Defund' the Left," *Raw Story*, October 31, 2009, *www.alternet.org/politics/143631/the_right_isn%5C%27t_only_trying_to_take_down_acorn,_it%5C%27s_got_a_25-year_project_to_%5C%27defund%5C%27_the_left?page=3.*
17. According to Media Matters, "*Washington Post* ombudsman Andrew Alexander criticized the newspaper for 'tardiness' in covering the ACORN videotape controversy, arguing that newspapers should pay more attention to right-wing media outlets and that the *Post's* purportedly slow reaction to the ACORN story is related to institutional liberal bias. In doing so, Alexander adopted the right-wing argument that the ACORN videos are a major story when, in fact, the government was not harmed as a result of ACORN's actions; the workers involved constituted a tiny fraction of ACORN's workforce; other organizations involved in scandal receive far more government funding than ACORN; and the videos are part of a longstanding effort by the right to use ACORN as a scapegoat and to distract from more important issues." See "*Post* Ombudsman Adopts Right-Wing Mantra That ACORN Videos Are a Major Story," September 20, 2009, *mediamatters.org/research/200909200015.*
18. Carol D. Leonnig and Alexi Mostrous, "For ACORN, Video Is Only Latest Crisis," *Washington Post*, September 20, 2009.
19. The *Post* reporters left the impression that ACORN was funded only by government grants and foundations, leaving out that ACORN was a dues-paying organization. When referring to the ACORN leadership's attitude toward Wade Rathke after the embezzlement, the reporters quoted minutes of a meeting saying, "Leadership has no faith in staff. Wade betrayed them," when in fact the leadership was divided over Rathke, with some board members fighting to keep him as head organizer. The *Post* claimed that ACORN had an "an expanding international presence," after it had ended its international organizing. In several articles the *Post* labeled ACORN "the liberal political organizing group," a characterization at odds with its populist and progressive tradition. Just as important were the facts the reporters left out. They failed to mention that ACORN has never been convicted of voter registration fraud. There was also no mention of Karl Rove's role in firing a U.S. attorney for failing to prosecute ACORN. The *Post* neglected to interview several scholars who had witnessed ACORN's work, written books and journal articles about it, and mostly praised it. One widely circulated Associated Press story falsely reported that $5 million, not $1 million, was embezzled from the community organization by Dale Rathke, relying on information supplied by the Louisiana attorney general Buddy Caldwell's office. The reporters did not check facts and failed to note that on June 10, 2008, ACORN issued a report grading most of the fifty state attorneys general on how they were helping consumers with the country's foreclosure crisis. Caldwell was one of the attorneys general to receive an "F," the lowest rating. See ACORN, "Statement Regarding False Assertions by Louisiana Attorney General Buddy Caldwell," press release, October 6, 2009; John O'Brian, "Dems Dominate Foreclosure Report," *LegalNewsline.com*, June 10, 2010, *legalnewsline.com/news/213359-dems-dominate-foreclosure-report*; John O'Brian, "ACORN: AG Caldwell Should Have Returned Questionnaire," *LegalNewsline.com*, June 16, 2010, *legalnewsline.com/news/213492-acorn-ag-caldwell-should-have-returned-questionnaire.*
20. Christina Hoag, "ACORN Activists Refuse to Buckle to Video Scandal," Associated Press, October 8, 2009; Judy Keen and William M. Welch, "For ACORN, Controversy Now a Matter of Survival," *USA Today*, September 24, 2009.
21. Separate from the family of connected organization, ACORN's core budget in 2008 was $25 million. The federal cuts equaled about 10 percent of that budget.
22. John O'Brian, "Dems Dominate Foreclosure Report," *LegalNewsline.com*, June 10, 2010, *legalnewsline.com/news/213359-dems-dominate-foreclosure-report*; John O'Brian, "ACORN: AG Caldwell Should Have Returned Questionnaire," *LegalNewsline.com*,

June 16, 2010, *legalnewsline.com/news/213492-acorn-ag-caldwell-should-have-returned-questionnaire.*

23. George Anastasia, "Supporters Turn Out for ACORN," *Philadelphia Inquirer*, September 26, 2009.
24. Press statement released by the Alliance for Justice, October 1, 2009.
25. Kate Linthicum, "Community Groups Band Together to Rally in Support of ACORN," *Los Angeles Times*," October 23, 2009.
26. Kareem Fahim, "ACORN Sues over Funding Voting in House, *New York Times*, November 12, 2009.
27. Scott Harshbarger and Amy Crafts, "An Independent Governance Assessment of ACORN: The Path to Meaningful Reform," December 7, 2009, *www.proskauer.com/files/uploads/report2.pdf.*
28. Joe Conason, "ACORN Videos Were Propaganda," *Salon*, December 11, 2009, *www.salon.com/opinion/conason/2009/12/11/acorn/index.html.*
29. Peter Dreier and Christopher R. Martin, "How ACORN Was Framed: Political Controversy and Media Agenda-Setting," unpublished document in author's possession.
30. Janie Lorber, "House Ban on Acorn Grants Is Ruled Unconstitutional," *New York Times*, December 11, 2009.
31. Representative John Conyers Jr., Democrat of Michigan and chairman of the House judiciary committee, requested the report along with Representative Barney Frank, Democrat of Massachusetts. Conyers released the report on Tuesday. Congressional Research Service Report, December 22, 2009, *www.scribd.com/doc/24424725/Congressional-Research-Service-Report-On-ACORN*; U.S. House of Representatives, Committee on the Judiciary, "Conyers Releases CRS Report on ACORN," press release, August 11, 2009, *judiciary.house.gov/news/091222.html*; Jake Sherman, "CRS Report: ACORN Didn't Break Law," *Politico*, December 22, 2009, *www.politico.com/news/stories/1209/30919.html.*
32. John Schwartz, "Review Finds Zero ACORN Wrongdoing," *New York Times*, December 23, 2009.
33. Peter Dreier and Christopher R. Martin, "How ACORN Was Framed: Political Controversy and Media Agenda-Setting," unpublished document in author's possession.
34. Belinda Luscombe, "Top 10 Scandals," *Time*, December 8, 2009, *www.time.com/time/specials/packages/article/0,28804,1945379_1944973_1945001,00.html*; Paul Bedard, "Top 10 Political Scandals of 2009," *U.S. News and World Report*, *www.usnews.com/news/washington-whispers/slideshows/top-10-political-scandals-of-2009/5.*
35. Pablo Eisenberg, "In Their Rush to Abandon ACORN, Many Are Ignoring Its Accomplishments," *Chronicle of Philanthropy*, October 29, 2009.
36. Katrina vanden Heuvel, "Extra, Extra—Read All about ACORN," *Nation*, January 5, 2010, *www.thenation.com/blogs/edcut/512453/extra_extra_read_all_about_acorn.*
37. Campbell Robertson and Liz Robbins, "4 Arrested in Phone Tampering at Landrieu Office," *New York Times*, January 26, 2010, *www.nytimes.com/2010/01/27/us/politics/27landrieu.html*; Ben Frumin, "Jon Stewart On James O'Keefe: 'This Guy's Getting All His Investigative Journalism Ideas From Porn Movie Plots,'" *Talking Points Memo*, January 28, 2010, *tpmlivewire.talkingpointsmemo.com/2010/01/stewart-on-acorn-sting-filmmaker-charged-in-phone-tampering-plot-this-guys-getting-all-his-investiga.php*; Robert Schlesinger, "James O'Keefe Arrested, Undercutting ACORN Allegations," *U.S. News and World Report*, January 26, 2010, *www.usnews.com/opinion/blogs/robert-schlesinger/2010/01/26/james-okeefe-arrested-undercutting-acorn-allegations.html.*

Epilogue

1. Randy Shaw, "ACORN's Problems Create Void for Community Organizing," *LA Progressive*, October 6, 2009, *www.laprogressive.com/2009/10/06/acorn%E2%80%99s-problems-create-void-for-community-organizing/.*
2. Lawrence Goodwyn, *The Populist Moment: A Short History of the Agrarian Revolt in America* (New York: Oxford University Press, 1978); Louise W. Knight, *Citizen: Jane*

Addams and the Struggle for Democracy (Chicago: University of Chicago Press, 2005); Jean Bethke Elshtain, *Jane Addams and the Dream of American Democracy: A Life* (New York: Basic Books, 2002); Jennifer Frost, *"An Interracial Movement of the Poor": Community Organizing and the New Left in the 1960s* (New York: New York University Press, 2001).

3. Peter Dreier and Christoper Martin, "Manipulating the Public Agenda: Why ACORN Was in the News, and What the News Got Wrong," Urban and Environmental Policy Institute, Occidental College, *departments.oxy.edu/uepi/acornstudy*.
4. On April 9, 2009, Media Matters for America released a well-researched report showing that conservatives have repeatedly resorted to blaming ACORN rather than engage in substantive discussions of causes and solutions, even where the organization has little or nothing to do with the issue at hand. See "Report: Conservative Media Consistently Scapegoat Undocumented Immigrants, ACORN," *mediamatters.org/reports/200904070005*.
5. Dan Eggen, "Groups on the Left Are Suddenly on Top; Obama's Election Has Elevated the Influence Industry's Liberal Side," *Washington Post*, June 4, 2009.
6. Matt Bai, *The Argument, Billionaires, Bloggers, and the Battle to Remake Democratic Politics* (New York: Penguin Press, 2007).
7. John Halpin and Ruy Teixeira, "Progressivism Goes Mainstream," *American Prospect*, April 20, 2009, *www.prospect.org/cs/articles?article=progressivism_goes_mainstream*.
8. Ibid.
9. Ruy Teixeira, "New Progressive America," Center for American Progress, March 11, 2009, *www.americanprogress.org/issues/2009/03/progressive_america.html*.
10. Dan Eggen, "Rise of Liberal Groups Shows in Court Nomination," *Washington Post*, June 3, 2009.
11. George Packer, "The New Liberalism: How the Economic Crisis Can Help Obama Redefine the Democrats," *New Yorker*, November 17, 2008.
12. Dan Eggen, "Rise of Liberal Groups."
13. Lisa Taddeo, "The Man Who Made Obama," *Esquire*, November 3, 2009, *www.esquire.com/features/david-plouffe-0309*.
14. Peter Dreier, "The Tide Is Turning on Healthcare Reform," *Nation*, October 23, 2009.
15. John Judis, "The Insider: Why Obama Needs to Make It Clearer to Democrats That He's on Their Side," *New Republic*, November 5, 2009, *www.tnr.com/article/the-insider*; John Judis, "Mixed Messages," *New Republic*, November 4, 2009.
16. Jonathan Alter, *The Defining Moment* (New York: Simon and Schuster, 2006).

Bibliography

Introduction

John McCain, Debate Transcript, "The Third McCain-Obama Presidential Debate." Commission on Presidential Debates, October 15, 2008, *www.debates.org/pages/trans2008d.html.*

Chapter 1
Wade Rathke and the Roots of ACORN

Adamson, Madeleine, and Seth Borgos. *This Mighty Dream*. New York: Routledge, 1984.
Alinsky, Saul D. *Reveille for Radicals*. Chicago: University of Chicago Press, 1945.
———. *Rules for Radicals*. New York: Random House, 1971.
Boyte, Harry. *The Backyard Revolution*. Philadelphia: Temple University Press, 1980.
Cloward, Richard, and Frances Piven. "The Weight of the Poor: A Strategy to End Poverty." *Nation*, May 2, 1966.
Delgado, Gary. *Organizing the Movement: The Roots and Growth of ACORN*. Philadelphia: Temple University Press, 1986.
Fisher, Robert. Let the People Decide. Boston: Twayne, 1984.
Flynn, Jack, "ACORN Grew from Springfield Riot." *Republican*, October 25, 2009.
Horwitt, Sanford D. *Let Them Call Me Rebel: Saul Alinsky—His Life and Legacy*. New York: Knopf, 1989.
Kotz, Nick A., and Mary L. Kotz. *Passion for Equality: George Wiley and the Movement*. New York: W. W. Norton, 1977.
Lieberman, Paul. "To Woodstock, on the 'Frankly Dankly' School Bus of '69." *LATimes.com*, August 15, 2009, *www.latimes.com/entertainment/news/arts/la-na-woodstock15-2009aug15,0,4911948,print.story.*
Moynihan, Daniel Patrick. *The Politics of a Guaranteed Income: The Nixon Administration and the Family Assistance Plan*. New York: Random House, 1973.
Piven, Frances Fox, and Richard Cloward. *Poor People's Movements*. New York: Vintage, 1979.
Rathke, Wade. "ACORN Organizing in Arkansas." *Southern Exposure* 2, 1, ACORN archives.
Russell, D. *Political Organizing in Grassroots Politics*. Lanham, Md.: University Press of America, 1990.
Silberman, Charles E. *Crisis in Black and White*. New York: Vintage, 1964.
Wiley, George. "Masking Repression As Reform." *Social Policy*, May–June 1972.
———. "The Nixon Family Assistance Plan: Reform or Repression?" *Back Law Journal*, Spring 1971.

Chapter 2
Stepping onto a Larger Stage

Adamson, Madeleine, and Seth Borgos. *This Mighty Dream*. New York: Routledge, 1984.
Boyte, Harry. *Community Is Possible*. New York: Harper-Colophon Books, 1984.

Delgado, Gary. *Organizing the Movement: The Roots and Growth of ACORN*. Philadelphia: Temple University Press, 1986.
Fisher, Robert. *Let the People Decide*. Boston: Twayne, 1984.
Horwitt, Sanford D. *Let Them Call Me Rebel: Saul Alinsky—His Life and Legacy*. New York: Knopf, 1989.
Kest, Steven, and Wade Rathke. "ACORN: An Overview of Its History, Structure, Methodology, Campaigns, and Philosophy as It Developed in Arkansas." *ACORN Community Organizing Handbook #2*, 3–13. Little Rock, Ark.: Institute for Social Justice, 1977.
Kotz. Nick A., and Mary L. Kotz. *Passion for Equality: George Wiley and the Movement*. New York: W. W. Norton, 1977.
Moynihan, Daniel Patrick. *The Politics of a Guaranteed Income: The Nixon Administration and the Family Assistance Plan*. New York: Random House, 1973.
Piven, Frances Fox, and Richard Cloward. *Poor People's Movements*. New York: Vintage, 1979.
Russell, Daniel M. "Alternatives in American Politics: A Study of the Association of Community Organizations for Reform Now." PhD diss., University of Massachusetts, 1986.
———. *Political Organizing in Grassroots Politics*. Lanham, Md.: University Press of America, 1990.
Silberman, Charles E. *Crisis in Black and White*. New York: Vintage, 1964.

Chapter 3
ACORN's Model T

Alinsky, Saul. *Rules for Radicals*. New York: Random House, 1975.
Astrachan, Anthony. "Working in the System." *New Republic*, July 3, 10, 1976.
Delgado, Gary. *Organizing the Movement: The Roots and Growth of ACORN*. Philadelphia: Temple University Press, 1986.
Freedberg, Robin. "ACSR May Weigh University's Role in Arkansas Environmental Dispute." *Harvard Crimson*, November 8, 1973, *www.thecrimson.com/article.aspx?ref=346381*.
Greenhouse, Linda. "White Plains: 'Downtown' for All Westchester; The Most Desirable' A Bank Boom Praise from Planners White Plains: New 'Downtown' Parking Is Ample Landmarks Fade," *New York Times*, April 30, 1973.
Harvard Crimson. "ACORN Asks 18 Additional Colleges to Help Fight Arkansas Power Plant." *Harvard Crimson*, February 14, 1974.
———. "Answer to ACORN?" *Harvard Crimson*, March 23, 1974.
———. "Citizens' Group Asks Bok to Aid Power Plant Fight." *Harvard Crimson*, November 7, 1973, *www.thecrimson.com/article.aspx?ref=345930*.
———. "Finally, a Word on AP&L." *Harvard Crimson*, April 27, 1974.
———. "Harvard and AP&L." *Harvard Crimson*, December 13, 1973.
Kest, Steven. "Who Is Responsible?" *Harvard Crimson*, November 13, 1973.
Kest, Steven, and Wade Rathke. "ACORN: An Overview of Its History, Structure, Methodology, Campaigns, and Philosophy as It Developed in Arkansas." *Community Organizing Handbook #2*. Little Rock, Ark.: Institute for Social Justice, 1977.
Kupferberg, Seth M. "ACSR Stalls AP&L Decision, Asks Professors for Opinions." *Harvard Crimson*, December 19, 1973.
———. Breaking with Precedent." *Harvard Crimson*, March 13, 1974.
———. "Study Attacks AP&L Plan." *Harvard Crimson*, December 7, 1973.
Lemann, Nicholas. "Acorn, Power and Light." *Harvard Crimson*, December 1, 1973.
———. "ACSR Active but Students Care Little. *Harvard Crimson*, June 13, 1974.
———. "ACSR to Meet, Discuss Proxy Votes, AP&L Plant." *Harvard Crimson*, March 5, 1974.
———. "Bok Receives Acorn Petition on Arkansas Power Facility." *Harvard Crimson*, November 20, 1973.
———. "Support Grows." *Harvard Crimson*, November 17, 1973.
———. "Uh . . . Let's Talk about It in January." *Harvard Crimson*, December 21, 1973.

Luxenberg, Steve. "Power Plant in a Nutshell." *Harvard Crimson*, November 14, 1973, *www.thecrimson.com/article.aspx?ref=110819*.

Meislin, Richard J. "Bumpers Predicts AP&L Will Control Its Pollution." *Harvard Crimson*, November 14, 1973.

———. "Farmers Square Off with a Utility." *Harvard Crimson*, November 10, 1973, *www.thecrimson.com/article.aspx?ref=106084*.

Rathke, Wade. "ACORN Organizing in Arkansas." *Southern Exposure* 2, 1. ACORN archives.

Chapter 4
The Innovation of Electoral Politics

Adamson, Madeleine, and Seth Borgos. *This Mighty Dream*. New York: Routledge, 1984.

Bradley, Bill. "A Party Inverted." *New York Times*, March 30, 2005.

Delgado, Gary. *Organizing the Movement: The Roots and Growth of ACORN*. Philadelphia: Temple University Press, 1986, chapter 5.

Horwitt, Sanford D. *Let Them Call Me Rebel: Saul Alinsky—His Life and Legacy*. New York: Knopf, 1989.

Howe, Irving, and B. J. Widick. *The UAW and Walter Reuther*. New York: Random House, 1949.

Institute for Social Justice. *ACORN Community Organizing Handbook* #2. Little Rock, Ark.: Institute for Social Justice, 1977.

Katz, Michael B. *The Undeserving Poor, from the War on Poverty to the War on Welfare*. New York: Pantheon, 1989.

Lichtenstein, Nelson. *The Most Dangerous Man in Detroit: Walter Reuther and the Fate of American Labor*. New York: Basic Books, 1995.

Powell, Lewis F., Jr. "Attack of American Free Enterprise System." Confidential Memorandum to the United States Chamber of Commerce, August 23, 1971

Chapter 5
Organizing a Union in the 'Hood

Burger King Corp. v. National Labor Relations Board, 725 F.2nd 1053 (6th Cir., 1984).

Cantor, Danny. "ACORN, the UAW, and the Teamsters." *Social Policy* 13, 4 (Spring 1983), 21.

Cloward, Richard, and Frances Fox Piven, "Who Should Be Organized? Citizen Action vs. Jobs for Justice." *Working Papers for a New Society*, May–June 1979.

Delgado, Gary. *Organizing the Movement: The Roots and Growth of ACORN*. Philadelphia: Temple University Press, 1986.

Detroit Free Press. "Having It Their Way: Fast Food Union Wins Burger King Vote." *Detroit Free Press*. March 16, 1980.

Fastfood Worker, SEIU Local 880 Records. March 1, 15, 16, and April 15, 1980. Author files.

Freedberg, Louis, "Behind the Counter: Teenage Workers Fuel Fast Food Assembly Line." Box 1, folder 6, SEIU Local 880 Records, 1983–1989.

"Goldman Workers Get Tough, Win Big." *United Labor News* 2, 1 (January 1981).

Howe, Irving. *The UAW and Walter Reuther*. New York: Da Capo Press, 1949.

Just Economics. "Union Drive Wins First Fastfood Election." *Just Economics* 3, 2 (March–April 1980). Author files.

Katznelson, Ira. *City Trenches: Urban Politics and the Patterning of Class in the United States*. New York: Pantheon Books, 1981.

Kelleher, Keith. "ACORN Organizing and Chicago Homecare Workers." *Labor Research Review* 8 (Spring 1986). Author files.

———. "From ACORN to ULU to SEIU: Building a Homecare Workers' Movement in the New Economy; The Illinois Model/Experience, 1983–2003." Word document. Author files.

Kest, Steven. "ACORN and Community-Labor Partnerships." August 10, 2002. Draft Word document. Author files.

Livingston, Victor. "Whose Renaissance?" *Detroit News Magazine*, July 27, 1980, 12.
Rose, Barbara. "Local 880 Success: Labor's New Up-and-Comer." *Chicago Tribune*, July 5, 2005.
Tait, Vanessa. *Poor Workers' Unions: Rebuilding Labor from Below.* Cambridge, Mass.: South End Press, 2005, chapter 4.
United Labor Unions and SEIU Local's Constitution and By-Laws. In author's possession.

Chapter 6
Partnering with the Enemy

Atlas, John. "And the World Keeps Changing: 25 Years of *Shelterforce*." *Shelterforce*, March–April 2000.
———. "Condomania: Causes and Solutions." *Shelterforce*, March 1980.
———. "Is It Time for a Populist Coalition of Low- and Middle-Income Americans for Affordable Housing?" *Shelterforce*, March–April 1994.
———. "Regulating the Banks; the Limits of Legislative Reform." *Shelterforce*, 1978.
Barnes, Julian E. "Reclaiming Our Cities, Block by Block: How a Little Rock Program Offers Hope for Countering Urban Decay—Arkansas." *Washington Monthly*, April 1996.
Brooks, Fred. "The Evolution of Community Organizing Campaigns at ACORN, 1970–2006." Paper presented at the annual meeting of the American Sociological Association, New York City, August 11, 2007. Author files.
Campen, Jim. "The Community Reinvestment Act: A Law That Works." *Dollars and Sense*, December–November 1977, *www.dollarsandsense.org/archives/1997/1197campen.html.*
Dedman, Bill. "The Color of Money. *Atlanta Journal-Constitution*, May 4, 1988.
Dreier, Peter. "Redlining Cities: How Banks Color Community Development." *Challenge: The Magazine of Economic Affairs* 34 (1991).
Lappe, Frances Moore. *Democracy's Edge: Choosing to Save Our Country by Bringing Democracy to Life*. San Francisco: Jossey Bass, 2006.
Lassen, Mary, and Madeline Adamson. "Erasing the Red-Line: The St. Louis Anti-Redlining Campaign." In *Actions and Campaigns: Community Organizing Handbook #3*. New Orleans: Institute for Social Justice, 1979.
Lender, Brad. "Cities Revive, but What About the People?" *Shelterforce*, November–December 2000, *www.shelterforce.org/online/issues/114/bookreview.html.*
National Community Reinvestment Coalition. *CRA Dollar Commitments since 1977.* Washington, D.C.: National Community Reinvestment Coalition, 1996.
———. *Models of Community Lending: Neighborhood Revitalization through Community-Lender Partnerships.* Washington, D.C.: National Community Reinvestment Coalition, 1997.
Ross, Stephen, and John Yinger. *The Color of Credit: What Is Known about Discrimination in Mortgage Lending*. Cambridge, Mass.: MIT Press, 2002.
Santilli, Tom. "Formalizing Poor People's Movements: Strategy, Power, and the Organizer in Acorn's Living Wage Campaigns." Master's thesis, William Paterson University of New Jersey, 2005.
Sidney, Mara. *Unfair Housing.* Lawrence: University Press of Kansas, 2003.
Squires, Gregory. *From Redlining to Reinvestment.* Philadelphia: Temple University Press, 1992.
———, ed. *Organizing Access to Capital.* Philadelphia: Temple University Press, 2003.
Swarts, Heidi. "Political Opportunity, Venue Shopping, and Strategic Innovation: ACORN's National Organizing." In *Transforming the City: Community Organizing and the Challenge of Political Change*, ed. Marion Orr. Lawrence: University of Kansas Press, 2006.
Walker, Christopher, and Mark Weinheimer. *Community Development in the 1990s.* Washington, D.C.: Urban Institute Press, 1998.
Wayne, Leslie. "A Special Report; New Hope in Inner Cities: Banks Offering Mortgages." *New York Times*, March 14, 1992.

Chapter 7
Urban Homesteading

Adamson, Madeline. "Need a House? Call ACORN." *Organizer*, 1981 Author files.

Borgos, Seth. "Low-Income Homeownership and the Acorn Squatters Campaign." In *Critical Perspectives on Housing*, ed. Rachel G. Bratt, Chester Hartman, and Ann Meyerson. Philadelphia: Temple University Press, 1986.

Gosse, Van, and Richard Moser, eds. *The World the Sixties Made: Politics and Culture in Recent America*. Philadelphia: Temple University Press, 2003.

Hartman, Chester, Dennis Keating, and R. LeGates. *Displacement: How to Fight It*. Berkeley, Calif.: National Housing Law Project, 1982.

Neuwirth, Robert. *Shadow Cities: A Billion Squatters, a New Urban World*. New York: Routledge, 2004.

Nussbaum, Paul. "A Long, Strange Trip for Milton Street." *Philadelphia Inquirer*, September 27, 2008.

Philadelphia Daily News. Editorial. August 8, 1977.

U.S. Department of Housing and Urban Development. *Evaluation of the Urban Homesteading Demonstration Program: Final Report*. Vol. 1, "Summary Assessment." Washington, D.C.: GPO, 1983.

———. *The Urban Homesteading Catalogue*. Vol. 3. Washington, D.C.: GPO, 1977.

Chapter 8
Political Ground Shifts

Bellah, Robert N., Richard Madsen, William M. Sullivan, Ann Swidler, and Steven M. Tipton. *Habits of the Heart: Individualism and Commitment in American Life*. Berkeley: University of California Press, 1986.

Cassidy, John. "The Ringleader," *New Yorker*, August 1, 2005.

Delgado, Gary. *Organizing the Movement: The Roots and Growth of ACORN*. Philadelphia: Temple University Press, 1986.

Easton, Nina. *Gang of Five: Leaders at the Center of the Conservative Ascendancy*. New York: Simon and Schuster, 2002.

Edsall, Thomas Byrne, and Mary D. Edsall. *Chain Reaction: The Impact of Race, Rights, and Taxes on American Politics*. New York: W. W. Norton, 1992.

Gitlin, Todd. *The Bulldozer and the Big Tent*. San Francisco: Wiley, 2007.

Goodwyn, Lawrence. *The Populist Moment: A Short History of the Agrarian Revolt in America*. New York: Oxford University Press, 1978.

Krugman, Paul. *The Conscience of a Liberal*. New York: W. W. Norton, 2009.

McGirr, Lisa. *Suburban Warriors: The Origins of the New American Right*. Princeton, N.J.: Princeton University Press, 2001.

Perlstein, Rick. *Before the Storm: Barry Goldwater and the Unmaking of the American Consensus*. New York: Hill and Wang, 2001.

Putnam, Robert. *Bowling Alone: The Collapse and Revival of American Community*. New York: Simon and Schuster, 2000.

Skocpol, Theda. *Diminished Democracy: From Membership to Management in American Civic Life*. Norman: University of Oklahoma Press, 2003.

Wilson, William Julius. *The Truly Disadvantaged: The Inner City, the Underclass, and Public Policy*. Chicago: University of Chicago Press, 1987.

Chapter 9
New York: A New Model

Cooper, Michael. "Neighborhood Report: Flatbush; Advocates Turn Tactics on Leader." *New York Times*, July 2, 1995.

Erlanger, Steven. "For a New Homesteader, Struggle Leads to Success." *New York Times*, October 12, 1987, *www.nytimes.com/1987/10/12/nyregion/for-a-new-homesteader-*

struggle-leads-to-success.html?n=Top%2fReference%2fTimes%20Topics%2fPeople%2fE%2f Erlanger%2c%20Steven.

———. "New York Turns Squatters into Homeowners." *New York Times*, October 12, 1987, *www.nytimes.com/1987/10/12/nyregion/new-york-turns-squatters-into-homeowners. html?n=Top%2fReference%2fTimes%20Topics%2fPeople%2fE%2fErlanger%2c%20Steven.*

Gonzalez, David. "Yesterday's Tenant Activist, Today's Landlord." *New York Times*, January 11, 2005.

Greer, William R. "Squatters and City Battle for Abandoned Buildings." *New York Times*, August 2, 1985.

Kugel, Seth. "Down at the Grass Roots, an Emotional Fight over Turf." *New York Times*, December 5, 2004.

Mollenkopf, John. *Phoenix in the Ashes: The Rise and Fall of the Koch Coalition in New York City Politics*. Princeton, N.J.: Princeton University Press, 1992.

Newfield, Jack, and Wayne Barrett. *City for Sale*. New York: Harper and Row, 1988.

Scott, Janelle, and Norman Fruchter. "Community Resistance to School Privatization: The Case of New York City." In *The People Shall Rule*, ed. Robert Fisher. Nashville: Vanderbilt University Press, 2009.

Siegal, Nina. "Neighborhood Report: East Harlem; Building Is Dangerous, but Tenants Cling." *New York Times*, March 19, 2000.

Siegel, Fred. *The Future Once Happened Here*. New York: Free Press, 1997.

Sleeper, Jim. *The Closest of Strangers: Liberalism and the Politics of Race in New York*. New York: W. W. Norton, 1990.

Thabit, Walter. *How East New York Became a Ghetto*. New York: New York University Press, 2003.

Chapter 10
A Living Wage

ACORN Living Wage Resource Center. "A Compilation of Living Wage Policies." Washington, D.C.: ACORN Living Wage Resource Center, June 2006.

Atlas, John. "In Red State Florida, Victory for Working People." *Shelterforce*, January/February 2005.

Atlas, John, and Peter Dreier. "Waging Victory." *American Prospect*, November 11, 2006.

———. "Voters Gave Big Thumbs Up to Minimum Wage Boost." *(Bergen County, N.J.) Record*, November 26, 2006.

Atlas, John, Peter Dreier, and Kelly Candaele. "Florida Gets It Right: Raising the Minimum Wage." *Commonweal*, June 3, 2005.

Berman, Richard. "Having It Both Ways." *Chicago Sun-Times*, March 6, 1996.

Bernstein, Jared, and Isaac Shapiro. *Buying Power of Minimum Wage at 51-Year Low: Congress Could Break Record for Longest Period without an Increase*. Washington, D.C.: Center on Budget and Policy Priorities, June 2006.

Boushet, Heather, Chauna Brocht, Bethney Gunderson, and Jared Bernstein. *Hardship in America: The Real Story of Working Families*. Washington, D.C.: Economic Policy Institute, 2001.

Brenner, Mark, Jeanette Wicks-Lim, and Robert Pollin. "Measuring the Impact of Living Wage Laws: A Critical Appraisal of David Neumark's 'How Living Wage Laws Affect Low-Wage Workers and Low-Income Families.'" Political Economy Research Institute Working Paper #43. 2002. *www.umass.edu/peri/pdfs/WP43.pdf.*

California Budget Project. "Making Ends Meet: How Much Does It Cost to Raise a Family in California?" Sacramento: California Budget Project. October 2001. *www.cbp.org/2001/ r0109mem.htm.*

Card, David, and Alan B. Krueger. *Myth and Measurement: The New Economics of the Minimum Wage*. Princeton, N.J.: Princeton University Press, 1995.

CBS News. "Low-Wage Workers Finding It Increasingly Difficult to Make Ends Meet." CBS News, September 2, 2001.

CounterMedia. "Living Wage Campaign in Chicago—Will the Real Democrats Stand Up?" *CounterMedia*, July 1966, *www.cpsr.cs.uchicago.edu/countermedia/briefings/livingwage.html.*

Crockett, Roger O. "From Projects to Progress in Chicago." *Business Week*, October 27, 2003.

Eckholm, Erik. "Chicago Orders 'Big Box' Stores to Raise Wage." *New York Times*, July 27, 2006.

Gertner, Jon. "What Is a Living Wage?" *New York Times Magazine*, January 15, 2006.

Graham, Kevin. "Election 2004, Late Registrations Disqualify 1,500 Voters; The Low-Income Voters Who Registered through a Third Party Will Be Allowed to Vote in the General Election on Nov. 2." *St. Petersburg Times*, August 19, 2004.

Hallifax, Jackie. "Group Pushing Ballot Measure to Raise Florida's Minimum Wage." Associated Press State and Local Wire, August 6, 2003.

———. "Proposal to Up the Minimum Wage Makes Florida Fall Ballot." Associated Press, July 27, 2004.

Herbert, Bob. "Suppress the Vote?" *New York Times*, August 16, 2004.

Huntley, Helen. "Minimum Wage Change: A Blip or a Bombshell?" *St. Petersburg Times*, September 23, 2004.

Kelleher, Keith, and Madeline Talbott. "Holding Public Officials Accountable in Chicago." *Shelterforce*, November–December 2000.

Kuttner, Robert. "Boston's 'Living Wage' Law Highlights New Grassroots Efforts to Fight Poverty." *American Prospect* (1997).

Langman, Brent. "Chicago Style. Vienna Beef Company Profile." *National Provisioner*, January 1, 2002, *www.accessmylibrary.com/coms2/summary_0286-25037653_ITM.*

Luce, Stephanie. "ACORN and the Living Wage Movement." In *The People Shall Rule: ACORN, Community Organizing, and the Struggle for Economic Justice*, ed. Robert Fisher. Nashville: Vanderbilt University Press, 2009.

———. *Fighting for a Living Wage*. Ithaca, N.Y.: Cornell University Press, 2004.

Madrick, Jeff. Scene: Battle over Living Wage Heats Up." *New York Times*, July 5, 2002.

Mayk, Lauren. "Living Wage Proposal Opposed." *Sarasota Herald-Tribune*, September 23, 2004.

Melita, Marie Garza. "Wage Warriors." *Chicago Tribune*, May 9, 1996.

Miller, Sabrina L., and Gary Washburn. "Aldermen Set to Vote Selves a Raise." *Chicago Tribune*, November 6, 2002.

Moberg, David. "Martha Jernegons's New Shoes." *American Prospect*, June 19 and July 3, 2000.

———. "What Do Students Think about Carleton College?" *www.edunetwork.com/student/PROF0042.htm.*

Murray, Bobbi. "The Living Wage Comes of Age." *Nation*, July 23, 2001.

Pollin, Robert, and Stephanie Luce. *The Living Wage: Building a Fair Economy.* New York: New Press, 2000.

Pollin, Robert, Mark Brenner, and Stephanie Luce. "Intended vs. Unintended Consequences: Evaluating the New Orleans Living Wage Proposal." *Journal of Economic Issues*, December 2002.

Pollin, Robert, Mark Brenner, Stephanie Luce, and Jeannette Wicks-Lim. *A Measure of Fairness: The Economics of Living Wages and Minimum Wages in the United States.* Ithaca, N.Y.: Cornell University Press, 2008.

Reich, M., P. Hall, and K. Jacobs. *Living Wages and Economic Performance.* Berkeley: Institute of Industrial Relations, University of California, March 2003.

Reynolds, David. "Living Wage Campaigns: An Activist's Guide to Organizing a Movement for Economic Justice." Labor Studies Center, Wayne State University, 2003, *www.laborstudies.wayne.edu/research/guide2002.pdf.*

Roggemann, Ellen. "ACORN's Minimum Wage Campaign 2004: Single Initiative or Social Movement?" December 29, 2004. Word document. Author files.

Roman, Bob. "The Jobs and Living Wage Ordinance: Commentary and Summary." *New Ground*, November–December 1996, *www.chicagodsa.org/ngarchive/ng62.html.*

Ruggless, Ron. "Minimum Wage Hike Bills Springing Up Nationwide." *Nation's Restaurant News*, February 3, 1997, *findarticles.com/p/articles/mi_m3190/is_n5_v31/ai_19089490.*

Santilli, Tom. "Formalizing Poor People's Movements: Strategy, Power, and the Organizer in Acorn's Living Wage Campaigns." Master's thesis, William Paterson University of New Jersey, August 2005.

Solomon, Deborah. "Weighing Minimum Wage Hikes: Oregon's Boost Didn't Curb Growth, but Did Squeeze Some Employers." *Wall Street Journal*, November 3, 2006.

Stern, Sol. "ACORN's Nutty Regime for Cities." *City Journal*, Spring 2003.

Swope, Christopher. "Living Wage Wars." December 1998, *governing.com/archive/1998/dec/wage.txt.*

Talbott, Madeline. "ACORN Organizes Public Housing Residents." *Shelterforce*, September–October 1994.

———. "Where Do We Begin." *Boston Review*, Summer 1996.

Thomas, Mike. "Wage Makes or Breaks Workers, Not Businesses." *Orlando Sentinel*, July 27, 2004.

Trigaux, Robert. "Push Is On for $6.15 State Minimum Wage." *St. Petersburg Times*, August 6, 2003.

Washburn, Gary, and Sabrina L. Miller. "Protest Seeks Boost in 'Living Wage.'" *Chicago Tribune*, May 2, 2002.

Weisbrot, Mark, and Michelle Sforza-Roderick. *Baltimore's Living Wage Law*. Washington, D.C.: Preamble Center, 1996.

Chapter 11
Never Borrow Money Needlessly

ACORN. *Separate and Unequal: Predatory Lending in America*. Washington, D.C.: Association of Community Organizations for Reform Now, 2000. Available at *www.acorn.org.*

Atlas, John, and Peter Dreier. "The Conservative Origins of the Sub-Prime Mortgage Crisis: Everything You Ever Wanted to Know about the Mortgage Meltdown but Were Afraid to Ask." *American Prospect*, December 18, 2007.

———. "Stemming the Red Tide, Greedy Bankers, Brokers, and Investors Abused Their Political Power and Forced Millions of Americans to Lose Their Homes. Now What Can We Do to Solve the Crisis?" *Shelterforce*, Spring 2008.

Atlas, John, Peter Dreier, and Gregory D. Squires. "Foreclosing on the Free Market: How to Remedy the Subprime Catastrophe." *New Labor Forum* 17, 3 (Fall 2008).

Coalition for Responsible Lending and Eric Stein. "Quantifying the Economic Cost of Predatory Lending." Durham, N.C.: Coalition for Responsible Lending, 2001.

Condon, Bernard. "Home Wrecker." *Forbes*, September 2, 2002.

Consumer Federation of America and National Insurance Consumer Organization. *Credit Life Insurance: The Nation's Worst Insurance Rip Off.* June 4, 1990; updated May 20, 1992 and July 25, 1995.

Davies, Paul D. "Drop City Stock in Predators." *Philadelphia Daily News*, May 9, 2001, *www.acorn.org/acorn10/household/press/drop.htm.*

Engel, Kathleen C., and Patricia A. McCoy. "A Tale of Three Markets: The Law and Economics of Predatory Lending." *Texas Law Review* 80, 6 (May 2002).

Eavis, Peter. "Lawsuits and Regulators Shadow Big Lender's Future." *New York Times*, August 17, 2002

Gilmer, Gary. "Household Is a Responsible Lender." *St. Petersburg Times*, May 12, 2001, *www.acorn.org/acorn10/household/press/letter.htm.*

Greising, David. "What Household International Became." *Chicago Tribune*, November 17, 2002.

———. Group Pickets Household in Florida." *Chicago Sun-Times*, May 9, 2001, *www.acorn.org/acorn10/household/press/picket.htm.*

Household Finance Corporation. *Financing the American Family*. Video. Chicago Film Laboratory, ca. 1935, *www.archive.org/details/Financin1935*.

Household International. *2000 Annual Report*. Prospect Heights, Ill: Household International, January 2001, *www.household.com/ffacts.html*.

Huber, Tim. "Household International to Pay Some $387 Million in Consumer Fraud Settlement." *Saint Paul Pioneer Press*, October 12, 2002.

HUD-Treasury Task Force on Predatory Lending. "Curbing Predatory Home Mortgage Lending." June 20, 2000.

Hurd, Maude. "Lending Looks Predatory." *St. Petersburg Times*, May 30, 2001, *www.acorn.org/acorn10/household/press/response.htm*.

Hurd, Maude, and Lisa Donner. "ACORN's Campaign against Household Finance." In *Roots to Power: A Manual for Grassroots Organizers*, ed. L. Staples. 2nd ed. Westport, Conn.: Praeger, 2004.

Hurd, Maude, and Lisa Donner, with Camellia Phillips. "Community Organizing and Advocacy: Fighting Predatory Lending and Making a Difference." In *Why the Poor Pay More*, ed. Gregory D. Squires. Westport, Conn.: Praeger, 2004.

Hurd, Maude, and Steven Kest. "Fighting Predatory Lending from the Ground Up: An Issue of Economic Justice." In *Organizing Access to Capital: Advocacy and the Democratization of Financial Institutions*, ed. Gregory D. Squires. Philadelphia: Temple University Press, 2003.

Julavits, Robert. "Protests at Household's Shareholders' Meeting." *American Banker*, May 9, 2001, *www.acorn.org/acorn10/household/press/protests.htm*.

Peacock, Sally. "How the Household Settlement Uncorked a Law Enforcement Bottleneck." National, States Attorneys General Program at Columbia Law School, n.d., *www.law.columbia.edu/center_program/ag/Library?exclusive=filemgr.download&file_id=92529&rtcontentdisposition=filename%3DPeacock,+S-+How+the+Household+Settlement+Uncorked+a+Law+Enforcement+Bottleneck.pdf*.

Stockfisch, Jerome R. "Protesters Say Lenders Prey." *Tampa Tribune*, May 9, 2001, *www.acorn.org/acorn10/household/press/lenders_prey.htm*.

Trigaux, Robert. "Florida Newest Turf in Lending Hostilities." *St. Petersburg Times*, May 9, 2001, *www.acorn.org/acorn10/household/press/newfla.htm*.

Chapter 12
ACORN's Family Party

Benson, Josh. "It's Mean Mark Green: Former Front Runner Jostles Freddy Ferrer." *New York Observer*, October 14, 2001.

Cantor, Daniel. "Friday IMterview: Dan Cantor." *New York Observer*, February 17, 2006.

———. "Minor Political Parties." Letter to the editor. *New York Times*, November 14, 2002.

Cooper, Michael. "Hevesi Speaks on Policing; His Rivals Show Off Support." *New York Times*, August 10, 2001.

Hernández, Daisy. "The 2002 Campaign: Voter Quiz; It's a Party, So Why Not Give Out Some Prizes?" *New York Times*, November 3, 2002.

Hicks, Jonathan P. "Third Party to Run a Candidate for Slain Councilman's Seat." *New York Times*, August 5, 2003.

Hu, Winnie, "A Third Party Makes Its First Mark." *New York Times*, November 9, Katz, Alyssa. "The Power of Fusion Politics." *Nation*, September 12, 2005.

Klein, etc., et al v. Garfinkle, Working Families Party. etc., et al., decisions.courts.state.ny.us/fcas/fcas_docs/2005jun/51002178720041sciv.pdf.

Lappe, Frances Moore. *Democracy's Edge: Choosing to Save Our Country by Bringing Democracy to Life*. San Francisco: John Wiley and Sons, 2005.

Long, Michael R. "State Chairman, New York State Conservative Party." Letter to the editor. *New York Times*, November 21, 2002.

Martin v. Alverez et. a1. Index No. 05-15985, *decisions.courts.state.ny.us/fcas/fcas_docs/2005aug/51001598520051sciv.pdf*.

Matter of New York Working Families Party v. Berman. 11 AD3d 646,764 NYS2d 557 (2d Dept 2004).
Newfield, J. "Working Families Party Takes Place at the Table." *New York Sun*, November 11, 2003.
Pérez-Peña, Richard. "McCall Rejects a Party; Cuomo Says It's Pre-emptive." *New York Times*, January 14, 2002.
Polett, Zach. "Fair Housing Drives New Party Growth." *Shelterforce*, September–October 1998.
Robbins, Tom. "Mark Green Exits, Stage Left." *Village Voice*, September 12, 2006.
Sargent, Greg. "First among Thirds." *American Prospect*, May 3, 2006.
Smith, Ben. "Is the Party Over for Working Families before It Starts?" *New York Observer*, November 2, 2003, *www.omgit.net/node/48273*.
Steinhauer, Jennifer. "Campaign Briefing, the Mayoral Race: Endorsement by Sunshade." *New York Times*, August 11, 2001.
Stern, Sol. "ACORN's Nutty Regime for Cities." *City Journal*, Spring 2003.
Working Families Party. "The WFP Strategy." n.d. *www.workingfamiliesparty.org/strategy.html*.

Chapter 13
Atlantic Yards, the Nets, and the Battle of Brooklyn

Angotti, Tom. "Atlantic Yards: Through the Looking Glass." *Gotham Gazette*, November 15, 2005, *www.gothamgazette.com*.
Atlas, John. "The Battle in Brooklyn." *Shelterforce*, Spring 2006.
Browne, J. Zamgba. "ACORN: Affordable Housing on Vacant Lots." *New York Amsterdam News*, March 5, 2003.
Griffith, M. W. "Calling the Question of ACORN." DMI Blog: Politics, Policy and the American Dream, December 30, 2005, *www.dmiblog.net/archives/2005/12/calling_the_question_of_acorn.html*.
Lipsky, M. *Protest in City Politics: Rent Strikes, Housing, and the Power of the Poor*. Chicago: Rand McNally, 1969.
Lobbia, J. A. "Wooten for the Wrong Team: Councilmember Quashes Hopes for Housing." *Village Voice*, February 3–9, 1999.
New York Times. "Fight for Bronx Building Is Moving to Courtroom." *New York Times*, July 25, 1988, *www.nytimes.com/1988/07/25/nyregion/fight-for-bronx-building-is-moving-to-courtroom.html?sec=&spon=&pagewanted=print*.
Pratt Center for Community Development, *www.prattcenter.net*.
Silverman, Justin Rocket. "The War for Brooklyn Battleground: Atlantic Yards." *Time Out New York*, July 27–August 2, 2006.
Smith, Chris. "Mr. Ratner's Neighborhood." *New York Magazine*, August 14, 2006.
Swarts, Heidi. *Organizing Urban America*. Minneapolis: University of Minnesota Press, 2008.
TimesRatnerReport, "More on the Observer's Roger Green Story: Challenging the 'Modern Blueprint,'" *timesratnerreport.blogspot.com/2005/12/more-on-observers-roger-green-story.html*.
Weiss, Philip. "The Lives They Lived: Fred C. Trump, b. 1905." *New York Times*, January 2, 2000.

Chapter 14
Then, Overnight, It Is Washed Away

Alpert, Bruce. "FEMA Chief Dawdled." *New Orleans Times-Picayune*, November 3, 2005.
Atlas, John, and Peter Dreier. "Katrina, the Missing Story." *Tikkun*, January–February 2007.
Baum, Dan. "The Lost Year: Behind the Failure to Rebuild." *New Yorker*, August 21, 2006.
Dao, James, "No Fixed Address." *New York Times*, September 11, 2005.
———. "Study Says 80% of New Orleans Blacks May Not Return." *New York Times*, January 27, 2006.

Davis, Mike. "Who Is Killing New Orleans?" *Nation*, April 10, 2006.
Dreier, Peter. "Katrina and Power in America." *Urban Affairs Review* 41, 1 (March 2006): 1–21.
Eggler, Bruce. "Lawsuit Seeks Change in N.O. Election Plans." *New Orleans Times-Picayune*, February 10, 2006.
Fletcher, M. A., and S. S. Hsu. "Storms Alter Louisiana Politics; Population Loss Likely to Reduce Influence of Black Voters." *Washington Post*, October 14, 2005.
Hartman, Chester, and Gregory Squires, eds. *There Is No Such Thing As a Natural Disaster: Race, Class, and Hurricane Katrina.* New York: Routledge, 2006.
Havemann, J. "A Shattered Gulf Coast; New Orleans' Racial Future Hotly Argued; The U.S. Housing Chief Expresses Doubts about Rebuilding, and Draws Anger and Concern." *Los Angeles Times*, October 1, 2005.
Lipton, Eric. "'Breathtaking' Waste and Fraud in Hurricane Aid." *New York Times*, June 27, 2006.
Rathke, Wade. *The Battle for the Lower 9th: ACORN and the Rebuilding of New Orleans.* London: Verso (in press).
Reich, Robert B., "Chickens and Eggs in New Orleans: How a Republican Congressman from Louisiana Plans to Rebuild New Orleans." *American Prospect*, February 16, 2006.
Remnick, David. "High Water." *New Yorker*, October 3, 2005.
Sontag, Deborah. "Months after Katrina, Bittersweet Homecoming in the 9th Ward." *New York Times*, December 2, 2005.

Chapter 15
A Rich Gumbo

Aqui, Reggie. "Some Katrina Evacuees Living in Houston Are in a Group of Buses Traveling East Tuesday." KHOU-TV, Houston. February 7, 2006.
Bates, Darien, and Rachel Kranz. "Spirit of Mardi Gras Shines through Katrina's Enduring Shadow in N.O." *Falls Church (Va.) News-Press*, March 9–15, 2006, *www.fcnp.com/601/mardi.htm.*
Baum, Dan. "The Lost Year: Behind the Failure to Rebuild." *New Yorker*, August 21, 2006.
Brinkley, Douglas. *The Great Deluge: Hurricane Katrina, New Orleans, and the Mississippi Gulf Coast.* New York: William Morrow, 2006.
Clark, Amy S. "Judge: FEMA Must Resume Katrina Payments, Agency Abruptly Ended 18-Month Housing Program in August." Associated Press, November 29, 2006.
Clark-Flory, Tracy. "Deficient Polling Places and Confusing Absentee Ballots Could Shut Thousands of Black Residents out of the City's Mayoral Election." *Salon*, April 15, 2006, *salon.com/news/feature/2006/04/15/neworleans_vote/index.html.*
Cobb, Kim, and Kristen Mack. "Nagin Headed into a Runoff: Incumbent to Face Lt. Gov. Landrieu to See Who Finishes Job of Rebuilding City." *Houston Chronicle*, April 23, 2006.
———. "New Orleans Mayoral Election, Black Voters Made Their Presence Felt. Predictions of Large Racial Shift In City Politics Prove Unfounded." *Houston Chronicle*, April 24, 2006.
Dao, James. "Study Says 80% of New Orleans Blacks May Not Return." *New York Times*, January 27, 2006.
Davis, Mike. "Who is Killing New Orleans." *Nation*, April 10, 2006.
Donze, Frank and Stephanie Grace, "ACORN plants its support in Pennington," *New Orleans Times-Picayune*, February 22, 2002
Dreier, Peter. "Katrina and Power in America." *Urban Affairs Review* 41, 1 (March 2006).
Dreier, Peter, and John Atlas. "Katrina, the Missing Story." *Tikkun*, January–February 2007.
Dvora, Petula. "Hurricane Victims Demand More Help." Washington Post, February 6, 2006.
Eggler, Bruce. "Lawsuit Seeks Change in N.O. Election Plans." *New Orleans Times-Picayune*, February 10, 2006.
Eliasoph, Nina. *Avoiding Politics: How Americans Produce Apathy in Everyday Life.* Cambridge: Cambridge University Press, 1998.

Gyan, Joe. "Groups Criticize Deadline to Fix or Board Up Houses." *Advocate*, August 4, 2006.
Hartman, Chester, and Gregory Squires, eds. *There Is No Such Thing As a Natural Disaster: Race, Class, and Hurricane Katrina*. New York: Routledge, 2006.
Kennedy, Rick. "Long Road Home." *Dallas Observer*, February 9, 2006.
Krupa, Michelle, and Frank Donze. "Leaders Stand United behind Recovery Plan: Blueprint Addresses Fears of Abandonment." *New Orleans Times-Picayune*, March 30, 2007.
Lipton, Eric. "'Breathtaking' Waste and Fraud in Hurricane Aid." *New York Times*, June 27, 2006.
Moreno, Sylvia. "Displaced Voters Make Wishes Known for New Orleans: Primary Election for Mayor." *Washington Post*, April 22, 2006.
Nossiter, Adam. "In New Orleans, Progress at Last in the Lower Ninth Ward." *New York Times*, February 23, 2007.
Ouroussoff, Nicolai. "History vs. Homogeneity in the New Orleans Housing Fight." *New York Times*, February 22, 2007.
———. "In New Orleans, Each Resident Is Master of Plan to Rebuild. *New York Times*, August 8, 2006.
Rathke, Wade. *The Battle for the Lower 9th: ACORN and the Rebuilding of New Orleans*. London: Verso (in press).
Roggemann, Ellen. "ACORN's Minimum Wage Campaign 2004: Single Initiative or Social Movement?" Word document. December 29, 2004. Author files.
Russell, Gordon, and Frank Donze. "Rebuilding Proposal Gets Mixed Reception: Critics Vocal, but Many Prefer to Watch and Wait." *New Orleans Times-Picayune*, January 12, 2006.
Saulny, Susan. "After Long Stress, Newsman in New Orleans Unravels." *New York Times*, August 10, 2006, *www.nytimes.com/2006/06/21/us/21depress.html?ex=1159675200&en=830c4ffbcac022fc&ei=5070*.
———. A Legacy of the Storm: Depression and Suicide." *New York Times*, June 21, 2006.
Sontag, Deborah. "Delery Street: Keepers of the Culture; When the Lower Ninth Posed Proudly." *New York Times*, February 9, 2006.
Thevenot, Brian. "Absentee Voters' Interest Is Brisk; But How Many Cast Ballot Is Big Question." *New Orleans Times-Picayune*, April 3, 2006.
Thomas, Cathy Booth. "New Orleans Mayor's Newest Foe Already Reeling from His Clumsy Race Remark, Ray Nagin Now Must Face a Tough Challenger in a Re-Election Bid." *Time*, February 1, 2006.
Thomas, Cathy Booth, and Russell McCulley. "Will Ray Nagin Win Redemption in New Orleans?" *Time*, April 10, 2006.
Tucker, Maria Luisa. "Hurricane Katrina's Emotional Hangover." AlterNet, February 6, 2006, *alternet.org/katrina/31637/*.

Chapter 16
The Right to Vote

ACORN. "ACORN Defeats Anti-Voter Legal Attacks; Group's Voter Registration Efforts Vindicated as Baseless Lawsuits Collapse." Press release, December 14, 2005.
American Center for Voting Rights. "Vote Fraud, Intimidation, AND Suppression in the 2004 Presidential Election." ACVR Legislative Fund Report, August 2, 2005. *www.ac4vr.com/reports/072005/080205report.pdf*.
Andersen, Shea. "Group Stands Firm in Bid for Sign-ups." *Albuquerque Tribune*, September 10, 2004.
———. "Mischief Reports Justify Probes." *Albuquerque Tribune*, September 9, 2004.
———. "More Glare on Voter Sign-ups." *Albuquerque Tribune*, August 25, 2004.
Asher, Ed. "Task force Will Eye Voter Fraud." *Albuquerque Tribune*, September 8, 2004.
Associated Press. "Court Orders Inspection of Voter Registrations." Associated Press, September 30, 2004.
Atlas, John. "Mock the Vote." *Shelterforce*, July 22, 2007.

———. "Out to Get ACORN." June 11, 2007, *www.tompaine.com*.
———. "US Attorneygate, Acorn, Voter Suppression and the Mainstream Press." *Op-Ed News*. June 21, 2007, *www.opednews.com*.
Becker, Jo, and Dan Eggen. "Voter Probes Raise Partisan Suspicions, Democrats, Allies See Politics Affecting Justice Department's Anti-Fraud Efforts." *Washington Post*, September 20, 2004.
Bleifuss, Joel. "The Fraudulence of Voter Fraud: The Bush Administration Purged U.S. Attorneys for Failing to Prosecute Crimes That Didn't Occur." *In These Times*, April 18, 2007.
Bobo, K., J. Kendall, and S. Max. *Organizing for Social Change: Midwest Academy Manual for Activists*. Santa Ana, Calif.: Seven Locks Press, 2001.
Brooks, Fred. "Resolving the Dilemma between Organizing and Services: Los Angeles ACORN's Welfare Advocacy." *Social Work*, July 1, 2005.
Brooks, Fred, and E. Brown. "A Program Evaluation of Los Angeles ACORN's Welfare Case Advocacy." *Journal of Human Behavior and the Social Environment* 12, 2–3 (2005), 185–204.
Charles Rousseau, et al. v. Acorn. U.S. District Court, Southern District of Florida, Miami Division, Case No. 04-61636-civ (2004).
Christopher, Drew, and Eric Lipton. "G.O.P. Anger in Swing State Eased Attorney's Exit." *New York Times*, March 18, 2007.
Clinton, Bill. *Giving: How Each of Us Can Change the World*. New York: Knopf, 2007.
Clyne, Meghan. "Acorn and the Money Tree." *National Review Online*, October 31, 2004, *www.nationalreview.com/comment/clyne200410311142*.as.
Cocco, Marie, "GOP's Unsubstantiated Voter Fraud Claims," *IndyStar.com*, May 19, 2007.
———. "The Real Voter Fraud," *Washington Post*, March 14, 2007.
Coleman, Michael. "Gripes about Iglesias Not New: E-Mails Show Long History of Complaints." *Albuquerque Journal*, March 15, 2007.
Davidson, Chandler. *Race and Class in Texas Politics*. Princeton, N.J.: Princeton University Press, 1992.
Employment Policies Institute. "Rotten ACORN: America's Bad Seed." Employment Policies Institute, July 2006, *www.rottenacorn.com/*.
Farrington, Brendan. "Accusations of Fraud, Wrongdoing Abound ahead of Nov. 2 Election." Associated Press, October 30, 2004.
Florida Department of Law Enforcement. "FDLE Investigates Statewide Voter Fraud." Press release, October 21, 2004.
Fund, John. "Grapes of Rathke: Acorn, a Liberal Activist Group, Comes under Scrutiny. About Time." *Wall Street Journal*, November 8, 2006.
———. "Whose Ox Is Gored? After Bush's Victory, Liberals Shouted 'Voter fraud!' Why Have They Changed Their Tune?" *Wall Street Journal*, July 30, 2007.
Gumbel, Andrew. *Steal This Vote*. New York: Nation Books, 2005.
Gisick, Michael. "Fired U.S. Attorney David Iglesias Embraces the Media in His Quest for Vindication." *Albuquerque Tribune*, May 10, 2007.
———. "GOP VIPs Ponder David Iglesias Fallout." *Albuquerque Tribune*, March 3, 2007.
Hajnal, Z., and J. Trounstine, "Turnout Matters: Voter Turnout and City Spending Priorities." Paper presented at the annual meeting of the Midwest Political Science Association, Chicago, April 15–18, 2004.
Hamburger, Tom. "Under Bush, the Department Has Been Tainted by Politics, Many Say." *Los Angeles Times*, March 25, 2007.
Holmes, Sue Major. "Voter ID Case Heads to Court, Could Affect Thousands." *Associated Press*, September 2, 2004.
Iglesias, David, with Davin Seay. *In Justice: An Insider's Account of the War on Law and Truth in the Executive Branch*. San Francisco: Wiley, 2008.
James, Joni. "Voter Fraud Charges Collapse, Judges' Rulings Negate a Fired Worker's Claims That the Grass Roots Group ACORN Mishandled Voter Registrations." St. Petersburg Times, December 15, 2005.

Kennedy, Robert F., Jr., and Greg Palast. "Block the Vote." *Rolling Stone*, October 7, 2008.

Larry Larranaga, et al. v. Mary E. Herrera, Bernalillo County Clerk and Rebecca Vigil-Giron, New Mexico Secretary of State. Second Judicial District Court, County of Bernalillo, State of New Mexico. District Court No. CV-2004–05391, September 8, 2004.

League of Women Voters of Florida v. Cobb, U.S. District Court, Southern District of Florida (Case 06-21265-CIV-JORDAN); U.S. Court of Appeals for the 11th Circuit (Case 06-14836-DD).

Lenderman, Andy. "3 GOP Candidates Want Voter Records." *Albuquerque Journal*, September 15, 2004.

———. "Court Gets Voter Registration Lawsuit." *Albuquerque Journal*, September 30 2004.

———. "Fight over Voter ID Heats Up." *Albuquerque Journal*, September 19, 2004.

Levine, Art. "The Republican War on Voting." *American Prospect*, April 1, 2008, *www.prospect.org/cs/articles?article=the_republican_war_on_voting.*

Lipton, Eric. "Missouri Prosecutor Says He Was Pushed to Resign." *New York Times*, May 10, 2007.

McKay, Dan. "Election 'Mischief' under Scrutiny." *Albuquerque Journal*, September 10, 2004.

———. "Too Young to Vote." *Albuquerque Journal*, August 20, 2004.

McKay, Dan, and Andy Lenderman. "County's Early-Polling Places 'Slammed' with Voters, Calls." *Albuquerque Journal*, October 19, 2004.

Meyerson, Harold. "The Cost of the 'Voter Fraud' Fraud." *American Prospect*, May 17, 2007.

Milarsky, Jeremy. "Ex-Worker Sues Activist Group." *South Florida Sun-Sentinel*, October 21, 2004.

Miller, Mark Crispin, ed. *Loser Take All: Election Fraud and the Subversion of Democracy, 2000–2008*. Brooklyn, N.Y.: IG Publishing, 2008.

Minnite, Lorraine. *The Myth of Voter Fraud.* Ithaca, N.Y.: Cornell University Press, forthcoming.

Minnite, Lorraine, Frances Fox Piven, and Margaret Groarke. *Keeping Down the Black Vote: Race and the Demobilization of American Voters*. New York: New Press, 2009.

Morgan, Lucy. "Group Faces Accusations of Broken Voting Laws." *St. Petersburg Times*, October 22, 2004.

Piven, Frances Fox, and Richard A. Cloward. *Why Americans Don't Vote and Why Politicians Want It That Way.* Boston: Beacon Press, 2000.

Polett, Zach. "2004 Voter Participation Campaign." Memorandum. Author files.

———. "Political Strategies 2005 and Beyond: Building on the 2004 Voter Participation Work." November 26, 2004. Author files.

Project Vote. "One Year Later: Results of 2004 Voter Fraud Investigations Give Vote Groups a Clean Slate, Community Group Vindicated as Baseless Lawsuits, Investigations Collapse." Press release, December 15, 2005.

Roth, Zachary. "Iglesias: 'I'm Astounded' by DOJ's ACORN Probe." *Talking Points Memo*, October 16, 2008, *tpmmuckraker.talkingpointsmemo.com/2008/10/iglesias_im_astounded_by_dojs.php.*

Roggemann, Ellen. "Tale of Two Organizers." Typescript. December 29, 2004. Author files.

Seper, Jerry, and Donald Lambro. "Anti-Bush Registration Drive Stirs Fraud Concerns; Party Memo Urges 'Pre-emptive Strikes' on GOP." *Washington Times*, October 15, 2004.

St. John, Paige. "Rumors of Vote Fraud Rampant." *Florida Today*, October 2, 2004.

Talev, Margaret. "Bush, Gonzales Reportedly Discussed Fired Prosecutor." McClatchy Newspapers, April 17, 2007.

U.S. Department of Justice. Office of the Inspector General. "An Investigation into the Removal of Nine U.S. Attorneys in 2006." September 2008, *www.usdoj.gov/oig/special/s0809a/final.pdf.*

Vigil, Adrian. "Voter ID Hearing Was Nothing More Than a Ruse." *Las Cruces Sun-News*, August 8, 2006.

Wallman, Brittany. "Group Sued over Alleged Disenfranchisement of Felons." *South Florida Sun-Sentinel*, October 29, 2004.

———. "Voter Registration Drive a Subterfuge, Lawsuit Claims." *South Florida Sun-Sentinel*, October 30, 2004.

Wallman, Brittany, and Alve James-Johnson. "Filled-In Voter Forms Surface." *South Florida Sun-Sentinel*, October 27, 2004.

Whelan, Kevin. "Acorn Statement on AP's Voter Registration Article." Press release. October 3, 2006.

Zucco, Tom. "Activist Group Blamed for Voter Roll Goofs." *St. Petersburg Times*, October 4, 2004.

Chapter 17
Growing Pains

ACORN. "Voter Registration Performance Verification Procedures." Accessed via *www.factcheck.org*, October 17, 2008.

Allen, J. Linn. "Banks, Activists Tailor Loans to Communities." *Chicago Tribune*, September 1, 1992.

Associated Press. "Pierce County to Pull 230 Names off Voter List." February 3, 2008.

Bliss, Jeff. "Obama Lawyer Asks for Probe Into Vote-Fraud Claims (Update1)." *Bloomberg News*, October 17, 2008.

Brown, David. "Obama to Amend Report on $800,000 in Spending." *Pittsburgh Tribune-Review*, August 22, 2008.

CNN. "Obama Camp Calls for Special Prosecutor in Fraud Investigation." October 18, 2008.

Dreier, Peter, and John Atlas, "The GOP's Blame-ACORN Game." *Nation*, October 22, 2008, *www.thenation.com/doc/20081110/dreier_atlas*.

Duncombe, Ted. "Drive Gains to Legally Place Homeless in Abandoned Buildings." Associated Press, December 1, 1987.

Falcone, Michael. "Acorn Replies to Questions about Role with Voters." *New York Times*, October 24, 2008.

Foulkes, Toni. "Case Study: Chicago—The Barack Obama Campaign." *Social Policy*, Winter 2003–Spring 2004.

Griffin, Drew, and Kathleen Johnston. "Thousands of Voter Registration Forms Faked, Officials Say." CNN, October 10, 2008.

Haynes, Colin. "Application and Affidavit for Search Warrant." Office of the Secretary of State, Nevada, October 2008.

Hoyt, Clark, "The Public Editor: The Tip That Didn't Pan Out." *New York Times*, May 16, 2009, *www.nytimes.com/2009/05/17/opinion/17pubed.html*.

Jordan, Lara Jakes. "Officials: FBI Investigates ACORN for Voter Fraud." Associated Press, October 16, 2008.

Lipton, Eric, and Ian Urbina. "In 5-Year Effort, Scant Evidence of Voter Fraud." *New York Times*, April 12, 2007.

McCain-Palin 2008. "Statement on Obama Campaign's Letter to Justice Department on Voter Fraud." Accessed via *www.factcheck.org*, October 17, 2008.

Minnite, Lorraine, *The Myth of Voter Fraud*. Ithaca, N.Y.: Cornell University Press, forthcoming.

Minnite, Lorraine, Frances Fox Piven, and Margaret Groarke. *Keeping Down the Black Vote: Race and the Demobilization of American Voters*. New York: New Press, 2009.

Munnell, Alicia H., et al. "Mortgage Lending in Boston: Interpreting HMDA Data." *American Economic Review*, March 1996.

Ringham, Bob. "The Loan Rangers." *Chicago Sun-Times*, September 23, 1993.

Swarts, Heidi, *Organizing Urban America: Secular and Faith- based Progressive Movements*. Minneapolis: University of Minnesota Press, 2008

Tayler, Etta, and Keith Herbert. "Chicago Streets Obama's Teacher." *Newsday*, March 2, 2008.

U.S. Department of Justice. Office of the Inspector General. "An Investigation into the Removal of Nine U.S. Attorneys in 2006." September 2008, *www.usdoj.gov/oig/special/s0809a/final.pdf*.

Vogrin, Bill. "Voice for the Needy Keeps Low Profile." *Colorado Springs Gazette*, April 18, 2005.

Chapter 18: The Prostitute and the Assault

Anastasia, George. "Supporters Turn Out for ACORN." *Philadelphia Inquirer*, September 26, 2009.
Anderson, Lincoln. "Right Has ACORN on Ropes, but Fight Isn't Over: Attorney." *Villager*, October 21–27, 2009, *www.thevillager.com/villager_338/righthas.html.*
Barrett, Barbara. "As ACORN Grew, So Did Its Clout and Its Problems." *McClatchy Newspapers*, September 18, 2009.
Brooks, Fred, Robert, Fisher, and Daniel Russell. "ACORN's Accelerated Income Redistribution Project: A Program Evaluation." *Research on Social Work Practice, 2006.* In author's possession.
Buell, John. "Stop the Vendetta against ACORN," *Progressive*, October 31, 2009.
Dreier, Peter, and Christoper Martin. "Manipulating the Public Agenda: Why ACORN Was in the News, and What the News Got Wrong." Urban and Environmental Policy Institute, Occidental College, *departments.oxy.edu/uepi/acornstudy.*
Fears, Darryl. "ACORN to Review Incidents, White House Joins Criticism over Hidden-Camera Videos." *Washington Post*, September 17, 2009.
Fessler, Pam. "ACORN Starts to Feel Funding Freeze." *National Public Radio*, October 16, 2009.
Fisher, Robert, ed. *The People Shall Rule.* Nashville: Vanderbilt University Press, 2009.
Flanagan, Jenna. "ACORN: Organization Will Continue with or without Federal Funds." *WNYC.org*, September 17, 2009, *www.wnyc.org/news/articles/by/jenna_flanagan.*
Hoag, Christina. "ACORN Activists Refuse to Buckle to Video Scandal." Associated Press, October 8, 2009.
Horner, Kim. "Despite National Controversy, Dallas ACORN Office Stays Focused on Mission." *Dallas Morning News*, September 26, 2009.
Huffstutter, P. J., and Kate Linthicum. "ACORN Scaling Back or Shutting Down in Many Cities." *Los Angeles Times*, September 19, 2009.
Kane, Muriel. "The Right Isn't Only Trying to Take Down ACORN, It's Got a 25-Year Project to 'Defund' the Left." *Raw Story*, October 31, 2009.
Lake, Celinda et al. Memo from Lake Research Partners to Bertha Lewis and Jeff Robinson, ACORN. "ACORN's Image among African American Voters," 2009. In Author's possession.
Linthicum, Kate. "Community groups band together to rally in support of ACORN." *Los Angeles Times*, October 23, 2009.
Marx, Greg. "Q & A: Rick Perlstein: The Liberal Historian on ACORN, the *Post*, and Wagging the Dog." *Columbia Journalism Review*, September 22, 2009.
O'Keefe, James. "Chaos for Glory: My Time with ACORN." *Big Government, biggovernment.com/2009/09/10/chaos-for-glory/.*
Olivarez-Giles, Nathan. "Activist group challenges mortgage lender in front of L.A. family's home." *Los Angeles Times*, August 19, 2009, *latimesblogs.latimes.com/laland/2009/08/activist-group-acorn-callsout-litton-loan-services-in-front-of-la-familys-home.html.*
Rodriguez, Cindy. "ACORN Funds Drop, Members Scramble to Fill Gap." *WNYC.org*, October 15, 2009.
Rutenberg, Jim. "ACORN's Woes Strain Its Ties to Democrats." *New York Times*, October 15, 2009, *www.nytimes.com/2009/10/16/us/politics/16acorn.html?pagewanted=3D1&_r=3D2&hp.*
Shaw, Randy. "ACORN's Problems Create Void for Community Organizing." *LA Progressive*, October 6, 2009, *www.laprogressive.com/2009/10/06/acorn%E2%80%99s-problems-create-void-for-community-organizing/.*
———. *Beyond the Fields.* Berkeley: University of California Press, 2008.

Swarts, Heidi. *Organizing Urban America: Secular and Faith-Based Progressive Movements.* Minneapolis: University of Minnesota Press, 2008.

Taranto, James. "Taking On the 'Democrat-Media Complex': The Conservative Internet Entrepreneur on Bringing down Acorn, Hollywood Liberals, and Embarrassing the Mainstream Media." *Wall Street Journal*, October 16, 2009.

Theimer, Sharon, and Pete Yost. "Did ACORN get too big for its own good?" *Associated Press*, September 20, 2009.

Weiner, Joann M. "ACORN Was Just Trying to Help." *Politics Daily*, September 17, 2009, *www.politicsdaily.com/2009/09/17/acorn-was-just-trying-to-help/.*

Additional Bibliography

Atlas, John. "The World as It Should Be." *Shelterforce*, September–October 2003.

Atlas, John, and Peter Dreier. "ACORN: Enraging the Right," *Shelterforce*, May–June 2003.

Boyte, Harry C. *Commonwealth: A Return to Citizen Politics.* New York: Free Press, 1989.

Brooks, Fred. "Innovative Organizing Practices: ACORN's Campaign in Los Angeles Organizing Workfare Workers." *Journal of Community Practice* 9, 4 (2001), 65–85.

———. "New Turf for Organizing: Family Child Care Providers." *Labor Studies Journal* 29, 4 (2005), 45–64.

Brooks, F., D. Russell, and R. Fisher. "ACORN's Accelerated Income Redistribution Project: A Program Evaluation." *Research on Social Work Practice* 16, no. 4, (2006), 369–81.

Freedman, Samuel G. *Upon This Rock: The Miracles of a Black Church.* New York: Harper Collins, 1993.

Fisher, R., F. Brooks, and D. Russell. "'Don't Be a Blockhead': ACORN, Direct Action, and Refund Anticipation Loans." *Urban Affairs Review*, 42 (2007).

Greider, William. *Who Will Tell the People: The Betrayal of American Democracy.* New York: Touchstone, 1993.

Hochschild, Adam. *Bury the Chains: Prophets and Rebels in the Fight to Free an Empire's Slaves.* New York: Houghton Mifflin, 2005.

Orr, Marion. *Transforming the City, Community Organizing and the Challenge of Political Change.* Lawrence: University of Kansas Press, 2007.

Roberts, Omar. *Streets of Glory: Church and Community in a Black Urban Neighborhood.* Chicago: University of Chicago Press, 2005.

Rogers, Mary Beth. *Cold Anger: A Story of Faith and Power Politics.* Denton: University of North Texas Press, 1990.

Warren, Mark. *Dry Bones Rattling: Community Building to Revitalize American Democracy.* Princeton: Princeton University Press, 2001.

Index